Digital Media and Early Child Development

Giana Bitencourt Frizzo
Editor

Digital Media and Early Child Development

Theoretical and Empirical Issues

Springer

Editor
Giana Bitencourt Frizzo
Developmental Psychology & Personality Department,
Psychology Graduation Program
Universidade Federal do Rio Grande do Sul
Porto Alegre, Rio Grande do Sul, Brazil

ISBN 978-3-031-69223-9 ISBN 978-3-031-69224-6 (eBook)
https://doi.org/10.1007/978-3-031-69224-6

This Springer imprint is published by the registered company Springer Nature Switzerland AG
The registered company address is: Gewerbestrasse 11, 6330 Cham, Switzerland

Contents

About the Contributors

Daniel Abs (ORCID: 0000-0001-8808-2773) Full Professor and Researcher at the Institute of Psychology of the University of São Paulo (USP), in the Department of Social and Work Psychology in the area of Socialization and Interaction in Virtual Environments. Coordinates the research laboratory in Psychology and Digital Processes. Psychologist, bachelor's degree from the University of Vale do Rio dos Sinos – Unisinos (Brazil). PhD in Psychology from the Federal University of Rio Grande do Sul (UFRGS/BRAZIL) and completed postdoctoral internships in Social Psychology at the Universitat de Girona (Spain) and UFRGS. His main research interests are Digital Interactions and Technologies, Games, Immersion and Engagement in Virtual Environments, Human-Computer Interaction, Artificial Intelligence, and Metaverses. E-mail: daniel.abs@usp.br

Fernanda Saraiva Almeida (ORCID: 0000-0002-6173-5188) Psychologist, undergraduated in Psychology at Universidade Federal do Rio Grande do Sul (UFRGS), Brazil. Master in Psychology at Pontifical Catholic University of Rio Grande do Sul (PUCRS). She works in clinical psychology, and is especially interested in anxiety disorders and mood disorders. She is a specialist in cognitive-behavioral psychotherapy with adults. E-mail: fernandasaraivaalmeida@gmail.com

Maira Lopes Almeida (ORCID: 0000-0002-6956-9858) Professor of Psychology at the Federal University of Goiás (UFG). BA and MS in Psychology from the Federal University of Uberlândia (UFU, Brazil). PhD in Psychology from the Federal University of Rio Grande do Sul (UFRGS). She completed a postdoctoral internship at Sherbrooke University (Québec, Canada). Associate member of the Assessment and Intervention in Child and Adolescent Development Research Group of the National Association for Research and Postgraduate Studies in Psychology (Anpepp). She is interested in how psychological factors, such as mental health and parental stress, can influence children's use of digital media. mairaalmeida@ufg.br

Adriane Xavier Arteche (ORCID: 0000-0002-2586-4900). Psychologist, PhD in Psychology at Universidade Federal do Rio Grande do Sul. Porto Alegre (UFRGS, Brazil). Professor at Pontifical Catholic University of Rio Grande do Sul (PUCRS). Productivity Research fellow CNPq PQ2. Main interests rely on social cognition and on parenting and its effects on child development. E-mail: adriane.arteche@pucrs.br

Rachel F. Barr (ORCID: 0000-0002-5855-9718) received her PhD from the University of Otago in New Zealand. She is Professor of Psychology at Georgetown University and Director of the Georgetown Early Learning Project. She is primarily interested in how children bridge the gap between what they learn from media and how they apply that information in the real world. She has published extensively on the effects of content and context of media on early learning. She has focused on dissemination of research findings to parents in coordination with the organization ZEROTOTHREE where she had earlier held a leadership fellowship. email. rfb5@georgetown.edu

Débora Becker (ORCID: 0000-0002-5556-2567) is a developmental psychologist with a master's degree in clinical psychology from UNISINOS University, São Leopoldo, Brazil (2020). She is a PhD student at UNISINOS University, with periods as a postgraduate fellow at Universität Heidelberg (2022) and Yale University (2022–2023). Since 2013, she has been focusing on the repercussions of screen exposure on child development and parenting. Her research interests include parent-infant interactions, early intervention programs, mentalization-based interventions, parental reflective functioning, parental mental health, child socioemotional development, and pretend play. E-mail: DEBBECKER@edu.unisinos.br

Mathieu Bégin (ORCID: 0009-0009-7141-6314) PhD (communication), University of Montréal, Québec; Postdoctoral (communication), Catholic University of Louvain, Belgium. Professor (digital media education), Department of preschool and primary education, University of Sherbrooke, Québec. Main interests: learning and communication practices of young people in digital media; discourses conveyed by educational resources for teachers and parents about misinformation and cyberbullying. E-mail: mathieu.begin3@usherbrooke.ca

Marie-Andrée Binet (ORCID: 0000-0002-9744-0517) received a bachelor's in Psychology and a master's in Health Sciences from the University of Sherbrooke, Canada. She currently pursues her studies in the Health Studies department as a PhD student. She is mainly interested in how digital media (durations, contents, and contexts of use) interacts with child cognitive, social, and physical development, as well as parental practices. E-mail: marie-andree.binet@usherbrooke.ca.

Dillon T. Browne (ORCID: 0000-0002-7445-6604) is a clinical psychologist. He received his Bachelor of Arts in Psychology from the University of Guelph, and his Master of Arts and PhD in School and Child Clinical Psychology from the Ontario Institute for Studies in Education at the University of Toronto. Dr. Browne completed clinical internship and postdoctoral fellowship in the Department of

Psychiatry, University of California, San Francisco. He is currently the Canada Research Chair in Child and Family Clinical Psychology and an Associate Professor in the Department of Psychology, University of Waterloo. His main research interests relate to adversity, child development, technology, and family therapy. Email: dillon.browne@uwaterloo.ca

Clarice Oliveira Campos (ORCID: 0000-0003-4488-3661) is a psychologist with a BA in Psychology from Universidade Federal de São João del Rei (UFSJ, Brazil) and an MS in Cognitive Neurosciences and Neuropsychology from the University of Algarve (UAlg), Portugal. She works as a clinical psychologist and as a researcher. Her research interests lie in the field of child development, psychological assessment, and cognitive processes in children. Email: cocampos@ualg.pt

Mélanie M. Couture (ORCID: 0000-0002-4919-573X) is an occupational therapist and received her MA in Child Study from Concordia University, her PhD in biomedical sciences (Université de Montréal), and specialized as a postdoctoral fellow (McGill University) with the autistic population. She is currently a professor at the Faculty of Medicine and Health Sciences at Sherbrooke University. She co-leads the provincial autism research network in Quebec and her research program focuses on the social participation and inclusion of autistic individuals. E-mail: Melanie.M.Couture@usherbrooke.ca

Laura Canani da Rosa (ORCID: 0000-0003-4956-6972) Psychologist, undergraduated in Psychology at Universidade Federal do Rio Grande do Sul (UFRGS), Brazil and Master student at the same university. Member of the Cognitive and Psychopathology Laboratory at UFRGS. She works with psychological evaluation, psychological diagnosis, and as a psychotherapist. She is interested in neurodivergencies and neurodiversity. E-mail: laura.canani@ufrgs.br

Mônia Aparecida da Silva (ORCID: 0000-0002-8840-7547) BA and MS in Psychology from Universidade Federal de São João del Rei (UFSJ, Brazil), specialist in Psychological Assessment from the Regional Psychology Council of Minas Gerais (CRP/MG). PhD and postdoctoral in Psychology from Universidade Federal do Rio Grande do Sul (UFRGS). Adjunct professor in the Psychology Department and coordinator of the Psychology Postgraduate Program at UFSJ. Associate member of the Brazilian Institute of Psychological Assessment (Ibap) and of the Assessment and Intervention in Child and Adolescent Development Research Group of the National Association for Research and Postgraduate Studies in Psychology (Anpepp). Email: monia@ufsj.edu.br.

Patricia Santos da Silva (ORCID: 0000-0002-4363-6821) Psychologist, undergraduated at Universidade Federal de Ciências da Saúde de Porto Alegre, PhD in Psychology at Universidade Federal do Rio Grande do Sul (UFRGS), Porto Alegre RS, Brasil. Postgraduate degree in Systemic Therapy with Individuals, Families and Couples at Centro de Estudos da Família e do Indivíduo de Porto Alegre. Psychologist in a private practice, with supervision and assistance for individuals, families, and couples. E-mail: patis.psico@gmail.com

Elisa Cardoso de Azevedo (ORCID: 0000-0002-7532-0602) Psychologist, undergraduated at Pontifícia Universidade Católica do Rio Grande Sul (PUCRS). She received her master's and PhD in Psychology from Universidade Federal do Rio Grande do Sul (UFRGS), Brazil. She was a member at the Center for Research and Intervention on families with infants and children, coordinated by Professor Giana Frizzo. She is a clinical and hospital psychologist. She is a specialist in Child Health and Hospital Psychology from Hospital de Clínicas de Porto Alegre. She is a child and adolescent psychotherapist with Psychoanalytic Guidance (CEAPIA).

Tagma Marina Schneider Donelli (ORCID: 0000-0003-3083-0083) Psychologist, BA in Psychology from Universidade do Vale do Rio dos Sinos (UNISINOS), Brazil. PhD in Psychology at Universidade Federal do Rio Grande do Sul (UFRGS), Brazil. Postdoctorate at the Department of Social Policy and Intervention from University of Oxford, UK. Professor at Universidade do Vale do Rio dos Sinos (UNISINOS), Brazil. Productivity research fellow by CNPq PQ2. She coordinates the Center for Baby Related Studies (CER Bebê). E-mail: tagmad@unisinos.br

Bruno Carlos Ferreira (ORCID: 0009-0004-8590-7636) is a psychologist with a degree in Psychology from Centro Universitário Faminas (Brazil) and a master's degree in Psychology from the Federal University of São João del Rei (UFSJ, Brazil). He works as a clinical psychologist. His main research interests are child development, psychological assessment, and the use of screens. E-mail: brunobps58@gmail.com

Caroline Fitzpatrick (ORCID: 0000-0002-9439-042X) is a professor of child development at the Université de Sherbrooke in the faculty of education and a visiting research fellow at the University of Johannesburg in the Department of Childhood Education. She is also the holder of the Tier 2 Canada research Chair on Digital media use by children and its implications for promoting togetherness: an ecosystemic approach. Her research aims to better understand the consequences of child and youth media habits on physical, cognitive, and social development.

Giana Bitencourt Frizzo (ORCID: 0000-0001-8106-4441) Psychologist, undergraduated at Universidade Federal de Santa Maria in the south of Brazil. PhD and Postdoctoral in Psychology at Universidade Federal do Rio Grande do Sul. Porto Alegre (UFRGS), RS, Brazil. Full professor at Universidade Federal do Rio Grande do Sul – UFRGS, Porto Alegre. Productivity Research fellow by CNPq PQ1D. She coordinates the Center for Research and Intervention on families with infants and childrenat UFRGS. Her main interests rely on infant and child development and intervention, family relations, and screen media use. E-mail: giana.frizzo@ufrgs.br

Giana Bitencourt Frizzo (ORCID: 0000-0001-8106-4441) Psychologist, undergraduated at Universidade Federal de Santa Maria in the south of Brazil. PhD and postdoctoral degree in Psychology at Universidade Federal do Rio Grande do Sul. Porto Alegre (UFRGS), RS, Brazil. Full professor at Universidade Federal do Rio Grande do Sul – UFRGS, Porto Alegre. Productivity Research fellow by CNPq PQ1D. She coordinates the Center for Research and Intervention on families with infants and children at UFRGS. Her main interests rely on infant and child development and intervention, family relations, and screen media use. E-mail: giana.frizzo@ufrgs.br

Gabrielle Garon-Carrier (ORCID: 0000-0002-9906-5247) Professor of developmental psychology in the Department of Psychoeducation at the Université de Sherbrooke, Québec (Canada). She holds a PhD in Psychology from the Université Laval and a postdoctoral fellowship in the Department of Psychology at Goldsmiths, University of London. Since 2020, she is the head of the Early Learning and Social Adjustment Research Lab (LilLab) and holds a Tier 2 Canada Research Chair in school readiness, inclusion, and social adjustment. Her work informs on the developmental mechanisms of child cognitive and mental health, and academic adjustment life-trajectory, and also advanced knowledge on the impact of social policies and services for families with young children. E-mail: gabrielle.garon-carrier@usherbrooke.ca

Bruna Cardoso Gerhardt (ORCID: 0000-0003-2815-838X) Pontifical Catholic University of Rio Grande do Sul (PUCRS). MSc in Psychology. Doctorate student in Psychology at Pontifical Catholic University of Rio Grande do Sul (PUCRS). Email: bruna.gerhardt@edu.pucrs

Elizabeth Harvey (ORCID: 0000-0002-5639-6986) holds a master's degree in psychology from Université Laval (Québec, Canada) and a PhD in psychoeducation from Université de Sherbrooke (Québec, Canada). She is Professor of Education at Université Sainte-Anne, Nova Scotia, Canada. Her work is in the framework of inclusive education and aims to understand the role of individual differences in temperament, family and school factors in children's academic success. She is particularly interested in contributing to the advancement of knowledge about temperament in school communities. E-mail: Elizabeth.harvey@usainteanne.ca

Letícia Carvalho Leão (ORCID: 0000-0002-5434-6088) holds BA and MS in Psychology from Universidade Federal de São João del Rei (UFSJ, Brazil). She is an associate member of the Brazilian Institute of Psychological Assessment (Ibap) and the Mental Health and Social Reintegration Research Group. Her research focuses on developmental psychology, cross-cultural adaptation, and childhood. Her research examines the interactions between several facets of digital media use and environmental aspects of child development. Email: leeh853@aluno.ufsj.edu.br

Manoela Yustas Mallmann (ORCID: 0000-0001-7774-4479) Psychologist, undergraduated at Pontifícia Universidade Católica do Rio Grande Sul. She is a PhD student in Psychology at Universidade Federal do Rio Grande do Sul (UFRGS), Porto Alegre, RS, Brazil. She is a member of the Center for Research and Intervention on families with infants and children at UFRGS and a child, adolescent and adult psychotherapist. She studies child development, parent-infant relations, and digital media use. E-mail: manoelaymallmann@gmail.com

Fernanda Martins Marques (ORCID: 0000-0002-5424-3513)—Psychologist, undergraduated and Master in Psychology at Universidade Federal do Rio Grande do Sul (UFRGS), Brazil. She is a psychologist, a public servant at UFRGS, and works with children, parents, and families in clinical and educational contexts. She is a doctoral student at UFRGS under the guidance of Dr. Giana Frizzo. Her research explores the subjective experiences and parental practices related to digital media throughout early childhood, before and during the COVID-19 pandemic. E-mail: martins.marques@ufrgs.br

Lauren J. Myers (ORCID: 0000-0001-9765-6118) holds BA in Psychology & Music from Furman University and MS and PhD in Psychology from The Pennsylvania State University. She is Associate Professor of Psychology at Lafayette College, where she has served as the inaugural Faculty Fellow for Engaged Scholarship at the Lafayette Landis Center for Community Engagement. She directs the Lafayette Kids Lab (https://sites.lafayette.edu/kidslab/), where she and her undergraduate research assistants conduct research on children's understanding and use of symbolic representations and interactive media (such as video chat). Her ongoing research examines how families and young children can use digital media in developmentally appropriate ways. Her research has been published in various developmental psychology journals and has been covered in major news outlets. E-mail: myersl@lafayette.edu

Bruna Gabriella Pedrotti (ORCID: 0000-0002-7910-9054)—Psychologist, received her bachelor's, master's, and PhD in Psychology from Universidade Federal do Rio Grande do Sul (UFRGS), Brazil. She was a member at the Center for Research and Intervention on families with infants and children, coordinated by Professor Giana Frizzo. She is a clinical psychologist, and she is interested in how the environment and parental practices influence child development, especially regarding the use of digital media. E-mail: brunagabriellapedrotti@gmail.com

Helena Silveira Riter (ORCID: 0000-0002-0068-820X) Psychologist, received her bachelor's and master's degree in Psychology from Universidade Federal do Rio Grande do Sul (UFRGS), Brazil. Specialist in psychotherapy with children and adolescents. She was a member of the Center for Research and Intervention on families with infants and children at UFRGS. Child, adolescent and adult psychotherapist. She studies child development, parent-infant relations, digital media use, and psychotherapy with children and adolescents. E-mail: helenariter@gmail.com

Meredith L. Rowe (ORCID: 0000-0002-0076-4161) received her BA (Psychology) and MS (Human Development) from the University of Rochester and her EdD from Harvard University. She is currently Professor of Education at the Harvard University Graduate School of Education. She leads a research program on understanding the role of parent and family factors in children's early language and literacy development. She is particularly interested in uncovering features of children's early communicative environments that contribute to language and cognitive development and applying this knowledge to the development of intervention strategies for caregivers. Email: Meredith_rowe@gse.harvard.edu

Lauren Schilling (ORCID: 0009-0004-3282-5653) holds BA in Psychology and Education Studies from the University of Wisconsin-Madison. She is a doctoral student at the Harvard Graduate School of Education working with Dr. Meredith Rowe. Her research explores how early language environments lay the foundation for literacy. She is particularly interested in the impacts of child-directed speech and semantics on visual word recognition. She is working toward developing a computational model of word reading with the goal of leveraging this model to identify linguistic inputs that can efficiently support young readers with wide ranges of early language experiences. E-mail: lschilling@g.harvard.edu

Sofia Sebben (ORCID: 0000-0001-8725-8482) PhD candidate in Psychology at the Federal University of Rio Grande do Sul (UFRGS, Brazil). BA and MS in Psychology from UFRGS. Member of the Center for Research and Intervention in Families with Babies and Children (NUFABE/UFRGS). She completed part of her master's degree at the Psychology Graduate Program at the University of Waterloo (Canada), as a visiting research fellow. Member of the International Society for the Study of Behavioural Development (ISSBD). Conducts research related to mentalization and parental reflective functioning, attachment theory, family interactions, and child development, especially in the contexts of screen use and adoption in childhood. E-mail: sofiasebben@hotmail.com

Indianara Sehaparini (ORCID 0000-0002-7552-0145) Psychologist, BA in Psychology from Faculdade da Serra Gaúcha (FSG), Brazil. MS in Psychology from Universidade Federal do Rio Grande do Sul (UFRGS), Brazil. Currently a PhD student in Psychology at UFRGS. Member of the Center for Research and Intervention in Families with Babies and Children (NUFABE/UFRGS). Clinical Psychologist. Her research focuses on investigating the interactions between various aspects of digital media use, particularly electronic games and social networks, and human development. E-mail: indianara.sehaparini@ufrgs.br

Gabrielle A. Strouse (ORCID: 0000-0002-6955-4955) received BA in Psychology from Northwestern University, and MS and PhD in Psychology from Vanderbilt University, USA. Associate Professor of Human Development and Educational Psychology at the University of South Dakota and Chair of the Division of Counseling and Psychology in Education. Her research focuses on understanding how adults can best support young children's learning in mediated contexts, such as from picture books, e-books, and videos, as well as how to create more supportive children's media. E-mail: Gabrielle.Strouse@usd.edu

Georgene L. Troseth (ORCID: 0000-0002-0333-1732) Professor of Psychology and Human Development, Emerita at Vanderbilt University. Troseth received BA from the University of Wyoming and PhD from the University of Illinois at Urbana-Champaign. Troseth has published research about very young children's symbolic development and their understanding and use of pictures, touchscreen images, video, and video chat. One focus is the importance of adult support or "scaffolding" for very young children's learning from traditional and digital media including e-books and educational applications. Troseth's research has informed the conversation about the effectiveness of very young children's learning from screens. E-mail: georgene.troseth@vanderbilt.edu

Gabriela Vescovi (ORCID: 0000-0001-6747-8744) received her PhD in Psychology from the Federal University of Rio Grande do Sul, Brazil, at Professor Giana Frizzo's lab. In 2022 she was a visiting fellow at Professor Meredith Rowe's Lab at the Harvard Graduate School of Education. She holds a master's and specialist degree in Health Psychology. She is interested in how early language environments shape children's language trajectories. Her research focuses on language input in a low-resource setting and how public policies and interventions can promote language-rich interactions in the home. She is also interested in how digital media such as television, smartphones, and tablets impact language environments and development. E-mail: gabriela-vescovi@saude.rs.gov.br

Rachelle Wakeham-Lewis (ORCID: 0009-0007-1071-3345) received her Bachelor of Arts (Honors) in Psychology from Memorial University of Newfoundland. She has worked as a research coordinator for the Nova Scotia Media use Study (NSMUS) and currently the Québec Preschooler Media Use Study (QPMUS). She is interested in the impact of screen time on children's cognitive, social, and physical development. Email: rachelle.wakehamlewis@usherbrooke.ca

Jasmine Zhang (ORCID: 0000-0001-8277-7283) holds Bachelor of Science (Honors) in Psychology from McMaster University and Master of Arts from the University of Waterloo. She is currently a doctoral student at the University of Waterloo, working with Dr. Dillon Browne. Her research explores how various aspects of digital media use interact with well-being outcomes in children, caregivers, and families. E-mail: jasmine.zhang@uwaterloo.ca

Jennifer M. Zosh (ORCID: 0000-0002-1698-4708) holds BA in Psychology from the University of Delaware, and MA and PhD in Psychological and Brain Sciences from Johns Hopkins University, USA. She is Professor of Human Development and Family Studies at Penn State University's Brandywine campus. As Director of the Brandywine Child Development Lab, she studies how infants and young children learn about the world around them. Most recently, her work has focused on (a) technology and its impact on children and families and (b) playful learning as a powerful pedagogy throughout childhood. E-mail: jzosh@psu.edu

Chapter 1
What Are the Current Challenges of Digital Media Use by Children Under Five?

Giana Bitencourt Frizzo

Children in the contemporary world are embedded in many digital contexts. But this is pretty recent in our lives since the first smartphones started to be commercialized only around 2007 and tablets around 2011. From there on, almost everywhere you go, you can see infants, toddlers, and children in general using some media device. Today's young children are unfamiliar with the world and relationships without the influence of digital media, as their access and use are part of their daily lives (Ashton & Beattie, 2019).

When the first articles began to be published, there was no consent for the right terms to use: media, media device, technology, screen media, screens, or touch-screen technology. The American Psychological Association in 2019 suggested the term digital media to encompass all set of devices, formats, and communication methods that convey digitized content through digital signals, such as on the Internet, television, computer networks, and telephony. Digital media include computer software, mobile applications, social networks, video games, web pages, digital images (photos and videos), and smartphones (American Psychological Association, 2019). At the moment, I am writing this chapter, and the literature suggests that we may not understand digital media as a whole package. However, we should now focus on understanding if they indeed have the same impact on child development.

Some authors, for example, started considering whether the use is passive or active, for instance, if the child is quiet, if he/she is watching a video on the TV, or if he/she is playing some games. But passive media, such as television and radio, are now accompanied by active media that promote instant and interactive access, such as cell phones, computers, tablets, and virtual games, indicating a significant increase in these new forms of digital media (Chassiakos et al., 2016; Radesky

G. B. Frizzo (✉)
Universidade Federal do Rio Grande do Sul, Porto Alegre, Brazil
e-mail: giana.frizzo@ufrgs.br

G. B. Frizzo (ed.), *Digital Media and Early Child Development*,
https://doi.org/10.1007/978-3-031-69224-6_1

et al., 2015). Besides that, touchscreen technology seemed to be a novelty, but in some studies already conducted by our research group (Mallmann & Frizzo, 2019; Pedrotti, 2019), the intense use of TV in families with infants and young children became quite evident, so we understand that this use also deserves investigation, especially because in recent years, TV has also become more interactive and remains one of the most used resources in families with young children (Bentley et al., 2016). Also, we have multiple devices turned on at the same time, so how can we measure the impact of each of them if we are embedded in different forms of technology every day? For some researchers, the immersion in technology is so intense that we probably should consider that we live in a digital context of human development (Abs, 2022).

Mothers, fathers, or legal caregivers play an essential role in children's relationship with digital media throughout childhood. In the early years of life, they rely on caregivers' mediation to access these devices and regulate their use (Kildare & Middlemiss, 2017). A big question depends on the forbidden use of digital media for children under 2 years old, as most guidelines of different pediatric societies suggest. Although most parents know about that, the truth is that infants are being exposed to digital media in their first months of life. Coyne et al. (2022) and Domoff et al. (2020) made an alert showing that digital media habits are formed very early in life, until toddlerhood, so this aspect deserves attention. Also, in infancy, we have the sensorimotor period (Piaget & Inhelder,1955/1976), where children learn most about the experience, so should digital media be one more way of stimulation in this era? Or, as WHO (2019) suggests, should we control digital media and not substitute daily routines of parent/adult–infant/child interaction?

Such guidelines still lack parameters with a consolidated scientific basis for families regarding media usage. Firstly, families tend not to adhere to these pediatric recommendations (Kucirkova et al., 2023; Radesky et al., 2015). Furthermore, Kucirkova et al. (2023) have recently made an important critique in the sense that much of what has been produced regarding media usage and childhood concerns predominantly white participants, mothers, and those with medium to high levels of education, leaving out a wide range of variability among families, such as socioeconomic differences, usage in non-first-world countries, racial issues, and families with low levels of education.

To some extent, it is important to problematize this, as other evidence demonstrates that parents' awareness of these recommendations has been associated with less time spent by children on digital media (Miguel-Berges et al., 2019). This topic is rarely addressed during routine medical consultations (Golden et al., 2020; Pedrotti, 2019). On the other hand, studies have found that pediatric association guidelines had no significant influence on parents' decisions to provide digital media to their infants (Golden et al., 2020; Pedrotti, 2019), and although caregivers agree to avoid exposing them to screens, they report difficulty in following this guidance (Brown & Smolenaers, 2018). Research also shows that while caregivers express concern about the negative effects of excessive digital media use in childhood, this does not always translate into more restrictive practices or reduced screen time (Mallmann & Frizzo, 2019; Mascheroni & Zaffaroni, 2023; Nikken, 2022).

By now, most studies focus on the potential harms digital media may bring. We need to be cautious because even though there is no consent yet for the early years about the benefits and damages it may lead to, especially in infancy and even toddlerhood, there is little evidence that digital media could benefit children (Fitzpatrick et al., 2023). Considering that the early years are the basis for the brain and all development domains, such as socioemotional, language, cognitive, and motor, it is urgent to reflect upon the influence digital media may have on children and also their families. Young children begin to use digital media at an earlier age, and their use increases as they grow older (Azevedo et al., 2022; Radesky et al., 2015). With the adoption of technology moving so quickly, research in the area also evolved, and theoretical and methodological issues also needed to change to understand this phenomenon. Besides taking only children into account, parents' usage may also be considered to understand the influence digital media has on families nowadays. Initially, studies focused almost exclusively on how much time a child was exposed to a screen. Going beyond, nowadays, studies are more concerned about the impacts of digital media use on child development; contexts of family routine, like bedtime and mealtime; and the influence of digital media use on family interactions (Barr et al., 2020; Browne et al., 2019).

For example, there is some consensus on the need for parent mediation in children's media usage, with co-viewing not associated with developmental delays. But if parents refer to using digital media to distract children when they are not available to work, do household chores, or rest (Azevedo et al., 2022; Pedrotti et al., 2022), consequently, most of the time children use digital media, they are not under supervision. Besides that, most apps are designed for children to use alone, which is not good for their development and may interfere with their digital rights (Radesky & Hiniker, 2022). In the Radesky et al. (2016a, b) qualitative study, participants reported conflicts regarding overload when trying to balance work tasks with household chores; they also reported cellphone use in the presence of their children as a potential factor both for generating interruptions during routine moments and being used as a strategy to reduce family tension. Yet, Mallmann and Frizzo (2019) also found similar results, with mothers stating that they offer children digital media because of their needs, not children's necessities. These studies can help us understand that digital media are often considered "nannies" for children due to family overload.

Guilting parents for that is unfair and does not help advance knowledge. Much needs to be understood in family lives to help them use digital media positively. Mallmann et al. (in press) suggested that mothers seek more favorable media usage that does not cause harm to their children. Mothers say they try not to replace important moments of care and interaction between mothers and babies when digital media is not the sole resource used to soothe or meet the baby's needs. They also said they observe signs of tiredness or boredom in children as a sign of stopping offering digital media and changing to another activity. Being connected to the emotional state of the babies is an important ability for parents to evolve, and it is through these processes that emotional development and regulation occur. So, it is not surprising that digital media should not be used to calm children, as suggested by Danet et al. (2022) and Radesky et al. (2016b), because screens, until now at least, cannot mirror emotional states and comfort children. If you, as an adult, are sad, do you prefer a hug, a comforting word, or watching a video on a smartphone to feel better?

Some more recent researchers have brought a very critical perspective regarding the investigation of media use in childhood, emphasizing excessively only the risks of use. Ashton and Beattie (2019) even question why studies have not evaluated harms as outcomes but also the advantages of children being digital natives, familiarized with the use of technologies so present in their lives from the beginning. In this line, Browne et al. (2019) suggest that certain families and children may be more susceptible to more problematic use, while others may reap more benefits from this use. In pursuing a more balanced scientific approach, these researchers advocate for considering both sides of the debate, addressing both risk factors and benefits associated with media use. Also, most studies emphasize screen time as the most important variable, even though this is a very problematic measure (Browne et al., 2021). If digital media is multilevel and many of them are used simultaneously, such as background TV, how can we say which time is being measured and for how long? Screen time is mostly based on self-report, a hard and inaccurate way to access time. The measure of usage is also difficult to understand since a lot of constructs are used and bring different outcomes. Media use in the everyday routine differs from problematic use or digital dependence (Browne et al., 2021). Besides that, screen time is a measure that puts individual responsibility on families. We can not be naïve about the design of the platforms that produce content for children nowadays with no or little regulations (Radesky & Hiniker, 2022). Together, these data reinforce the importance of a broad view of the phenomenon, which should not be restricted to an exclusively negative position on media use in childhood, as we expect you to have while reading this book.

It is urgent to reflect on social, educational, and socioeconomic aspects, the social desirability factor, and cultural differences in research on the use of digital media. The COVID-19 pandemic also played an important role in the use of digital media with children and their families, and this issue also needs to be addressed in publications nowadays. In this sense, this e-book aims to discuss five topics: *digital media: theoretical and methodological issues*; *digital media and early child development*; *digital media, COVID-19 pandemic, and early child development*; *digital media and parenthood*; and *digital media, early child development, and possible interventions*. Together, these topics may help professionals and researchers better understand the complexity of digital media usage in early childhood and families.

References

Abs, D. (2022). *Contextos digitais: encontros, pesquisas e práticas*. UFRGS. Available at: https://lume.ufrgs.br/handle/10183/245521

American Psychological Association. (2019). Digital media. Thesaurus of psychological index terms. Retrieved from https://psycnetapa.ez45.periodicos.capes.gov.br/thesaurus/item?term=digital%20media

Ashton, J. J., & Beattie, R. M. (2019). Screen time in children and adolescents: Is there evidence to guide parents and policy? *The Lancet. Child & Adolescent Health, 3*(5), 292–294. https://doi.org/10.1016/S2352-4642(19)30062-8

Azevedo, E. C., Riter, H. S., Pieta, M. A. M., & Frizzo, G. B. (2022). Digital media use on interactions between mother and child: Differences in infants' early years. *Paidéia (ribeirão Preto), 32*, e3210. https://doi.org/10.1590/1982-4327e3210

Barr, R., Kirkorian, H., Radesky, J., Coyne, S., Nichols, D., Blanchfield, O., Rusnak, S., Stockdale, L., Ribner, A., Durnez, J., Epstein, M., Heimann, M., Koch, F. S., Sundqvist, A., Birberg--Thornberg, U., Konrad, C., Slussareff, M., Bus, A., Bellagamba, F., & Fitzpatrick, C. (2020). Beyond screen time: A synergistic approach to a more comprehensive assessment of family media exposure during early childhood. *Frontiers in Psychology, 11*, 1–17. https://doi.org/10.3389/fpsyg.2020.01283

Bentley, G. F., Turner, K. M., & Jago, R. (2016). Mothers' views of their preschool child's screen--viewing behaviour: A qualitative study. *BMC Public Health, 16*(718), 1–11. https://doi.org/10.1186/s12889-016-3440-z

Brown, A., & Smolenaers, E. (2018). Parents' interpretations of screen time recommendations for children younger than 2 years. *Journal of Family Issues, 39*(2), 406–429. https://doi.org/10.1177/0192513X16646595

Browne, D., Thompson, D. A., & Madigan, S. (2019). Digital media use in children: Clinical vs scientific responsibilities. *JAMA Pediatrics, 174*, 111. https://doi.org/10.1001/jamapediatrics.2019.4559

Browne, D. T., May, S. S., Colucci, L., Hurst-Della Pietra, P., Christakis, D., Asamoah, T., et al. (2021). From screen time to the digital level of analysis: A scoping review of measures for digital media use in children and adolescents. *BMJ Open, 11*(5), e046367. https://doi.org/10.1136/bmjopen-2020-046367

Chassiakos, Y. R., Radesky, J., Christakis, D., Moreno, M. A., & Cross, C. (2016). Children and adolescents and digital media. *American Academy of Pediatrics, 138*(5). https://doi.org/10.1542/peds.2016-2593

Coyne, S. M., Holmgren, H. G., Shawcroft, J. E., Barr, R., Davis, E., Ashby, S., Stockdale, L., & Domoff, S. (2022). Special collection: Behavioral addiction to technology ABCs or attack—Boom—Crash ? A longitudinal analysis of associations between media content and the development of problematic media use in early childhood. *Technology, Mind, and Behavior, 3*(4). https://doi.org/10.1037/tmb0000093

Danet, M., Miller, A. L., Weeks, H. M., Kaciroti, N., & Radesky, J. (2022). Children aged 3-4 years were more likely to be given mobile devices for calming purposes if they had weaker overall executive functioning. Acta Paediatrica, February, 1–7. https://doi.org/10.1111/apa.16314

Domoff, S. E., Borgen, A. L., & Radesky, J. S. (2020). Interactional theory of childhood problematic media use. *Human Behavior & Emerging Technologies, 2*, 343–353. https://doi.org/10.1002/hbe2.217

Fitzpatrick, C., Binet, M. A., Cristini, E., Almeida, M. L., Bégin, M., & Frizzo, G. B. (2023). Reducing harm and promoting positive media use strategies: New perspectives in understanding the impact of preeschooler media use on health and development. *Psicologia: Reflexão e Crítica, 36*, 19. https://doi.org/10.1186/s41155-023-00262-2

Golden, S. L., Blake, J. W. C., & Giuliano, K. K. (2020). Infant behavior and development parental decision-making : Infant engagement with smartphones. *Infant Behavior and Development, 61*(February), 101497. https://doi.org/10.1016/j.infbeh.2020.101497

Kildare, C. A., & Middlemiss, W. (2017). Impact of parents mobile device use on parent-child interaction: A literature review. *Computers in Human Behavior, 75*, 579–593. https://doi.org/10.1016/j.chb.2017.06.003

Kucirkova, N. I., Livingstone, S., & Radesky, J. S. (2023). Faulty screen time measures hamper national policies: Here is a way to address it. *Frontiers in Psychology, 14*. https://doi.org/10.3389/fpsyg.2023.1243396

Mallmann, M. Y., & Frizzo, G. B. (2019). O uso das novas tecnologias em famílias com bebês: um mal necessário? *Revista Cocar. Edição Especial. Dossiê: Crianças, mídias e mediações, 7*, 26–46.

Mascheroni, G., & Zaffaroni, L. (2023). From "screen time" to screen times: Measuring the temporality of media use in the messy reality of family life. *Communications*, 1–22. https://doi.org/10.1515/commun-2022-0097

Miguel-Berges, M. L., Santaliestra-Pasias, A. M., Mouratidou, T., Flores-Barrantes, P., Androutsos, O., De Craemer, M., & OBOTS Group. (2019). Parental perceptions, attitudes and knowledge on European preschool children's total screen time: The ToyBoxstudy. *European Journal of Public Health., 30*(1), 105–111. https://doi.org/10.1093/eurpub/ckz151

Nikken, P. (2022). The touchscreen generation: Trends in Dutch parents' perceptions of young children's media use from 2012–2018. *Communications, 47*(2), 286–306. https://doi.org/10.1515/commun-2020-0028

Pedrotti, B. G., Mallmann, M. Y., Almeida, C. R. S., Marques, F. M., Vescovi, G., da Riter, H. S., Almeida, M. L., Pieta, M. A. M., & Frizzo, G. B. (2022). Infants' and toddlers' digital media use and mothers' mental health: A comparative study before and during the COVID-19 pandemic. *Infant Mental Health Journal, 43*(1), 24–35. https://doi.org/10.1002/imhj.21952

Piaget, J., & Inhelder, B. (1955/1976). *Da lógica da criança à lógica do adolescente*. Pioneira.

Pedrotti, B. G. (2019). *Como prescindir das novas tecnologias no cuidado e na interação com os bebês?*. Dissertação de Mestrado, Instituto de Psicologia, Universidade Federal do Rio Grande do Sul, Porto Alegre. Available at https://lume.ufrgs.br/handle/10183/202058

Radesky, J., & Hiniker, A. (2022). From moral panic to systemic change: Making child-centered design the default. *International Journal of Child-Computer Interaction, 31*, e100351. https://doi.org/10.1016/j.ijcci.2021.100351

Radesky, J. S., Schumacher, J., & Zuckerman, B. (2015). Mobile and interactive media use by young children: The good, the bad, and the unknown. *Pediatrics, 135*(1), 1–3. https://doi.org/10.1542/peds.2014-2251

Radesky, J. S., Kistin, C., Eisenberg, S., Gross, J., Block, G., Zuckerman, B., & Silverstein, M. D. (2016a). Parent perspectives on their mobile technology use: The excitement and exhaustion of parenting while connected. *Journal of Developmental & Behavioral Pediatrics, 37*(9), 694–701. https://doi.org/10.1097/DBP.0000000000000357

Radesky, J., Peacock-Chambers, E., Zuckerman, B., & Silverstein, M. (2016b). Use of mobile technology to calm upset children: Associations with social-emotional development. *JAMA Pediatrics, 170*(4), 397–399. Retrieved from http://jamanetwork.com/pdfaccess.ashx?url=/data/journals/peds/935110/

World Health Organization WHO. (2019). *Guidelines on physical activity, sedentary behaviour and sleep for children under 5 years of age*. World Health Organization. Retrieved from http://www.who.int/iris/handle/10665/311664.

Chapter 2
Challenges in Research on Screen Media Use in Early Childhood: Conceptual, Practical, and Measurement Aspects

Letícia Carvalho Leão, Mônia Aparecida da Silva, Elisa Cardoso Azevedo, and Giana Bitencourt Frizzo

Introduction

The first years of life are crucial for development and extremely important in the long term, being influenced by several factors. The digital media use in childhood has been the target of interest of several scientific associations and public agencies, aiming to guide families on safe guidelines for their use and thus avoid harm to development (American Academy of Pediatrics (AAP), 2016; Royal College of Paediatrics and Child Health (RCPCH), 2019; World Health Organization (WHO), 2019). Screen use has intensified in all age groups over the past decades, resulting in possible consequences for children's development. There is a broad academic interest in understanding the use and effects of digital media, especially on developmental outcomes. However, there are still theoretical and methodological challenges that need to be clarified. This chapter aims to discuss them in the light of international findings.

Overview of Screen Media Use Prevalence by Children in Early Childhood

Estimates on mobile apps and tablets used by children aged zero to eight were made by the US report The Common Sense Census: Zero to Eight (Rideout & Robb, 2020). This report covers both older media platforms, such as television and

L. C. Leão (✉) · M. A. da Silva
Universidade Federal de São João del Rei, São João del Rei, Brazil
e-mail: leeh853@aluno.ufsj.edu.br; monia@ufsj.edu.br

E. C. Azevedo · G. B. Frizzo
Universidade Federal do Rio Grande do Sul, Porto Alegre, Brazil
e-mail: giana.frizzo@ufrgs.br

G. B. Frizzo (ed.), *Digital Media and Early Child Development*,
https://doi.org/10.1007/978-3-031-69224-6_2

computers, and more current ones, such as streaming and smartphones. The results for a sample of 5700 participants indicated that children between the ages of zero and eight use digital media on average for two 2 and a half hours a day. The daily use is about 3 hours among children aged five to eight, and the number one choice of the children's audience is television, with 79% of the preference. Between 2017 and 2020, there was an increase of 20 minutes per day dedicated to online videos, on platforms such as YouTube and TikTok (Rideout & Robb, 2020). According to a UK report, nearly 80% of children in the age range of 3–7 use video-sharing platforms or watch TV and videos. However, the report also notes that preschoolers are at a different life stage than older children, with significantly less autonomy and more parental supervision (Ofcom, 2022).

In Brazil, Rocha et al. (2021) analyzed a total of 3155 children aged 0–60 months. The average total screen exposure time was 2.6 hours per day, with 1.5 hours for TV and 0.6 hours for tablets/smartphones. Another study carried out in Brazil between 2018 and 2019 uncovered several intriguing insights regarding technology usage among children and families. Shockingly, the study found that over half, specifically 54%, of infants were already engaging with computers or various mobile devices. As children grew older, the prevalence of personal device ownership increased, indicating a trend toward earlier and more independent technology usage. Additionally, a significant portion of mothers, around 33%, had downloaded applications specifically tailored for their children, with a notable preference for entertainment platforms like YouTube and Netflix, constituting 61.1% of the downloads, while educational apps accounted for 32.9%. Disturbingly, 43% of mothers admitted that the television remained on in their households even when no one was actively watching, the so-called background TV. However, amidst these trends, there was evidence of a balanced approach to television consumption, with 61% of families alternating between programming designed for adults and that catered to children's interests. These findings shed light on the evolving landscape of technology integration within Brazilian households and underscore the need for further research and awareness regarding its potential impacts on early childhood development (Azevedo et al., 2022). Data collections made during the periods of relaxation of social distancing measures and after the end of the pandemic have shown that when compared to the pre-lockdown period, screen time increased and remained consistent throughout lockdowns, implying that the disturbance induced by lockdown procedures may have impacted habitual kid watching behaviors (Pedrotti et al. 2022). A priori, it can be said that the pandemic has changed children's habits about screen media use (Hedderson et al., 2023; Gueron-Sela et al., 2023).

Historical Overview

Research investigating the effects of children's digital media use dates back to the launch of this media. For instance, the first studies on television can be traced back to the 1950s, coinciding with the advent of color broadcasts. A PubMed search, restricted to full texts and combining the terms "television," "children," and

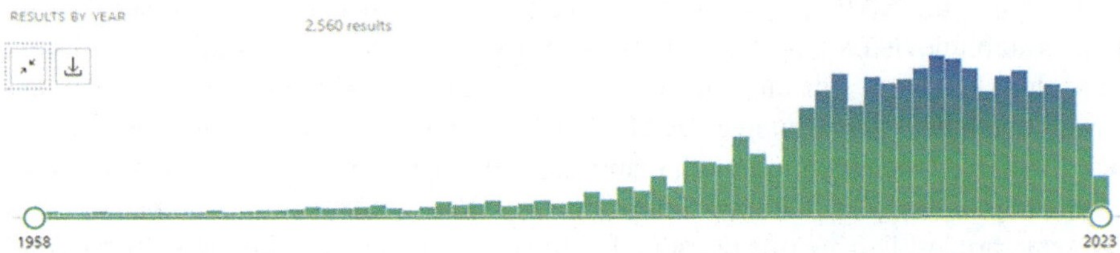

Fig. 2.1 Beginning and expansion of studies related to exposure to television in children. (From PubMed, by the National Center for Biotechnology Information (NCBI), 2023 (https://pubmed.ncbi.nlm.nih.gov/?term=television+AND+children+AND+effects&filter=years.1951-2023&timeline=expanded). In the public domain)

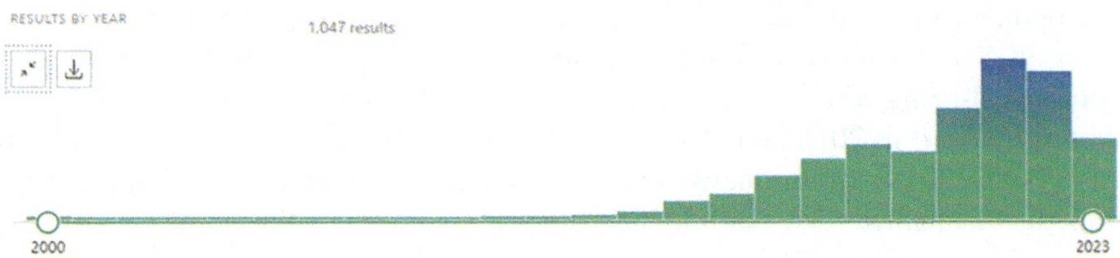

Fig. 2.2 Beginning and expansion of studies related to exposure to smartphones in children. (From PubMed, by the National Center for Biotechnology Information (NCBI), 2023 (https://pubmed.ncbi.nlm.nih.gov/?term=smartphone+AND+children+AND+effects&filter=years.2000-2023&timeline=expanded). In the public domain)

"effects," showcases the beginning and progression of studies related to television exposure in children (see Fig. 2.1). The primary research focus was on investigating the effects of television viewing on children, as television was the dominant media platform during that time (Anderson, 1998; Anderson et al., 1985; Huston et al., 1990; Collins & Wiens, 1983; Rudolf, 1959).

Rudolf's (1958) study on the relationship between television viewing habits and aggressive behaviors in children was one of the pioneering works. From there, research expanded in a slow progression, with less than ten publications per year until the 1990s, when the number of studies relating TV exposure and effects on children began to expand more intensely. This occurred concurrently to the American Academy of Pediatrics' (AAP, 1999) first guidelines. In the 1990s, the AAP shared a statement that recommended no screen time for children under 2 years old and limited screen time for older children, establishing that there were risks and benefits from exposure to mass media. For example, researchers emphasized the importance of limiting screen time for young children, once excessive screen time was associated with potential negative effects on social development (Vessey et al., 1998). Researchers also investigated the content of children's television programming, especially violent ones, and its potential influence on behavior and learning.

Related to the effects of exposure to smartphones, a similar search on PubMed crossing the terms "smartphone," "children," and "effects" shows that the emergence of studies occurred around 2000, but expanded around the 2010s, which coincides with the popularization of social media (see Fig. 2.2).

By 2001, the AAP updated its guidelines, claiming that children and adolescents who watch television may have potential negative health effects such as aggressive or violent behavior, substance usage, sexual activity, obesity, poor body image, and lower academic performance (AAP, 2001). Some years later, the AAP (2016) acknowledged the changing media landscape and have encouraged parents to establish a media use plan for their children, including guidelines on screen time and content choices. During this decade, the introduction of smartphones and tablets led to increased accessibility to digital media, raising concerns about its impact on young children's development.

In the 2010s, as digital media technologies became more prevalent, research expanded to encompass a wider range of media devices and interactive apps. Studies aimed to understand digital media effects on various aspects of early childhood development, including cognitive, socio-emotional, and language skills (Allan & Smith, 2020). The effects of screen time on sleep patterns, physical health, and overall well-being also became areas of interest (Duch et al., 2013), which was advised by AAP in 2016 and also by the World Health Organization guidelines in 2019 (WHO, 2019). Additionally, studies explored the potential of educational digital media to enhance early learning and literacy skills (Ramadhan et al., 2019).

Conceptual Issues

Enhancing Conceptual Clarity in Research on Media Use: Defining Key Terms and Concepts

Conceptual clarity holds paramount importance in academic research, entailing the provision of well-defined terms and a clear research scope. It ensures unambiguous communication, guides the formulation of focused research questions, facilitates data collection and analysis, and enhances the validity and reliability of research outcomes. Upholding conceptual clarity enables researchers to contribute to cumulative knowledge-building and strengthen the impact and rigor of their studies within the broader scientific community (Kahn & Zeidler, 2017).

In the scientific literature, the most diverse names are found to designate digital media (Kaye et al., 2020). Digital media is the set of communication devices, formats, and methods that deliver digitized content, including text, graphics, audio, and video, through digital signals, such as on the Internet, TV, computer, and telephone networks. Examples of digital media include computer software, mobile applications, social networks, video games, web pages, digital images (photos and videos), and smartphones (APA, 2019). Numerous investigations have explored the associations between digital media usage and psychological, educational, and health outcomes, particularly after the 2000s, as discussed previously in this chapter. However, since the beginning, various descriptors have been employed to characterize the utilization, manipulation, or behaviors pertaining to digital media and their respective effects. Common terminology encompassing the domain of digital media usage includes "screen time," "digital media use," "screen media use," "screen media usage," "screen use," "touchscreen technology," and "screen media habits." These terms are often utilized to describe and categorize the extent and nature of individuals' engagement with digital media platforms, considering their potential implications on psychological, educational, and health-related outcomes.

In the scientific literature, various terms have been used to refer to digital media (Kaye et al., 2020). Digital media encompasses a range of communication devices, formats, and methods that deliver digitized content, including text, graphics, audio, and video, through digital signals found on the Internet, TV, computer, and telephone networks. Examples of digital media include computer software, mobile applications, social networks, video games, web pages, digital images (photos and videos), and smartphones (APA, 2019).

The presence of these numerous descriptors reflects the ever-changing and evolving nature of this field. Consequently, studies in this area encounter challenges when investigating the use of digital media, primarily due to the absence of well-established terminology (Davidson et al., 2022). Researchers frequently utilize different terms to describe and categorize individuals' engagement with digital media platforms, considering their potential implications on psychological, educational, and health-related outcomes.

As mentioned earlier, the original emphasis was on quantifying the time spent using screens, and the term "screen time" served as a suitable representation of this aspect. However, researchers came to recognize the necessity for a more comprehensive conceptualization to understand screen media use and its effects on various aspects of children's lives, especially as the landscape of screen media evolved with the emergence of new portable touchscreen-based devices (Klakk et al., 2020). Consequently, there has been a shift, now viewed as a meaningful activity influenced by various contextual factors such as connections, content, purpose, timing, and communication (Barr et al., 2020). Within this context, descriptors like "digital media use," "screen media use," and "screen media usage" have been employed to better grasp the potential benefits and effects of screen use. This transition in descriptors may indicate a change in emphasis, particularly concerning screen time, and has played a vital role in addressing the limitations present in earlier literature. These limitations encompass issues related to poor conceptualization and the use of non-standardized metrics. As a result, researchers have advocated for a more user-focused approach (Kaye et al., 2021).

The descriptor "screen use" is sometimes used as an abbreviation for "screen media use" and is employed in various ways. Its earliest records of use in PubMed date back to 1980, and it serves as a descriptor for the utilization or interaction with devices that have a screen. Additionally, it is used to describe touch screen use in research or the type of screen utilized in equipment or devices, such as those used by doctors. Consequently, while the term "screen use" is more commonly found in research on digital media, it can also be associated with other areas of research. The term "screen media habits" is less commonly used compared to the other descriptors mentioned earlier. However, it has been increasingly appearing in recent studies, particularly from the 2020s, indicating a trend toward growth. This descriptor is frequently employed in research investigating the influence of screen use on aspects such as physical activity, sleep patterns, recreational screen media engagement, household rules related to screen use, and related subjects. Many different descriptors have emerged to refer to screen usage, some of which may not have been mentioned here. This diversity of terms reflects the expanding and multifaceted interest in this field of research.

Finally, it has been observed that certain studies associate clinical criteria, particularly "addiction" and "dependence," with the previously mentioned terms related to media behaviors. Consequently, this often results in an overemphasis on the negative aspects of these behaviors (Browne et al., 2021). Among the descriptors used in such research are "digital media addiction/dependence" and "screen media addiction/dependence." Past research has underscored the importance of differentiating between compulsive and habitual social media use since they originate from distinct underlying mental processes and elicit different effects. Habitual social media use is characterized by known automaticity indicators, such as a lack of awareness and immediate control, conscious intention, and mental efficiency. In contrast, compulsive social media use tends to be more detrimental, linked to adverse effects like connection overload and poor sleep (Davidson et al., 2022; Koban et al., 2023). Therefore, it is crucial for researchers to clarify the nature of individuals' media habits to avoid drawing misleading or unwarranted conclusions.

Evaluating and Selecting Appropriate Theoretical Frameworks to Guide the Research: The Context Role

Theoretical frameworks serve as organized systems of concepts and theories derived from existing knowledge in a specific field, guiding researchers' thinking and interpretation of their research topic. Their primary functions include providing explanations for phenomena, predicting behaviors or outcomes of variables, contextualizing the research within existing knowledge, and establishing conceptual connections between different elements of the study. Acting as an overarching lens, theoretical frameworks offer systematic understanding and a roadmap for researchers to explore relationships and identify relevant variables in their investigations (Elhai & Montag, 2020).

Contextual theorists (Vygotsky, 1978; Bronfenbrenner and Morris, 2006) talk about the importance of measuring the interaction between contexts and how children develop. Current research on digital media has been based on family context using the concept of family media ecology, considering the importance of assessing the use that the whole family makes of digital media (Barr, 2019; Barr et al., 2020). Family media ecology is a set of parental decisions about the use, characteristics (behaviors, affects, and cognitions) of all family members related to the use, availability, and role that media plays in the home environment (Levine et al., 2019). It proposes that it is essential to focus on how digital media are used by the family, such as caregivers' media time, the use of screens as a parenting tool (Wartella et al., 2014), and how media standards can collaborate or interfere with healthy use and potentially promote learning (Barr, 2019). Knowing it allows understanding the pattern of use and exposure of the family and, therefore, also of the child to the media (Barr, 2019).

Children's media habits are shaped first in the family context (Vandewater, 2013). Therefore, thinking about all family dynamics represents a broader and more accurate view than previous research that focused only on digital media use time. When evaluating the context of the use of digital media, it is possible to access demographic and environmental issues, characteristics of the house, and parental mediation.

Studies have discussed the way parents use digital media with their children, describing mediation styles of use that parents make with their children (Clark, 2011). One is active mediation, when there is some kind of conversation and discussion about media use; another is restrictive mediation, where some rules are established to restrict time or content; and the last one is shared use, which occurs when parents and children share media experiences (Shin, 2015; Valkenburg et al., 1999). There are also other styles of mediation, such as monitoring the child's online activities or using resources to restrict the use of media devices (Livingstone & Helsper, 2008). Some research has identified that the style of family mediation varies according to the cultural context. For example, American parents often use active mediation (Austin, 1993); Dutch parents prefer co-viewing (Valkenburg et al., 1999); Korean parents apply restrictive mediation (Lee, 2012); and in Belgium, France, and Sweden, parents use technical resources to restrict the use of media devices (Livingstone et al., 2011).

Despite several styles of mediation pointed out in the literature, the experience of using digital media in the presence of someone is different from using it in interaction with someone. The use of digital media by children only in the presence of an adult does not require involvement, nor exchanges or interaction, but only some kind of distance supervision or even no supervision at all. There are families that rely on technological resources to free themselves from their children, in order to handle their own tasks. This can lead to a completely solitary use of digital media by children, which is not recommended (Azevedo et al., 2022). However, a shared and active use, mediated by exchanges of looks and affection, with constant presence and interaction of the parents in the use that the child is making of the media, can be considered a healthier use. If there is no participation and interaction of a caregiver willing to mediate the technological experience, digital media alone will not fulfill an adequate function of exchange and education.

Studies evaluating digital media use, by including the context, are able to register the use of simultaneous screens and the different uses that the same device provides. While the video game can be used for socializing, it can also be used alone; a child can use YouTube to watch educational videos while communicating with peers at school (Browne et al., 2021). So, the presence of devices can interrupt the interaction between parents and children (Barr et al., 2020). In contrast, it is reported that simultaneous use or switching between devices can have cognitive impacts, particularly on attention. It is indicated that exposure to video games is positively associated with selective attention in young children, but the effects depend on the characteristics of the users, the form that digital technologies take, and the circumstances in which use occurs (Samson et al., 2021; Vedechkin, & Borgonovi, 2021).

Developing or Utilizing Conceptual Frameworks That Organize and Structure the Research: The Content Role

Conceptual frameworks are specific and focused frameworks that guide the research design and data analysis within a particular study. These frameworks also help in generating hypotheses or research questions by highlighting relationships between identified variables, serving as a basis for formulating testable statements. Lastly, they provide guidance for selecting appropriate data analysis techniques by specifying relationships between variables, enabling a structured approach to analyzing and interpreting collected data. Overall, conceptual frameworks complement broader theoretical frameworks and focus on the specific aspects of a research project. In the study on digital media in early childhood, the operationalization of the content accessed assisted in clarifying their definitions and measurements (Van der Waldt, 2020).

Early research related to the content offered by digital media emphasized, above all, those linked to television, since it was for a period of time the only device that provided something to the children's audience, whether it was aimed at entertainment or education (Lerner, 2016). However, with the advance of electronic devices, there has been rapid progress in the creation of content on digital platforms. Currently, discussions focus on whether the content offered by digital media is appropriate for children's development and well-being (Lerner, 2016). Although there are applications and platforms already created to promote development, access to these is still low since they need the mediation of parents or teachers, and, in the Brazilian context, the application of these technologies to advance knowledge still finds barriers in basic education, such as an inadequate physical infrastructure (Bielschowsky, 2023). Given this reality, it remains for researchers to worry about the role of content distributed by the media in investigating the exposure of the children's audience to them (Lauricella et al., 2017).

For instance, US and British preschoolers consume mostly videos on social media platforms, such as YouTube and TikTok (Dormedy, 2023; Ofcom, 2022). Eighty-nine percent of children between 3 and 4 years old and 93% of kids between 5 and 7 years old use video platforms (Ofcom, 2022). In the Brazilian study by Pedrotti et al. (2022), most mothers have downloaded YouTube for their under 3-year-old children. Besides, social networks are constantly changing, as are the features that each has, so some authors have proposed operationalizing the content consumed by adopting the dichotomic terms passive and active use of digital media.

Passive use (PSMU) refers to the consumption of social media content (SMU) without the person participating directly in social interactions, such as reading other people's profiles, text or audiovisual posts, short videos (popularly known as reels), or comments (Meier & Krause, 2022; Verduyn et al., 2017). Meanwhile, all digital actions that encourage social interaction with third parties, such as sending messages, leaving comments on other people's content, and transmitting the content itself, are considered active use (ASMU) (Meier & Krause, 2022; Verduyn et al., 2017).

Primarily, the dichotomy between the concepts active and passive allows for a more detailed analysis of social media by explaining part of the complexity of these and is applicable to various existing platforms and future creations by being in contact with elements and central features of social media (Meier & Krause, 2022; Verduyn et al., 2017). It also provides valuable insights for translational research practices by taking the negative bias of social media and balancing the benefits and risks of SMU, allowing for a more flexible and generalized view of their impact on children (Parry et al., 2022). Furthermore, the advantage of using the active/passive arrangement in studies is that it presents several important methodological strengths, in particular when using a consistent SMU measurement (Trifiro & Gerson, 2019).

Measurement Challenges

Measuring Digital Media: Collection Tools and Their Strengths and Limitations

Studying digital media use in early childhood is crucial but demands careful attention due to developmental limitations and ethical concerns. As technology becomes more prevalent in young children's lives, understanding their interactions with digital devices and media is essential. This chapter outlines two common methods to measure digital media use in early childhood research: parental reporting and data collected from apps. By using these approaches, researchers can gather valuable information about young children's digital media habits and their impact on early development while prioritizing participant safety and well-being.

Parental Reporting

One of the main benefits of parent-report measures is their capacity to offer a detailed evaluation of aspects of young children's screen media use. These measurements consider not only how often children use screens but also attitudes toward media consumption and the types of media children engage with (Klakk et al., 2020). Thus, by using those methods, researchers can learn more about the general trends in screen media use and how it may affect children's development (Barr et al., 2020). Moreover, measures based on parent reports also permit the inclusion of pertinent variables that may affect young children's use of screens, such as family social dynamics, parent–infant play, emotional qualities, and home environment characteristics (Barr et al., 2020).

Parent-report measures can also be valuable as research instruments because of their internal reliability and consistency (Dubay & Watson, 2019). By demonstrating good internal consistency, these measures demonstrate a level of coherence and stability in assessing screen media use over time and across different settings, enhancing the reliability of the data obtained (Dubay & Watson, 2019). Another advantage is that these measures are quite affordable and accessible. Then, they provide a convenient way to obtain information on the use of screen media by large groups of young children, once they may be delivered through surveys or interviews. This practicality makes it possible to conduct more in-depth and diverse research (Dubay & Watson, 2019).

By involving parents in reporting their children's screen media use, researchers can promote parental awareness of the potential implications of excessive or inappropriate media consumption. Therefore, more aware parents can make safer and intentional choices regarding screen use in the home environment. Lastly, parent-report measures can serve as a basis for further research and investigations into screen media use in early childhood. While they offer valuable insights, they can be complemented by other data sources, such as direct observation or device-based tracking, to provide a more comprehensive and triangulated understanding of children's media habits (Barr et al., 2020). However, it is crucial to acknowledge that parent-report measures have limitations and should be complemented with other methods to achieve a comprehensive understanding of screen media use in young children (Barr et al., 2020).

One of the primary limitations of this method is the potential for recall bias (Duch et al., 2013). Parents may not accurately remember or report the exact amount of time their child spends with screens, leading to inaccuracies in data, especially since these behaviors are extremely linked to the participants' daily lives, as are digital media (Geyer et al., 2021; Radesky et al., 2020). This limitation can distort research findings and difficult the formulation of effective guidelines and interventions. In addition, social desirability bias is a relevant issue when assessing parents' reported screen media use (Duch et al., 2013), since in a society increasingly concerned about the possible negative effects of excessive screen time, parents may feel pressured to minimise the amount of screen exposure their children receive. Consequently, this bias can lead to an underreporting of screen time, making it difficult to obtain a true representation of a child's media consumption (Duch et al., 2013).

Additionally, parent-report measures may fail to capture the full extent of a child's screen media exposure (Barr et al., 2020). Children often have access to screens outside of their home environment, such as in school, where parents may not be able to supervise or accurately report usage. Moreover, these types of measures are unable to provide detailed information about the content and context of screen media use (Barr et al., 2020). As previously illustrated, understanding what kind of content a child is exposed to is crucial in assessing its potential effects on their development.

In conclusion, parent-report measures may provide valuable data, though they are susceptible to recall bias and social desirability bias and they may not accurately reflect a child's broad exposure to screen media or provide specific context information. Researchers can get over these restrictions and develop a more thorough picture of young children's screen media use by adding metrics like direct observation through parent-report and device-based tracking. This information can help people make informed decisions, which will help kids create constructive media habits and promote their overall development.

Data Collected from Apps

By contrast, apps-based measures can provide a more accurate and objective assessment of children's media use compared to parent-report (Geyer et al., 2021; Radesky et al., 2020). By using apps to track screen media use, researchers can obtain precise data, ensuring a more valid representation of a child's mobile device usage (Parry et al., 2021). Apps can capture not only the duration of media exposure but also the content in which it occurs (Barr et al., 2020). Similarly, they can provide insights into whether children are exposed to age-appropriate and educational content or potentially harmful material, contributing to a better understanding of the impact of media on young minds. Understanding the content of media exposure, for instance, is essential, especially in early childhood when children's brains are rapidly developing (Ismail et al., 2017).

Apps are particularly appropriate for measuring short bursts of mobile device usage, which has become common in today's digital age (Barr et al., 2020). Traditional methods may struggle to capture these intermittent periods of screen time, but apps can efficiently track such usage patterns, providing a more comprehensive picture of media consumption behavior. Moreover, the flexibility of apps allows researchers to gather data from multiple devices and combine it to get a more complete picture of how people use media in their homes (Geyer et al., 2021). This integration can also include data from web-based questionnaires, time-use diaries, and passive-sensing apps, creating a richer dataset and generating deeper insights into screen media use within the family context.

Furthermore, apps-based measures are versatile and can capture screen media use both inside and outside the home (Geyer et al., 2021). This flexibility offers a more comprehensive view of a child's overall media exposure, taking into account a variety of contexts where mobile devices are available. Apps can also facilitate monitoring changes in media consumption over time (Zimmermann, 2021). Thus, researchers can gain a dynamic notion of how media habits change in early infancy by following the use of screen media across time and identifying trends, seasonality, or variations in usage patterns (Zimmermann, 2021). Finally, the use of apps in measuring screen media use is in line with technological advancements and the digital nature of modern society, ensuring that data collection methods remain relevant in an increasingly digital world (Kaye et al., 2021).

On the other hand, when using apps or similar, data security and privacy are crucial considerations, especially when these are associated with other psychological assessments or sensitive demographic variables (Kaye et al., 2021). In the context of digital media and its impact on individuals, researchers should pay attention to the potential risks associated with the processing of personal data, especially when parents' data is mixed with children's data, depending on device sharing (Matthews et al., 2016). Besides, while raw data, such as total smartphone usage time, may not raise immediate security concerns, more specific information about individual apps or usage patterns may reveal personal issues that people may want to keep private. Therefore, researchers should implement additional security procedures, such as the use of encrypted cloud services, to protect the confidentiality of participants (Geyer et al., 2021; Kaye et al., 2020). Another problem using apps is that they are unable to consider multi-screen use, which is also very frequent considering we are embedded in a digital world.

To make significant progress in this domain, it is recommended that researchers combine objective measures of behavior with open research practices, such as parent-report. By adhering to these practices, it can be ensured that findings are verifiable and contribute to the advancement of knowledge. In addition, it is suggested to use novel parent-report methods to extract meaningful information from the data collected. These analytical approaches that go beyond simple device-level measures can provide valuable additional insights into technology-related behaviors. Hence, by using both measures and innovative analytical techniques, researchers can improve their understanding of the causal effects of digital media in early childhood (Geyer et al., 2021; Kaye et al., 2020).

Implications, Future Directions, and Concluding Thoughts

The screen media use investigation and its correlates and impacts in early childhood have several significant implications for research and practice. Recognizing the conceptual and measurement challenges in this rapidly evolving field is fundamental for advancing our understanding of young children's digital media habits and their potential impact on development. In this chapter, we emphasized the importance of conceptual clarity in academic research, stressing the need for well-defined terms and a clear research scope to ensure robust and reliable outcomes.

An important aspect that emerged from our discussions is the existence of different descriptors used to characterize digital media habits and behaviors. The ever-changing nature of technology and media consumption has led researchers to adapt their terminology to encompass a wide range of digital experiences. Descriptors such as "screen time," "digital media use," "screen media use," "screen media usage," "screen use," "touchscreen technology," and "screen media habits" have been employed. To foster effective communication and comparability across studies, it is essential for scholars to establish consensus on standardized terminology by using "digital media," recommended by the American Academy of Pediatrics (APA) (APA, 2019). Doing so will be pivotal in consolidating findings, addressing research gaps, and informing evidence-based practices for promoting healthy media habits in early childhood.

One important discussion of this chapter is the significance of using multiple assessment methods to gain a comprehensive understanding of screen media use in young children. While parent-report measures provide valuable insights into children's media habits and usage patterns, they should be complemented with other approaches to create a more holistic picture. Apps-based measures offer great potential in capturing screen media use both inside and outside the home, enabling researchers to monitor changes in media consumption over time and consider various environments where mobile devices are accessible, even though they still lack the multi-screen reality. As technology evolves, researchers need to count on a set of media assessment tools needed to assess media usage in a rapidly changing media landscape (Barr et al., 2020).

As the digital media landscape continues to evolve, future research directions should focus on developing more standardized and validated measures to assess screen media use in early childhood. Enhancing the reliability and validity of measurement tools will aid in comparing results across studies and advancing our understanding of the impact of digital media on young children's development.

In summary, for a more complete understanding of media use and child development, researchers must investigate not only the duration of media use but also the content and the contexts where the child is using media (e.g., family routines). There is a growing literature demonstrating that factors like mediation of child media use, and parents' own media use, can be related to children's access and use of media (Barr et al., 2020). According to Barr et al. (2020) the greatest challenge is to provide a reliable media measure sensitive enough to evaluate child and household media exposure in a cost-effective way.

In conclusion, the assessment of screen media use in early childhood presents both conceptual and measurement challenges. Nevertheless, with a commitment to conceptual clarity, the integration of various assessment methods, and a focus on future research directions, we can navigate these challenges and expand our knowledge in this important area of study. By taking a comprehensive and thoughtful approach, we can ensure the well-being and healthy development of young children in an increasingly digital world.

References

Allan, A., & Smith, S. (2020). Digital media and sleep in children. In *The Routledge companion to digital media and children* (pp. 403–413). Routledge.

American Academy of Pediatrics Committee on Public Education. (1999). Media education. *Pediatrics, 104*(2), 341–343.

American Academy of Pediatrics Committee on Public Education. (2001). American Academy of Pediatrics: Children, adolescents, and television. *Pediatrics, 107*(2), 423–426. https://doi.org/10.1542/peds.107.2.423

American Academy of Pediatrics, Council on Communications and Media. (2016). Media and young minds. *Pediatrics, 138*(5), 1–8. https://doi.org/10.1542/peds.2016-2591

American Psychological Association. (2019). Thesaurus of psychological index terms. Recuperado de: https://psycnetapaorg.ez25.periodicos.capes.gov.br/thesaurus/item?term=digital%20 media.

Anderson, D. R., Field, D. E., Collins, P. A., Lorch, E. P., & Nathan, J. G. (1985). Estimates of young children's time with television: a methodological comparison of parent reports with time-lapse video home observation. *Child Development, 56*(5), 1345–1357. https://doi.org/10.2307/1130249

Anderson, D. R. (1998). Educational television is not an oxymoron. *The Annals of the American Academy of Political and Social Science, 557*(1), 24–38.

Austin, E. W. (1993). Exploring the effects of active parental mediation of television content. *Journal of Broadcasting & Electronic Media, 37*, 147–158. https://doi.org/10.1080/08838159309364212

Azevedo, E. C., Riter, H. S., Pieta, M. A. P., & Frizzo, G. B. (2022). Digital media use by mothers and infants. *Paideia (Ribeirão Preto), 32*, e3210. https://doi.org/10.1590/1982-4327e3210

Barr, R. (2019). Growing up in the digital age: Early learning and family media ecology. *Current Directions in Psychological Science, 28*(4), 341–346. https://doi.org/10.1177/0963721419838245

Barr, R., Kirkorian, H., Radesky, J., Coyne, S., Nichols, D., Blanchfield, O., Rusnak, S., Stockdale, L., Ribner, A., Durnez, J., Epstein, M., Heimann, M., Koch, F.-S., Sundqvist, A., Birberg-Thornberg, U., Konrad, C., Slussareff, M., Bus, A., Bellagamba, F., & Fitzpatrick, C. (2020). Beyond screen time: A synergistic approach to a more comprehensive assessment of family media exposure during early childhood. *Frontiers in Psychology, 11*, 1283. https://doi.org/10.3389/fpsyg.2020.01283

Bielschowsky, C (2023). *CONECTA: Tecnologias na Educação: desafios e dificuldades*. Rede Nacional de Ciência para a Educação. https://cienciaparaeducacao.org/blog/2023/03/27/tecnologias-na-educacao-desafios-e-dificuldades/

Bronfenbrenner, U., & Morris, P. A. (2006). The bioecological model of human development. In R. M. Lerner & W. Damon (Eds.), *Handbook of child psychology: Theoretical models of human development* (pp. 793–828). John Wiley & Sons Inc.

Clark, L. S. (2011). Parental mediation theory for the digital age. *Communication Theory, 21*(4), 323–343. https://doi.org/10.1111/j.1468-2885.2011.01391.x

Collins, W. A., & Wiens, M. (1983). Cognitive processes in television viewing: Description and strategic implications. In *Cognitive strategy research: Psychological foundations* (pp. 179–201). New York, NY, Springer New York.

Davidson, B. I., Shaw, H., & Ellis, D. A. (2022). Fuzzy constructs in technology usage scales. *Computers in Human Behavior, 133*, 107206. https://doi.org/10.1016/j.chb.2022.107206

Dormedy, K. (2023). [New Report] Kids & the Screen USA. Precise TV and Giraffe Insights. https://blog.precise.tv/blog/report-kids-and-the-screen-usa

DuBay, M., & Watson, L. R. (2019). Translation and cultural adaptation of parent-report developmental assessments: Improving rigor in methodology. *Research in Autism Spectrum Disorders, 62*, 55–65. https://doi.org/10.1016/j.rasd.2019.02.005

Duch, H., Fisher, E. M., Ensari, I., & Harrington, A. (2013). Screen time use in children under 3 years old: A systematic review of correlates. *International Journal of Behavioral Nutrition and Physical Activity, 10*, 1–10. http://www.ijbnpa.org/content/10/1/102

Elhai, J. D., & Montag, C. (2020). The compatibility of theoretical frameworks with machine learning analyses in psychological research. *Current Opinion in Psychology, 36*, 83–88. https://doi.org/10.1016/j.copsyc.2020.05.002

Geyer, K., Ellis, D. A., Shaw, H., & Davidson, B. I. (2021). Open-source smartphone app and tools for measuring, quantifying, and visualizing technology use. *Behavior Research Methods, 54*(1), 1–12. https://doi.org/10.3758/s13428-021-01585-7

Gueron-Sela, N., Shalev, I., Gordon-Hacker, A., Egotubov, A., & Barr, R. (2023). Screen media exposure and behavioral adjustment in early childhood during and after COVID-19 home lockdown periods. *Computers in Human Behavior, 140*, 107572. https://doi.org/10.1016/j.chb.2022.107572

Hedderson, M. M., Bekelman, T. A., Li, M., Knapp, E. A., Palmore, M., Dong, Y., et al. (2023). Trends in screen time use among children during the COVID-19 pandemic, July 2019 through august 2021. *JAMA Network Open, 6*(2), –e2256157. https://doi.org/10.1001/jamanetworkopen.2022.56157

Huston, A. C., Wright, J. C., Rice, M. L., Kerkman, D., & St Peters, M. (1990). Development of television viewing patterns in early childhood: A longitudinal investigation. *Developmental Psychology, 26*(3), 409.

Ismail, F. Y., Fatemi, A., & Johnston, M. V. (2017). Cerebral plasticity: Windows of opportunity in the developing brain. *European Journal of Paediatric Neurology, 21*(1), 23–48. https://doi.org/10.1016/j.ejpn.2016.07.007

Kahn, S., & Zeidler, D. L. (2017). A case for the use of conceptual analysis in science education research. *Journal of Research in Science Teaching, 54*(4), 538–551. https://doi.org/10.1002/tea.21376

Kaye, L. K., Orben, A., Ellis, D. A., Hunter, S. C., & Houghton, S. (2020). The conceptual and methodological mayhem of "screen time". *International Journal of Environmental Research and Public Health, 17*(10), 3661. https://doi.org/10.3390/ijerph17103661

Kaye, L. K., Kuss, D. J., & Rumpf, H. J. (2021). Conceptual and methodological considerations of gaming disorder and internet gaming disorder. In N. el-Guebaly, G. Carrà, M. Galanter, & A. M. Baldacchino (Eds.), *Textbook of addiction treatment* (pp. 967–977). Springer. https://doi.org/10.1007/978-3-030-36391-8_68

Koban, K., Stevic, A., Matthes, J. (2023). A tale of two concepts: differential temporal predictions of habitual and compulsive social media use concerning connection overload and sleep quality, *Journal of Computer-Mediated Communication, 28*(2). https://doi.org/10.1093/jcmc/zmac040

Klakk, H., Wester, C. T., Olesen, L. G., Rasmussen, M. G., Kristensen, P. L., Pedersen, J., & Grøntved, A. (2020). The development of a questionnaire to assess leisure time screenbased media use and its proximal correlates in children (SCREENS-Q). *BMC Public Health, 20*, 1–12. https://doi.org/10.1186/s12889-020-08810-6

Lauricella, A. R., Blackwell, C. K., & Wartella, E. (2017). *The "new" technology environment: The role of content and context on learning and development from mobile media* (pp. 1–23). The effects of content and context on learning and development.

Lee, B. (2012). An exploratory study on early childhood smart device usage at home. *Child Education Studies, 16*(6), 511–532.

Lerner, C. (2016). Context matters: How co-using screen media impacts young children-commentary on chapter 11. In *Media exposure during infancy and early childhood: The effects of content and context on learning and development*. https://doi.org/10.1007/978-3-319-45102-2_12

Levine, L. E., Waite, B. M., Bowman, L. L., & Kachinsky, K. (2019). Mobile media use by infants and toddlers. *Computers in Human Behavior, 94*, 92–99. https://doi.org/10.1016/j.chb.2018.12.045

Livingstone, S., & Helsper, E. J. (2008). Parental mediation of children's internet use. *Journal of Broadcasting & Electronic Media, 52*(4), 581–599.

Livingstone, S., Haddon, L., Görzig, A., & Ólafsson, K. (2011). Risks and safety on the internet: the perspective of European children: full findings and policy implications from the EU Kids Online survey of 9-16 year olds and their parents in 25 countries. http://eprints.lse.ac.uk/33731/

Matthews, T., Liao, K., Turner, A., Berkovich, M., Reeder, R., & Consolvo, S. (2016). " She'll just grab any device that's closer". A Study of Everyday Device & Account Sharing in Households. In *Proceedings of the 2016 CHI Conference on Human Factors in Computing Systems*. https://doi.org/10.1145/2858036.2858051

Meier, A., & Krause, H. (2022, October). Does passive social media use harm well-being? An adversarial review. https://doi.org/10.1027/1864-1105/a000358

Ofcom. (2022). Children and parents: media use and attitudes report. https://www.ofcom.org.uk/__data/assets/pdf_file/0024/234609/childrens-media-use-and-attitudes-report-2022
Parry, D. A., Davidson, B. I., Sewall, C. J., Fisher, J. T., Mieczkowski, H., & Quintana, D. S. (2021). A systematic review and meta-analysis of discrepancies between logged and self-reported digital media use. *Nature Human Behaviour, 5*(11), 1535–1547. https://doi.org/10.1038/s41562-021-01117-5
Parry, D. A., Fisher, J. T., Mieczkowski, H., Sewall, C. J. R., & Davidson, B. I. (2022). Social media and well-being: A methodological perspective. *Current Opinion in Psychology, 45*, 101285. https://doi.org/10.1016/J.COPSYC.2021.11.005
Pedrotti, B. G., Mallmann, M. Y., Almeida, C. R. S., Marques, F. M., Vescovi, G., da Riter, H. S., Almeida, M. L., Pieta, M. A. M., & Frizzo, G. B. (2022). Infants' and toddlers' digital media use and mothers' mental health: A comparative study before and during the COVID-19 pandemic. *Infant Mental Health Journal, 43*(1), 24–35. https://doi.org/10.1002/imhj.21952
Radesky, J. S., Weeks, H. M., Ball, R., Schaller, A., Yeo, S., Durnez, J., et al. (2020). Young children's use of smartphones and tablets. *Pediatrics, 146*(1). https://doi.org/10.1542/peds.2019-3518
Ramadhan, S., Sukma, E., & Indriyani, V. (2019). Teacher competence in utilizing digital media literacy in education. *In Journal of Physics: Conference Series, 1339*(1), 012111. IOP Publishing.
Rideout, V., & Robb, M. B. (2020). *The common sense census: Media use by kids age zero to eight, 2020*. Retrieved from https://www.commonsensemedia.org/sites/default/files/uploads/research/2020_zero_to_eight_ census_final_web.pdf
Rocha, H. A. L., Correia, L. L., Madeiro Leite, L. J., Tavares Machado, M. M., Lindsay, A. C., Maia Oliveira Rocha, S. G., Campos, J. S., de Silva, A. C., & Sudfeld, C. R. (2021, November 11). Screen time and early childhood development in Ceará, Brazil: A population-based study. *BMC Public Health. BioMed Central, 21*, 1–8. https://doi.org/10.1186/s12889-021-12136-2
Royal College of Paediatrics and Child Health RCPCH. (2019). *The health impacts of screen time: a guide for clinicians and parents*. Retrieved from:https://www.rcpch.ac.uk/resources/health-impacts-screen-time-guide-cliniciansparents
Rudolf, G. D. M. (1958). The effect of children's television on behaviour. *Mental Health, 17*(2), 55.
Rudolf, G. (1959). Effect of children's television on behaviour. *Mental Health, 18*(1), 34. Retrieved from https://www.ncbi.nlm.nih.gov/pmc/articles/PMC5081801/
Samson, A. D., Rohr, C. S., Park, S., Arora, A., Ip, A., Tansey, R., et al. (2021). Videogame exposure positively associates with selective attention in a cross-sectional sample of young children. *PLoS One, 16*(9), e0257877. https://doi.org/10.1371/journal.pone.0257877
Shin, W. (2015). Parental socialization of children's internet use: A qualitative approach. *New Media & Society, 17*(5), 649–665. https://doi.org/10.1177/1461444813516833
Trifiro, B. M., & Gerson, J. (2019). Social media usage patterns: Research note regarding the lack of universal validated measures for active and passive use. *Social Media+ Society, 5*(2), 2056305119848743. https://doi.org/10.1177/2056305119848743
Valkenburg, P. M., Krcmar, M., Peeters, A. L., & Marseille, N. M. (1999). Developing a scale to assess three styles of television mediation: "Instructive mediation," "restrictive mediation," and "social coviewing". *Journal of Broadcasting & Electronic Media, 43*(1), 52–66. https://doi.org/10.1080/08838159909364474
Van der Waldt, G. (2020). Constructing conceptual frameworks in social science research. *TD: The Journal for Transdisciplinary Research in Southern Africa, 16*(1), 1–9.
Vandewater, E. A. (2013). Ecological approaches to the study of media and children. In D. Lemish (Ed.), *The Routledge international handbook of children, adolescents and media* (pp. 72–79). Routledge.
Vedechkina, M., & Borgonovi, F. (2021). A review of evidence on the role of digital technology in shaping attention and cognitive control in children. *Frontiers in Psychology, 12*, 611155. https://doi.org/10.3389/fpsyg.2021.611155
Verduyn, P., Ybarra, O., Résibois, M., Jonides, J., & Kross, E. (2017). Do social network sites enhance or undermine subjective well-being? A critical review. *Social Issues and Policy Review, 11*(1), 274–302. https://doi.org/10.1111/sipr.12033

Vessey, J. A., Yim-Chiplis, P. K., & MacKenzie, N. R. (1998). Effects of television viewing on children's development. *Pediatric Nursing, 24*(5), 483–487.

Vygotsky, L. S. (1978). *Mind in society: The development of higher psychological processes*. Harvard University Press.

Wartella, E., Rideout, V., Lauricella, A. R., & Connell, S. (2014). *Parenting in the age of digital technology*. Report for The Center on Media and Human Development School of Communication Northwestern University.

World Health Organization WHO. (2019). *Guidelines on physical activity, sedentary behaviour and sleep for children under 5 years of age*. World Health Organization. Retrieved from http://www.who.int/iris/handle/10665/311664

Zimmermann, L. (2021). "Your screen-time app is keeping track": Consumers are happy to monitor but unlikely to reduce smartphone usage. *Journal of the Association for Consumer Research, 6*(3), 377–382. https://doi.org/10.1086/714365

Chapter 3
The Digital Level of Analysis: A Systemic Framework for Exploring Child Development in a Technology-Saturated World

Jasmine Zhang, Sofia Sebben, and Dillon T. Browne

Rapid advancements in the technology industry have drastically altered the nature of human development in recent decades. As the world grows increasingly digitized, Internet-connected screen-based devices (e.g., computers, smartphones, televisions, and tablets) have become indispensable in the twenty-first century. These developments raise complex, novel issues in the fields of developmental psychopathology and family science. There are growing concerns that spending time on screens (i.e., *screen time*) is detrimental to young people's physical and mental wellbeing. This discourse has permeated both scientific and popular conversations, propagating calls for robust policies that foster positive development in the digital world (Kucirkova et al., 2023). Yet, ongoing efforts to develop evidence-based strategies continue to be thwarted by conceptual and methodological limitations in the current literature. These issues stem from an overemphasis on the amount of time that children and youth spend on screens, which condenses all media activities into a one-dimensional factor.

The construct of screen time overlooks the complex infrastructure of the digital world and its myriad interactions with developmental systems. Increasing acknowledgment of this challenge has incited a paradigm shift to move "beyond screen time" (Barr et al., 2020). Accordingly, we propose the "Digital Level of Analysis" as a conceptual frame of reference that facilitates nuanced, ecologically valid studies of children's media use. Following a summary of the extant screen time literature, we review relevant theories of children's media use and developmental

J. Zhang · D. T. Browne (✉)
Department of Psychology, University of Waterloo, Waterloo, ON, Canada
e-mail: jasmine.zhang@uwaterloo.ca; dillon.browne@uwaterloo.ca

S. Sebben
Department of Psychology, University of Waterloo, Waterloo, ON, Canada

Universidade Federal do Rio Grande do Sul, Porto Alegre, Brazil
e-mail: sscolognese@uwaterloo.ca

G. B. Frizzo (ed.), *Digital Media and Early Child Development*,
https://doi.org/10.1007/978-3-031-69224-6_3

processes. We also expand upon the "multiple levels of analysis" notion from developmental psychopathology (Cicchetti & Dawson, 2002) and describe ways to incorporate technology into extant frameworks via the Digital Level of Analysis. Finally, we present recommendations that aim to facilitate multilevel, multidisciplinary studies that inform a refined understanding of how technology shapes the modern-day developmental landscape.

The Rise of Screen Time

At the turn of the millennium, television sets, video game consoles, and computers were commonplace in homes across developed nations (Roberts et al., 1999). Internet access has since become ubiquitous, garnering attention as a social determinant of health with significant repercussions for individual and public well-being (Benda et al., 2020). In contrast to previous generations, who were tasked with adapting to technology later in life, interactions with digital media now begin in infancy (Christakis, 2009) and increase exponentially with age. Recent estimates of device ownership in the United States indicate that nearly all children and youth have access to screen-based electronics and the Internet (Rideout et al., 2022). Accordingly, large-scale surveys report that school-aged children use devices for approximately 4–6 hours each day, and over half (i.e., 7–9 hours) of adolescents' daily waking hours are spent on screens (Rideout et al., 2022). These trends intensified as countries around the globe mandated shelter-in-place orders during the COVID-19 pandemic, rendering screens more indispensable to daily life than ever before (McArthur et al., 2021; Nagata et al., 2022).

Alarmingly high screen time estimates have propagated significant apprehension among caregivers and pediatric clinicians. Their concerns emerged long before the pandemic and skyrocketed thereafter (Mcclain, 2022; Sultana et al., 2020). Most worries center on the ostensibly harmful effects that devices cast on children's social, emotional, and physical development. In response, influential child health organizations from around the world (Canadian Paediatric Society Digital Health Task Force, 2019; Committee on Public Education, 1999; World Health Organization, 2019) published guidelines on screen time limits for children of different age groups. The American Academy of Pediatrics (AAP) touted the "2 × 2 rule"—preventing screen use in children under 2 years old and limiting screen use to 2 hours per day thereafter (Committee on Public Education, 1999)—for nearly two decades. As these rules gained traction, screen time became an umbrella term that captured all children's activities on technology.

The Screen Time Debate

Screen time guidelines rest on the assumption that technology use harms children and youth. This stance lies at the crux of messaging from government and professional organizations, who tend to broadcast the risks associated with digital media use more than the potential benefits (Blum-Ross & Livingstone, 2018). However, the notion that empirical evidence wholly supports the negative impacts of screen time, and thereby media in general, has come under scrutiny in recent years. Many studies indeed demonstrate that screen time is associated with worse psychological well-being in nationally representative, high-quality datasets (McAllister et al., 2021; Roberston et al., 2022; Twenge & Campbell, 2018, 2019). Specific correlates include (but are not limited to) increased feelings of loneliness, low mood, suicidality, anxiety, and behavioral problems, sometimes at levels constituting clinical impairment (Roberston et al., 2022). In contrast, other studies report contradictory findings (Johannes et al., 2022; Orben & Przybylski, 2019; Przybylski & Weinstein, 2019) and argue that any negative consequences of screen use are "too small to warrant policy change" (Orben & Przybylski, 2019, p. 1). As debates ensued among researchers and policymakers, caregivers were left worried and confused about how best to manage their children's screen time.

Beyond a lack of consistent empirical support, the 2 × 2 rule also presents various practical limitations. It seems easy for parents to monitor their children's screen time via built-in functions on modern devices, but "unplugging" for most of the day has become increasingly unfeasible. Indeed, a lack of access to devices may lead children and youth to miss opportunities for socialization, self-discovery, learning, and mastery of cognitive and academic skills (LeBlanc et al., 2017; Reid & Weigle, 2014; Rideout & Katz, 2016). As such, screen time rules were and continue to be misaligned with the lived experiences of children and families in today's media-saturated society (Kucirkova et al., 2023).

Moving Beyond Screen Time

Given ongoing acknowledgment of the notion that digital media now play "multifunctional and multifaceted" (Kucirkova et al., 2023, p. 3) roles in children and youth's lives, there have been attempts to revise screen time guidelines. In 2016, a widely publicized rebranding of recommendations from the American Academy of Pediatrics called for more family-based strategies such as creating a family media plan, encouraging co-viewing, and reminding parents to act as models of positive media use habits, whereas other components remained time-based (Livingstone, 2016). Although these guidelines were better allied with life in a digitized society, *attention to the effects of digital media on children remained scattered and overemphasized screen time.* Studies conducted several years after the release of the AAP's new guidelines suggest that most caregivers (86%) continued to enforce time-based rules for their children's electronic device use (Auxier et al., 2020; Konca, 2022). Hence, despite increased recognition that the effects of digital media vary across content and contexts, general trends illustrate that time remains at the root of perceived challenges related to digital media. Empirical studies have been similarly inundated with "'isolated, uncoordinated studies' without a long-term or collaborative focus" (Pecora et al., 2009, p. 1, as cited in Orben, 2020, p. 8), hindering the success of *efforts to reconcile discrepancies in the media use literature* (Browne et al., 2021; Kaye et al., 2020).

In sum, arguments that screen time is either "good" or "bad" both oversimplify a highly mixed body of literature and lack ecological validity as they fail to capture the complex role of digital media in modern life. These realizations have led researchers to abandon screen time as the only relevant variable in understanding technological phenomena. Electronic media will continue to grow in complexity, and theoretical models of child development must account for these advancements to facilitate studies of digital media use as a multidimensional construct. In doing so, researchers must contextualize research questions concerning media in extant models of child development. Below, we review notable theoretical models and explore their strengths and limitations. We also highlight similarities and differences between models. In doing so, we hope to convey that the literature is now in need of a unifying framework, such as the Digital Level of Analysis, to facilitate knowledge translation and consolidation across theoretical orientations and disciplines.

Developmentally Oriented Models of Digital Media Use

The Three Cs of Media Use

Although screen time has only received increasing public scrutiny in the past decade, researchers and scholars began to question the validity of this construct in the 2000s. Guernsey (2007) raised important questions regarding the AAP's 2 × 2 rule, pointing out that although this advice was highly debated among child health professionals, both supporters and opponents "admitted that there was very little evidence of harm or benefit to screen time" (p. 23). Hence, the rule likely inspired unnecessary panic and fear among caregivers. To redress this issue, Guernsey undertook extensive research and consultation with academics, parents, and members of the media industry. The resulting concept of the three Cs—content, context, and the child—was a more nuanced framing of children's TV and DVD viewing activities.

"Content" describes the importance of considering *what* children are viewing. Guernsey (2007) urges caregivers to seek age-appropriate and educational media that may enhance their child's development by encouraging learning, critical thinking, and creativity. For instance, the popular children's TV program *Sesame Street* has been linked to long-lasting positive outcomes in school readiness, prosocial behavior, and literacy (Fisch et al., 1999), supporting a "quality over quantity" perspective. The second factor, "context", encompasses the environments or settings in which children's screen use takes place. Caregivers must consider *who* their children consume media around and the nature of their conversations about the contents viewed. This underscores the interpersonal components of media use, such as caregiver guidance and co-use with siblings and peers. Examples include asking questions to stimulate critical thinking about the content of television programs or co-playing video games with friends to facilitate bonding. Importantly, Guernsey does not recommend that caregivers fully abandon considerations of screen time, as the context factor also comprises the extent to which media use dominates a child's day. The third and final factor of the three Cs encourages caregivers to consider their child's developmental needs, characteristics, and interests, which should inform individualized selections of media content. For instance, children with Autism Spectrum Disorder may face more discrimination and cyberbullying on popular social media platforms (Carrington et al., 2017), but they can derive substantial benefits from specialized online gaming servers (e.g., Autcraft) that facilitate identity expression (Ringland, 2019). The "child" factor can also inform the contexts of media use. For instance, Coyne et al. (2011) demonstrated gender differences in outcomes associated with video game co-play between adolescents and their parents, such that benefits (i.e., decreased levels of internalizing symptoms and aggression, increased prosocial behavior, and improved parent–child connectedness) were only observed in girls. Sibling video game co-play outcomes also vary based on both gender and the contents (violent vs. prosocial) of the video game being played (Coyne et al., 2016).

Guernsey's (2007) three Cs represent an important early step in overturning a "one-size-fits-all" approach to children's media use. Each of the factors encourages parents and caregivers to shift their focus away from their child's screen time and instead consider the extent to which specific facets of media use interact with developmental needs and environments. Although the media landscape has grown exponentially more complex since the model's inception, the three Cs continue to hold significant practical implications by providing a simple yet robust set of questions for caregivers to ask themselves about the place of media in their children's lives. For researchers, the three Cs also set the foundation for ongoing efforts to move beyond screen time as a standalone indicator of children's media use. Its tenets, however, are quite broad, and there lacks a systematic framework for organizing the myriad influences that can fall within the scope of each of the three Cs. Models that integrate these factors into extant organizational frameworks of developmental science will likely prove more effective for generating research questions and testing hypotheses. To date, researchers have formulated many theories with close relevance to the three Cs. We summarize several noteworthy models in the following sections.

Differential Susceptibility to Media Effects Model

The Differential Susceptibility to Media Effects Model (DSMM; Valkenburg & Peter, 2013) applies differential susceptibility—the notion that some children are more strongly impacted by environmental influences than others, for better *and* for worse (Belsky et al., 2007)—to understanding variation in changes how individuals experience and respond to media use. Hence, the DSMM posits that the strength and valence of media effects vary across individuals. Although this model does not focus exclusively on children and families, its principles naturally align with the individualized nature of the three Cs, providing theory-grounded approaches for studying interactions between development and complex aspects of media use.

The DSMM builds upon four integrated propositions. Most relevant to the present discussion is the notion that "media effects are conditional" (Valkenburg & Peter, 2013, p. 226) upon three groups of variables that confer differential susceptibility to media effects. *Dispositional factors* comprise "all person dimensions that predispose the selection of and responsiveness to media" (Valkenburg & Peter, 2013, p. 227). These include both transient states (e.g., mood) and traits that are stable across time and settings (e.g., demographic characteristics). *Developmental susceptibility* captures variation in how individuals use and respond to media according to their cognitive, emotional, and social growth (Valkenburg & Peter, 2013). The authors acknowledge that these factors are most prominent early in life. As such, the DSMM includes a strong developmental orientation that calls attention to the notion that media use can accentuate risks and opportunities during childhood and adolescence. Finally, *social susceptibility* factors range from the effects of specific socialization agents (e.g., parents, peers, and educators) to expansive societal contexts (e.g., schools and neighborhoods) that impact how one chooses and experiences digital media (Valkenburg & Peter, 2013). Each of these differential susceptibility variables that Valkenburg and Peter (2013) propose adds nuance to Guernsey's (2007) three Cs. Dispositional and developmental factors define specific ideas to consider when tailoring media based on the child component. Social susceptibility, on the other hand, closely mirrors well-established developmental frameworks (e.g., ecological systems theory; Bronfenbrenner, 1977) and provides opportunities for exploring how the multilevel contexts surrounding a child may color their media use choices, experiences, and associated outcomes.

Beyond conceptualizing media effects as conditional, the three other propositions within the DSMM further add cohesion to the three Cs. It is important to consider the three Cs as interdependent constructs. For example, educational television programs can often promote language development, but a child with underdeveloped verbal skills may miss out on these benefits unless they are accompanied by an adult who actively directs their viewing. The DSMM accounts for these synergistic interactions by proposing that (1) the cognitive, emotional, and excitatory effects of media effects often operate via indirect pathways; (2) differential susceptibility variables can be both predictors and moderate individuals' experiences of media;

and (3) the links between media effects and responses to them, in the context of differential susceptibility variables, are transactional (Valkenburg & Peter, 2013).

The various components of the DSMM draw upon key principles of developmental science to explain why and how some individuals are more influenced by media content than others. However, as the DSMM was not specifically designed to understand digital media use in children and youth, it includes relatively limited consideration of developmental processes and trajectories and places less emphasis on a direct representation of change over time, which may present limitations for research questions that target how media influences on developmental outcomes evolve. Moreover, the DSMM does not assign particular importance to specific social influences, particularly those within the family system. Given ongoing calls to adopt family-wide perspectives in research on child development in the digital age (Barr et al., 2020; Jennings, 2017), incorporating consideration of the family media ecology and examining whether media effects operate at between- or within-person levels of analysis will further strengthen models such as the DSMM.

Bronfenbrenner's Bioecological Model

Systems-based models emphasize that growth occurs within various contexts that surround developing organisms. Among the most influential of these models is Bronfenbrenner's bioecological model (Bronfenbrenner, 1977), which places great emphasis on the dynamic interactions between individual characteristics and their surrounding environments. That is, developmental trajectories are guided by individual biological and psychological factors, and these form within the confines of contextual influences. Following several reformulations, the final bioecological model builds upon the process-person-context-time model as a working operationalization (Rosa & Tudge, 2013; Xia et al., 2020). Proximal processes—the primary mechanisms of development—represent the increasingly complex interactions between an organism and its immediate environments over the course of development. Personal characteristics refer to the unique features that individuals bring to social interactions. The most well-known component of the bioecological theory is perhaps the five interconnected, concentric systems that describes different environmental contexts that surround an organism. The developing child's traits, identities, and characteristics lie at the core of the system. This is engulfed in the microsystem—the immediate environments in which children directly experience face-to-face interactions, such as with family members, peers, teachers, and neighbors (Bronfenbrenner, 1977). The next layer, the mesosystem, refers to interactions between microsystems. The exosystem pertains to distal events that indirectly influence environment, whereas macrosystems involve broad sociocultural influences. Finally, the chronosystem addresses sociohistorical conditions and longitudinal changes that affect all other layers of the model (Bronfenbrenner, 1977; Rosa & Tudge, 2013; Xia et al., 2020).

The bioecological model remains one of the most prominent theories within developmental psychology. Although Bronfenbrenner developed and refined this model several decades before rapid global digitization, it nonetheless holds strong utility for understanding and analyzing how present-day technologies permeate environmental influences and interact with biopsychosocial processes. The following sections review attempts to form "technologized" versions of bioecological theories. These collectively elucidate multilevel perspectives on the synergistic interactions between media use patterns and child development.

The Technosubsystem

Some scholars have focused on inserting technology into extant levels of Bronfenbrenner's framework. Johnson and Puplampu (2008) proposed the ecological techno-subsystem as a dimension that mediates interactions between the child and their immediate surrounding environments (i.e., the microsystem). This environmental "layer" comprises children's access to the Internet and the ways in which social and solitary online activities impact them. In keeping with the bidirectional nature of nested ecological levels, the techno-subsystem also considers how children influence their environments via the Internet (Johnson & Puplampu, 2008). The authors cite early evidence indicating that Internet use in childhood differs across contexts (Kerawalla & Crook, 2002; Murphy & Beggs, 2003) to sustain that "ecological analysis requires simultaneous consideration of all contexts of child development and Internet use" (Johnson & Puplampu, 2008, p. 6). The techno-subsystem further suggests that understanding *what* children do online is essential to the model's ecological validity, pointing to studies that illustrate different Internet use patterns and their interactions with learning and cognitive outcomes. As such, Johnson and Puplampu's model compellingly integrates the three Cs into a well-established theory of child development.

Can the techno-subsystem thoroughly facilitate a "holistic exploration of the developmental consequences of Internet use during childhood" (Johnson & Puplampu, 2008, p. 7)? The model indeed acknowledges that the Internet brings the features of the microsystem into the virtual realm, though Navarro and Tudge (2022) argue that these are already accounted for in the bioecological model. However, children's digital media activities also undoubtedly interact with components at other ecological layers (McHale et al., 2009). Exposure to mass media can directly shape young people's emotions, beliefs, and ideologies, representing influences from the macrosystem (Srivastava et al., 2018). Conversely, youth can easily engage with societal issues virtually by signing online petitions for social causes or joining virtual activist communities (Elliott & Earl, 2018). These examples illustrate that digital media does not solely reside at microsystemic levels. Accordingly, we stand to gain a more comprehensive and refined understanding of the interactions between child development and media use interaction by incorporating more extensive modifications to the bioecological theory.

Neo-bioecological Theory

Recently developed by Navarro and Tudge (2022), the neo-bioecological theory expands the bioecological model to include changes brought about by the digital age. In particular, the authors propose amendments to the micro- and macrosystems, which have been highlighted as particularly important contexts to consider in understanding technology and its interactions with child development.

The microsystem functions as the foundation for social interactions, and in recognizing that technology has drastically altered modern-day relationships, the neo-ecological theory includes three adaptations to this key developmental context. First, Navarro and Tudge propose two microsystems, present across physical and virtual realms. This distinction is essential as it acknowledges that social experiences are no longer bound by physical space. For instance, a child partaking in a family WhatsApp chat group can contact and interact with loved ones daily, despite a complete lack of physical contact. Hence, the physical and virtual microsystems each possess distinct features and can confer different effects on various aspects of development. Notwithstanding, the physical and virtual microsystems are not mutually exclusive. Social interactions often occur simultaneously in both contexts and lead to complementary and opposing effects. For instance, adolescents are often socially engaged with the digital microsystem by texting with friends or sharing posts on social media while surrounded by very different interactions in their physical setting (e.g., school).

The neo-ecological theory further considers how social interactions can occur in multiple digital microsystems but a single physical microsystem, such as a child who is video chatting with peers (digital microsystem number one) while playing a mobile phone game (digital microsystem number two). This illustrates the third alteration to traditional views of microsystems: the flexible opening and closing of virtual microsystems. According to the neo-ecological model, these actions are determined by the interactions that a child engages in during these digital microsystems. For instance, a child may be playing a game on a smartphone and suddenly switch to a different platform or app, thereby "shutting down" the previous microsystem and "turning on" a new one. Defining physical and virtual microsystems therefore more accurately depicts the malleable nature of social interactions in the twenty-first century, enabling studies that explore relationships across a diverse set of environments.

Interactional Theory of Childhood Problematic Media Use

As trends in screen media use have shown exponential increases in recent years, there have been mounting efforts to understand progressions from normative to "addictive" or "problematic" technology use. This work has informed accounts of how multilevel factors could exacerbate children's vulnerability to leading an overly screen-based life, such as the Interactional Theory of Childhood Problematic Media

Use (IT-CPU; Domoff et al., 2020). Domoff et al. (2020) suggest that problematic media use (PMU) arises when digital media impairs the child's well-being and overall development and interferes with their academic, social, and/or physical functioning. However, PMU has yet to be recognized as a disorder in major diagnostic systems such as the Diagnostic and Statistical Manual of Mental Disorders, Fifth Edition (American Psychiatric Association, 2022). Nonetheless, its core symptomatology has been identified as falling across clusters of excessive use, addictive behaviors, social withdrawal, problems with emotional regulation, negative emotions, and academic or psychosocial deficits linked to digital media (Domoff et al., 2020).

The IT-CPU model addresses the etiology of PMU by exploring a wide range of individual and environmental risk and protective factors. Like the DSMM model, the IT-CPU theory emphasizes the dynamic interplay between the individual, their surrounding contexts, and the contents of their media consumption to understand PMU. The model refers specifically to Bronfenbrenner's person-process-context-time model (Domoff et al., 2020); Rosa & Tudge, 2013) to emphasize the interplay between individual characteristics, the environment, and longitudinal changes in relation to PMU.

Domoff et al. (2020) further discuss how proximal and distal risk factors situated across layers of the developmental sphere may increase an individual's propensity for media use and contribute to the development and maintenance of PMU. Key proximal factors include child, family, and social characteristics, which have immediate influences on engagement with media and susceptibility to problematic use. For instance, Coyne et al. (2021) reported positive associations between PMU and relying on media for emotion regulation in toddlers with challenging temperaments, which they hypothesized was due to the development of dependence and overreliance on media to achieve affective equilibrium. Proximal social influences (e.g., parental stress or beliefs regarding media use, peers' access to technology) also shape children's preferences and experiences with digital media and subsequently influence contextual factors that increase one's disposition to inappropriate or excessive media use. The IT-CPU model further posits that the early risks for PMU in children are related to distal factors, which bidirectionally interact with proximal factors. Examples of distal risks include poverty, parental problematic media use, and digital settings. Domoff et al. (2020) indicate that although individual distal risks for childhood PMU are unlikely to confer strong impacts on their own, their influence can increase significantly through cumulative effects or interactions with proximal factors. This aligns well with the foundational principles of developmental theory and represents a strong application of the three Cs and neo-ecological theory. Yet, the IT-CPU model is narrower in scope given its focus on media use associated with clinical impairment and focuses on the potential harms associated with digital media use. Although this restricts the model to a narrow range of outcomes, it continues to represent an important area of inquiry, with noteworthy implications for both child development and public health.

The theories described above were selected for their relevance and close applicability to developmental orientations that provide insight on human growth in a digitized society. As each model has unique strengths, it would be difficult to nominate a particular one as an optimal theory that fulfills the needs of every research question and experiment. There are also other relevant models and research tools that have important contributions but were not described in detail in the present chapter (e.g., Edwards et al., 2017; Jordan, 2004; Wang et al., 2010; Williams & Merten, 2011). Moreover, restricting empirical questions to fit within a single model or theory would likely limit the scope of hypotheses and deter researchers from designing complex studies that span multiple aspects of development and extend across disciplines. Hence, we suggest the need for a framework that retains the core principles of developmental science and offers researchers conceptual flexibility.

The Digital Level of Analysis

First introduced by Browne et al. (2021), the Digital Level of Analysis conceptualizes the myriad interactions between media use and child development as "a distinct layer of organization in which digital developmental phenomena can be conceptualized, measured, modeled, and studied to best understand the influences and consequences of child well-being in the digital age." This framework stems from the notion that every aspect of modern development, no matter how big or small, potentially impacts and is impacted by technology. It further seeks to provide a frame of reference for researchers to study the complex associations between child development and media use. Fundamentally, the Digital Level of Analysis expounds on the "multiple levels of analysis" principle within developmental psychopathology (Cicchetti & Dawson, 2002). In pioneering the "multiple levels of analysis" framework, Cicchetti (2023) identified a long-standing issue—that studies of pediatric mental health challenges rely on a narrow set of predictors and outcomes to draw far-reaching conclusions. This, in turn, hinders the scope and clinical utility of research findings. Understanding the etiology, prognosis, and role of risk/protective factors associated with psychopathology requires the integration of developmental phenomena across different scales or levels of detail (Cicchetti, 2023). At the most minute levels lie microscopic biological events (e.g., gene expression; neural development), followed by observable changes in physical growth. Broader levels capture the development of one's internal experiences and external expressions (temperament, social cognition, and emotional response patterns). These psychobiological processes and outcomes are embedded in social influences that operate in a "top–down" manner. These range from proximal effects such as a child's home environment (e.g., parenting, sibling relationships, family socioeconomic status), peer relationships, and school settings, to mesosystemic influences linked to neighborhoods (e.g., safety, access to resources). Even broader cultural values and practices, as well as major societal events that bring about widespread changes, are typically considered the topmost levels of the social infrastructure (Cicchetti, 2023). As summarized by Cicchetti and Toth (2009), researchers must strike interdisciplinary collaborations to understand mental health difficulties as "in a more dynamic fashion that reflects the probabilistic, bidirectional, and transactional nature of genetic, neurobiological, social, psychological, and pre- and postnatal environmental influences over the life course" (p. 20).

The Digital Level of Analysis fits squarely into principles of developmental psychopathology, capturing media use activities as an extensive collection of risk and protective factors that interact with mechanisms from "neurons to neighborhoods" (National Research Council, 2000; Thompson, 2016). Although this framing shares features with modern adaptations of Bronfenbrenner's work, it is wider and more dynamic in scope. The bioecological theory places significant emphasis on proximal influences, as these "serve as the conduit for synergistic interrelations between the characteristics of the person and their environments across time" (Navarro & Tudge, 2022, p. 11). Accordingly, technologized renditions have largely tended to alterations or additions to the microsystem (Johnson & Puplampu, 2008; Navarro & Tudge, 2022). While the Digital Level of Analysis certainly includes proximal processes and outcomes, it directs equal or greater attention to distal phenomena. Furthermore, it provides a general lens for studying digital media and development instead of operating within a specific theoretical framework. Below, we outline an example that illustrates how studies spanning multiple levels of evidence can be integrated to help understand a complex digital developmental issue.

Recent decades have witnessed the rapid uptake of video gaming in children and youth. This, in turn, has spurred attempts to understand the contribution of gaming to developmental processes and outcomes, for better or for worse. Creating a thorough and valid theory of video game play and children's mental health requires knowledge integration across findings that address multiple levels of development, yielded from different disciplines. Correlations between video gaming time and mental health symptoms alone cannot adequately inform theory building. We must also integrate psychological studies indicating that video games can offer a host of cognitive and emotional benefits, particularly for children with pre-existing challenges (Granic et al., 2014; Ringland, 2019). The extent to which children reap these benefits varies according to technical components of the game, which may require input from studies involving game developers. Whether gaming reduces or promotes physical activity is another important factor (Sween et al., 2014). Furthermore, contextual factors can simultaneously promote and hinder social processes and outcomes; co-playing video games with siblings and caregivers is associated with family bonding (Musick et al., 2021), but problematic gaming in adolescents is linked to indicators of poor family functioning (Bonnaire & Phan, 2017). These findings illustrate a range of proximal influences and their interrelationships.

Distal influences also have active contributions. For instance, video game platforms can be tailored to form accessible macrosystemic social spaces for youth with specialized needs such as autism (e.g., Autcraft; Ringland et al., 2016). At even broader societal levels, the benefits of video games must be considered in the context of predatory monetization techniques within games, which are associated with gambling outcomes (Zendle & Bowden-Jones, 2019) and addictive gaming behavior (King & Delfabbro, 2018). These associations may vary by country-level regulatory practices (or lack thereof; McCaffrey, 2019). Moreover, particularly salient effects may emerge for individuals who are biologically predisposed to impulsivity and addictions (Rapinda et al., 2023). As illustrated in the present example, the Digital Level of Analysis identifies numerous processes that highlight the effects of a seemingly simple digital activity. Accordingly, theory building and testing becomes an iterative process that helps create knowledge that is congruent with evidence at different levels of analysis.

Applying the Digital Level of Analysis framework redresses several challenges that have plagued the field for many years. These include (1) restrictively focusing on unidirectional and linear associations, (2) using unidimensional variables (typically screen time) to proxy far more complex digital activities, and (3) drawing and interpreting associations without directly assessing the contexts in which they emerge. Ameliorating these issues requires researchers to conduct studies that span "multiple domains of variables, both inside and outside the developing person" (Cicchetti, 2023, p. 32). Table 3.1 depicts media-related influences and levels of analysis in detail and offers potential areas of exploration in association with digital media use. The consideration of single aspects of media use (e.g., screen time) would be unlikely to have a powerful and causal impact on outcomes (e.g., anxiety), and such a hypothesis would stand at odds with a fundamental principle in developmental psychopathology: Complexity is the rule, not the exception. Situating contradictory research findings within this perspective offers grounds for further exploration rather than disputes over which results are "correct." For instance, researchers operating within the Digital Level of Analyses may find that contradictory studies addressed outcomes at different level(s) of development or different findings could be accounted for by an alternative construct at a different level of analysis. Hence, this framework affords researchers greater flexibility and enables much more comprehensive accounts of the links between different facets of media use and child development.

In summary, the Digital Level of Analysis operates on the principle that media influences decussate all other levels of the modern developmental landscape. It encompasses principles of extant models that situate digital media use within the developmental landscape, but studies conducted via this frame of reference need not be constrained to a particular theoretical orientation. It is possible, and oftentimes beneficial, to conduct studies that are not housed within extant models. The Digital Level of Analysis therefore provides an interdisciplinary and transtheoretical frame of reference that accounts for influences captured across both general models of child development (e.g., ecological systems theory, social learning theory, and family systems theory; Bandura, 1977; Bavelas & Segal, 1982; Bronfenbrenner, 1977) and those specific to digital media use (e.g., neo-Bronfenbrenner theory, ecological techno-subsystem; Johnson & Puplampu, 2008; Navarro & Tudge, 2022). Its implications are therefore wide-ranging and incorporate knowledge from not only developmental psychology but also public health, biological psychiatry, and pediatric medicine, to name a few.

Table 3.1 Sample research questions that fit within the Digital Level of Analysis

Level of analysis	Relevant processes and outcomes	Potential research questions and relevant articles
Biological	Microbiology Genetic predispositions and disorders Neurodevelopmental progress Age and sex	To what extent do neurodevelopmental disorders interact with children's exposure to educational and prosocial media content? (Ringland, 2019; Takahashi et al., 2023) Does early media use interact with brain development processes (e.g. synaptic pruning) and relevant cognitive outcomes throughout the lifespan? (Crone & Konijn, 2018)
Psychological	Personality and temperament Intelligence Sense of identity Self-esteem and self-efficacy	Are children drawn to specific contents of media use based on differences in personality and temperament? (Shin et al., 2021) Are individuals who show more impulsive tendencies at higher risk of developing gambling-like behaviors virtually by interacting with in-game purchasing mechanisms? (Rapinda et al., 2023) Are differences in media access in children and families from underrepresented groups linked with different well-being outcomes? (Hampton & Shin, 2022)
Familial	Socioeconomic status Parenting practices and caregivers' media use habits Family structure, relationships, and dynamics	Might parental media use in front of their children impede the development of positive, healthy relationships in the family? (Coyne et al., 2016) What aspects of children's media use are the most prominent sources of conflict within families? Does video game co-play encourage positive relationships at different subsystems within the family? (Coyne et al., 2011; Musick et al., 2021) If so, do benefits carry over dyads and subsystems?
Communal	Peer relationships and influences Neighborhood safety Access to community resources and healthcare	How might the availability of mass media facilitate or hinder children's understanding of and reactions to global events? (Stainback et al., 2020) Does Internet access bolster youth's access to community resources and healthcare services? (Kauer et al., 2014) Is this mediated by indices of neighborhood risk?
Cultural/ societal	Public policy Racial and economic disparity Activism and political climate	What kinds of mass media coverage encourage youth to engage with activism movements, instead of inciting feelings of anxiety and distress? (Stainback et al., 2020)

Implementing the Digital Level of Analysis

The Digital Level of Analysis is an expansive frame of reference that aims to facilitate theory-grounded studies of child development and well-being in a technologized world. It remains untethered to highly specific theories and instead focuses on providing general organizing principles to consider when designing research questions and operationalizing variables. Hence, it offers flexibility in the methodological and analytical strategies available to researchers. However, this raises an important question concerning practical applications: How can researchers feasibly operationalize variables and design studies that align with such a complex, multilevel framework? Studies that attempt to encompass interactions across every aspect of the Digital Level of Analysis would be unrealistic due to both conceptual constraints and practical barriers (e.g., limited funding, lack of opportunities for interdisciplinary work, oversaturated models, and unduly complex analyses). Rather, we suggest that the Digital Level of Analysis should act as a guiding framework that encourages researchers to follow several principles at each stage of the scientific method. We discuss each of these below, organized from higher-level conceptual ideas to more specific and concrete recommendations.

Studies of child development and digital media must be grounded within theories of development At its core, the Digital Level of Analysis acknowledges that interactions with technology early in life could alter short- and long-term trajectories and outcomes (Browne et al., 2021). Accordingly, *studies of digital media in children and youth must be informed by relevant theories and conceptual models.* We do not endorse specific theories or models to allow researchers to maintain a high degree of flexibility, recognizing that different research questions may uniquely draw from different models. We further suggest that studies should not be bound by extant models. Revising current models to better reflect modern-day media influences as well as developing and testing new models is critical to knowledge advancement. For example, a study that aims to examine the associations between parent–child digital media use and family functioning outcomes may draw from the family systems theory (Bavelas & Segal, 1982) and focus on how each family member's device use influences their relationships with others and the formation or dissipation of subunits within the family. In contrast, researchers wishing to investigate the risk factors of Internet gaming addiction may rely on the differential susceptibility theory to elucidate individual differences ranging from biological influences (e.g., genetic disposition to addiction) to broader social–contextual factors (e.g., the role of online gaming in fulfilling one's social needs) and legislations surrounding potentially addictive properties of games (e.g., microtransactions and loot boxes). These examples demonstrate the importance of conducting theory-grounded studies to achieve results with strong ecological validity and useful clinical implications.

Pursue interdisciplinary collaborations Developmental science is inherently interdisciplinary (Cicchetti & Toth, 2009). However, given that experts hold highly specialized knowledge across subfields, most studies of media use and child development have remained narrow in scope. To overcome this issue, we suggest that *studies must engage interdisciplinary teams of researchers*. Ideally, studies that align with the Digital Level of Analysis should be designed with multilevel models and hypotheses in mind. This subsequently leads to the assessment of processes and outcomes residing across multiple levels of analysis. In crossing traditional interdisciplinary boundaries, we stand to gain much stronger knowledge about the assessment of processes and outcomes residing relevant to digital media use.

Operationalize digital media use as multidimensional variables Developmental scientists examine constellations of risk and protective factors and their interactions across multilevel formulations of the developmental ecology (Cicchetti, 2023). Similarly, the Digital Level of Analysis asserts that the links between digital media and child development are much more intricate and dynamic than can be captured by studies that selectively focus on screen time and specific indicators of development. We suggest that *studies of digital developmental phenomena should assess the contents and contexts of children's media use*. This bolsters ecological validity and strengthens the practical utility of findings. For example, asking parents and caregivers to enforce screen time limits has become increasingly unfeasible given the pervasive nature of device use, but helping them understand and manage the contents of their children's media consumption provides a more feasible avenue to mitigate associated risks. This requires a thorough empirical understanding of the kinds of content that children are viewing (Huang et al., 2022), how they are engaging in them (e.g., passive vs. active use; Khan et al., 2022), and the extent to which environmental factors may mediate or moderate associated outcomes. These factors are best captured with multi-method, multi-informant tools with strong ecological validity. In recent years, techniques such as daily diaries and ecological momentary assessments have gained traction in media research. We support the use of such measurements, as well as the uptake of novel measures such as the Comprehensive Assessment of Family Media Exposure tools (Barr et al., 2020), to achieve multimodal data on media activities in the family. Such data effectively speaks to inter- and intra-level influences present within the digital developmental landscape as captured by the digital level of analysis.

Conclusion

As the technology industry continues to grow and evolve, it will become increasingly difficult to disentangle life in the virtual realm from in-person activities. This is particularly the case for children and youth, whose lives are deeply immersed in screen-based activities from a very young age. Accordingly, empirical studies must shift their focus away from isolating the impacts of screen time. Researchers should engage in concerted efforts to unpack the dynamic, reciprocal associations between various aspects of media use and outcomes in different developmental domains, situated across multiple levels of analysis in a child's surrounding environment. The Digital Level of Analysis provides an expansive and flexible framework for researchers to undertake this research. Studies that follow this framework investigate hypotheses grounded in theories of children's media use and involve multiple forms of measurement across several levels of organization within the developmental ecology. Striving to meet these standards will help researchers progress toward unified theoretical knowledge. This will further bolster the clinical utility of empirical studies. By pursuing research questions using methods and protocols that inform the Digital Level of Analysis, we ultimately stand to gain an in-depth understanding of how technology shapes the lives of children and youth in the twenty-first century and beyond.

References

American Psychiatric Association. (2022). *Diagnostic and statistical manual of mental disorders: Diagnostic and statistical manual of mental disorders* (5th ed., Text Revision). American Psychiatric Association. https://doi.org/10.1176/appi.books.9780890425596

Auxier, B., Anderson, M., Perrin, A., & Turner, E. (2020). *Parenting children in the age of screens*. Pew Research Centre. https://www.pewresearch.org/internet/2020/07/28/parenting-children-in-the-age-of-screens/

Bandura, A. (1977). *Social learning theory* (Vol. 1). Prentice Hall. http://www.asecib.ase.ro/mps/Bandura_SocialLearningTheory.pdf

Barr, R., Kirkorian, H., Radesky, J., Coyne, S., Nichols, D., Blanchfield, O., Rusnak, S., Stockdale, L., Ribner, A., Durnez, J., Epstein, M., Heimann, M., Koch, F.-S., Sundqvist, A., Birberg-Thornberg, U., Konrad, C., Slussareff, M., Bus, A., Bellagamba, F., & Fitzpatrick, C. (2020). Beyond screen time: A synergistic approach to a more comprehensive assessment of family media exposure during early childhood. *Frontiers in Psychology, 11*, 1283. https://doi.org/10.3389/fpsyg.2020.01283

Bavelas, J. B., & Segal, L. (1982). Family systems theory: Background and implications. *Journal of Communication, 32*(3), 99–107. https://doi.org/10.1111/j.1460-2466.1982.tb02503.x

Belsky, J., Bakermans-Kranenburg, M. J., & van IJzendoorn, M. H. (2007). For better and for worse: Differential susceptibility to environmental influences. *Current Directions in Psychological Science, 16*(16). https://doi.org/10.1111/j.1467-8721.2007.00525.x

Benda, N. C., Veinot, T. C., Sieck, C. J., & Ancker, J. S. (2020). Broadband internet access is a social determinant of health! *American Journal of Public Health, 110*(8), 1123–1125. https://doi.org/10.2105/AJPH.2020.305784

Blum-Ross, A., & Livingstone, S. (2018). The trouble with "screen time" rules. In G. Mascheroni, C. Ponte, & A. Jorge (Eds.), *Digital parenting. The challenges for families in the digital age*. Nordicom. https://www.nordicom.gu.se/sites/default/files/kapitel-pdf/16_blum-ross_livingstone.pdf

Bonnaire, C., & Phan, O. (2017). Relationships between parental attitudes, family functioning and internet gaming disorder in adolescents attending school. *Psychiatry Research, 255*, 104–110. https://doi.org/10.1016/j.psychres.2017.05.030

Bronfenbrenner, U. (1977). Toward an experimental ecology of human development. *American Psychologist, 32*(7), 513. https://doi.org/10.1037/0003-066X.32.7.513

Browne, D. T., May, S. S., Colucci, L., Hurst-Della Pietra, P., Christakis, D., Asamoah, T., Hale, L., Delrahim-Howlett, K., Emond, J. A., Fiks, A. G., Madigan, S., Perlman, G., Rumpf, H.-J., Thompson, D., Uzzo, S., Stapleton, J., Neville, R. D., & Prime, H. (2021). From screen time to the digital level of analysis: A scoping review of measures for digital media use in children and adolescents. *BMJ Open, 11*(5), e046367. https://doi.org/10.1136/bmjopen-2020-046367

Canadian Paediatric Society Digital Health Task Force. (2019). Digital media: Promoting healthy screen use in school-aged children and adolescents. *Paediatrics & Child Health, 24*(6), 402–408. https://doi.org/10.1093/pch/pxz095

Carrington, S., Campbell, M., Saggers, B., Ashburner, J., Vicig, F., Dillon-Wallace, J., & Hwang, Y.-S. (2017). Recommendations of school students with autism spectrum disorder and their parents in regard to bullying and cyberbullying prevention and intervention. *International Journal of Inclusive Education, 21*(10), 1045–1064. https://doi.org/10.1080/13603116.2017.1331381

Christakis, D. A. (2009). The effects of infant media usage: What do we know and what should we learn? *Acta Paediatrica, 98*(1), 8–16. https://doi.org/10.1111/j.1651-2227.2008.01027.x

Cicchetti, D. (2023). A multiple levels of analysis developmental psychopathology perspective on adolescence and young adulthood. In *APA handbook of adolescent and young adult development* (pp. 487–503). American Psychological Association. https://doi.org/10.1037/0000298-030

Cicchetti, D., & Dawson, G. (2002). Editorial: Multiple levels of analysis. *Development and Psychopathology, 14*(3), 417–420. https://doi.org/10.1017/S0954579402003012

Cicchetti, D., & Toth, S. L. (2009). The past achievements and future promises of developmental psychopathology: The coming of age of a discipline. *Journal of Child Psychology and Psychiatry, 50*(1–2), 16–25. https://doi.org/10.1111/j.1469-7610.2008.01979.x

Committee on Public Education. (1999). Media education. *Pediatrics, 104*(2 Pt 1), 341–343. https://pubmed.ncbi.nlm.nih.gov/10429023/

Coyne, S. M., Padilla-Walker, L. M., Stockdale, L., & Day, R. D. (2011). Game on… girls: Associations between co-playing video games and adolescent behavioral and family outcomes. *Journal of Adolescent Health, 49*(2), 160–165. https://doi.org/10.1016/j.jadohealth.2010.11.249

Coyne, S. M., Jensen, A. C., Smith, N. J., & Erickson, D. H. (2016). Super Mario brothers and sisters: Associations between coplaying video games and sibling conflict and affection. *Journal of Adolescence, 47*(1), 48–59. https://doi.org/10.1016/j.adolescence.2015.12.001

Coyne, S. M., Shawcroft, J., Gale, M., Gentile, D. A., Etherington, J. T., Holmgren, H., & Stockdale, L. (2021). Tantrums, toddlers and technology: Temperament, media emotion regulation, and problematic media use in early childhood. *Computers in Human Behavior, 120*, 106762. https://doi.org/10.1016/j.chb.2021.106762

Crone, E. A., & Konijn, E. A. (2018). Media use and brain development during adolescence. *Nature Communications, 9*(1), 588. https://doi.org/10.1038/s41467-018-03126-x

Domoff, S. E., Borgen, A. L., & Radesky, J. S. (2020). Interactional theory of childhood problematic media use. *Human Behavior and Emerging Technologies, 2*(4), 343–353. https://doi.org/10.1002/hbe2.217

Edwards, S., Henderson, M., Gronn, D., Scott, A., & Mirkhil, M. (2017). Digital disconnect or digital difference? A socio-ecological perspective on young children's technology use in the home and the early childhood Centre. *Technology, Pedagogy and Education, 26*(1), 1–17. https://doi.org/10.1080/1475939X.2016.1152291

Elliott, T., & Earl, J. (2018). Organizing the next generation: Youth engagement with activism inside and outside of organizations. *Social Media + Society, 4*(1), 2056305117750722. https://doi.org/10.1177/2056305117750722

Fisch, S. M., Truglio, R. T., & Cole, C. F. (1999). The impact of sesame street on preschool children: A review and synthesis of 30 years' research. *Media Psychology, 1*(2), 165–190. https://doi.org/10.1207/s1532785xmep0102_5

Granic, I., Lobel, A., & Engels, R. C. M. E. (2014). The benefits of playing video games. *American Psychologist, 69*(1), 66–78. https://doi.org/10.1037/a0034857

Guernsey, L. (2007). *Into the minds of babes: How screen time affects children from birth to age five* (pp. xvi, 287). Basic Books.

Hampton, K. N., & Shin, I. (2022). Disconnection more problematic for adolescent self-esteem than heavy social media use: Evidence from access inequalities and restrictive media parenting in rural America. *Social Science Computer Review*, 626–647. https://doi.org/10.1177/08944393221117466

Huang, S., Lai, X., Zhao, X., Dai, X., Yao, Y., Zhang, C., & Wang, Y. (2022). Beyond screen time: Exploring the associations between types of smartphone use content and adolescents' social relationships. *International Journal of Environmental Research and Public Health, 19*(15), 8940. https://doi.org/10.3390/ijerph19158940

Jennings, N. (2017). Media and families: Looking ahead. *Journal of Family Communication, 17*(3), 203–207. https://doi.org/10.1080/15267431.2017.1322972

Johannes, N., Dienlin, T., Bakhshi, H., & Przybylski, A. K. (2022). No effect of different types of media on well-being. *Scientific Reports, 12*(1). https://doi.org/10.1038/s41598-021-03218-7

Johnson, G. M., & Puplampu, K. P. (2008). Internet use during childhood and the ecological techno-subsystem. *Canadian Journal of Learning and Technology, 34*(1). https://doi.org/10.21432/T2CP4T

Jordan, A. (2004). The role of media in children's development: An ecological perspective. *Journal of Developmental & Behavioral Pediatrics, 25*(3), 196. https://journals.lww.com/jrnldbp/fulltext/2004/06000/the_role_of_media_in_children_s_development__an.9.aspx. https://doi.org/10.1097/00004703-200406000-00009

Kaye, K. L., Orben, A., A. Ellis, D., C. Hunter, S., & Houghton, S. (2020). The conceptual and methodological mayhem of "screen time". *International Journal of Environmental Research and Public Health, 17*(10), 3661. https://doi.org/10.3390/ijerph17103661

Kauer, S. D., Mangan, C., & Sanci, L. (2014). Do online mental health services improve help-seeking for young people? A systematic review. *Journal of Medical Internet Research, 16*(3), e3103. https://doi.org/10.2196/jmir.3103

Kerawalla, L., & Crook, C. (2002). Children's computer use at home and school: Context and continuity. *British Educational Research Journal, 28*(6), 751–771. https://doi.org/10.1080/0141192022000019044

Khan, A., Lee, E.-Y., Janssen, I., & Tremblay, M. S. (2022). Associations of passive and active screen time with psychosomatic complaints of adolescents. *American Journal of Preventive Medicine*, S0749379722000630. https://doi.org/10.1016/j.amepre.2022.01.008

King, D. L., & Delfabbro, P. H. (2018). Predatory monetization schemes in video games (e.g. 'loot boxes') and internet gaming disorder. *Addiction, 113*(11), 1967–1969. https://doi.org/10.1111/add.14286

Konca, A. S. (2022). Digital technology usage of young children: Screen time and families. *Early Childhood Education Journal, 50*(7), 1097–1108. https://doi.org/10.1007/s10643-021-01245-7

Kucirkova, N. I., Livingstone, S., & Radesky, J. S. (2023). Faulty screen time measures hamper national policies: Here is a way to address it. *Frontiers in Psychology, 14*, 1243396. https://doi.org/10.3389/fpsyg.2023.1243396

LeBlanc, A. G., Gunnell, K. E., Prince, S. A., Saunders, T. J., Barnes, J. D., & Chaput, J.-P. (2017). The ubiquity of the screen: An overview of the risks and benefits of screen time in our modern world. *Translational Journal of the American College of Sports Medicine, 2*(17), 104–113. https://doi.org/10.1249/TJX.0000000000000039

Livingstone, S. (2016, October 21). *New 'screen time' rules from the American Academy of Pediatrics*. London School of Economics and Political Science. https://blogs.lse.ac.uk/medialse/2016/10/24/new-screen-time-rules-from-the-american-academy-of-pediatrics/

McAllister, C., Hisler, G. C., Blake, A. B., Twenge, J. M., Farley, E., & Hamilton, J. L. (2021). Associations between adolescent depression and self-harm behaviors and screen media use in a nationally representative time-diary study. *Research on Child and Adolescent Psychopathology, 49*(12), 1623–1634. https://doi.org/10.1007/s10802-021-00832-x

McArthur, B. A., Racine, N., Browne, D. T., McDonald, S., Tough, S., & Madigan, S. (2021). Recreational screen time before and during COVID-19 in school-aged children. *Acta Paediatrica, 110*(10), 2805. https://doi.org/10.1111/apa.15966

McCaffrey, M. (2019). The macro problem of microtransactions: The self-regulatory challenges of video game loot boxes. *Business Horizons, 62*(4), 483–495. https://doi.org/10.1016/j.bushor.2019.03.001

Mcclain, C. (2022, April 28). *How parents' views of their kids' screen time, social media use changed during COVID-19*. Pew Research Center. https://www.pewresearch.org/short-reads/2022/04/28/how-parents-views-of-their-kids-screen-time-social-media-use-changed-during-covid-19/

McHale, S. M., Dotterer, A., & Kim, J.-Y. (2009). An ecological perspective on the media and youth development. *The American Behavioral Scientist, 52*(8), 1186–1203. https://doi.org/10.1177/0002764209331541

Murphy, C., & Beggs, J. (2003). Primary pupils' and teachers' use of computers at home and school. *British Journal of Educational Technology, 34*(1), 79–83. https://doi.org/10.1111/1467-8535.00307

Musick, G., Freeman, G., & McNeese, N. J. (2021). Gaming as family time: Digital game co-play in modern parent-child relationships. *Proceedings of the ACM on Human-Computer Interaction, 5*(251), 1–25. https://doi.org/10.1145/3474678

Nagata, J. M., Cortez, C. A., Cattle, C. J., Ganson, K. T., Iyer, P., Bibbins-Domingo, K., & Baker, F. C. (2022). Screen time use among us adolescents during the COVID-19 pandemic: Findings from the Adolescent Brain Cognitive Development (ABCD) study. *JAMA Pediatrics, 176*(1), 94–96. https://doi.org/10.1001/jamapediatrics.2021.4334

National Research Council. (2000). From neurons to neighborhoods: The science of early childhood development. https://doi.org/10.17226/9824.

Navarro, J. L., & Tudge, J. R. H. (2022). Technologizing Bronfenbrenner: Neo-ecological theory. *Current Psychology*. https://doi.org/10.1007/s12144-022-02738-3

Orben, A., & Przybylski, A. K. (2019). The association between adolescent well-being and digital technology use. *Nature Human Behaviour, 3*(2), 173–182. https://doi.org/10.1038/s41562-018-0506-1

Pecora, N., Murray, J. P., & Wartella, E. A. (Eds.). (2009). The changing nature of children's television: Fifty years of research. In *Children and television* (pp. 23–62). Routledge. https://doi.org/10.4324/9781410618047-8

Przybylski, A. K., & Weinstein, N. (2019). Digital screen time limits and young children's psychological Well-being: Evidence from a population-based study. *Child Development, 90*(1). https://doi.org/10.1111/cdev.13007

Rapinda, K. K., Edgerton, J. D., & Keough, M. T. (2023). Impulsivity moderates the association between anxiety and problem gambling among Canadian undergraduates. *Journal of Gambling Studies*. https://doi.org/10.1007/s10899-023-10238-7

Reid, D., & Weigle, P. (2014). Social media use among adolescents: Benefits and risks. *Adolescent Psychiatry, 4*. https://doi.org/10.2174/221067660402140709115810

Rideout, V., & Katz, V. S. (2016). Opportunity for all? Technology and learning in lower-income families. https://www.joanganzcooneycenter.org/wp-content/uploads/2016/01/jgcc_opportunityforall.pdf, DOI: https://doi.org/10.15766/mep_2374-8265.10468

Rideout, V., Peebles, A., & Robb, M. B. (2022). *The Common Sense Census: Media use by tweens and teens, 2021*. https://www.commonsensemedia.org/sites/default/files/research/report/8-18-census-integrated-report-final-web_0.pdf

Ringland, K. E. (2019). "Autsome": Fostering an autistic identity in an online Minecraft community for youth with autism. In N. G. Taylor, C. Christian-Lamb, M. H. Martin, & B. Nardi (Eds.), *Information in contemporary society* (Vol. 11420, pp. 132–143). Springer. https://doi.org/10.1007/978-3-030-15742-5_12

Ringland, K. E., Wolf, C. T., Boyd, L. E., Baldwin, M. S., & Hayes, G. R. (2016). Would you be mine: Appropriating Minecraft as an assistive technology for youth with autism. In *Proceedings of the 18th International ACM SIGACCESS Conference on Computers and Accessibility* (pp. 33–41). https://doi.org/10.1145/2982142.2982172

Roberts, D. F. (1999). Kids & media @ the new millennium: A Kaiser Family Foundation Report. A Comprehensive National Analysis of Children's Media Use. https://www.kff.org/wp-content/uploads/2013/01/kids-media-the-new-millennium-executive-summary.pdf

Roberston, L., Twenge, J. M., Joiner, T. E., & Cummins, K. (2022). Associations between screen time and internalizing disorder diagnoses among 9- to 10-year-olds. *Journal of Affective Disorders*. https://doi.org/10.1016/j.jad.2022.05.071

Rosa, E. M., & Tudge, J. (2013). Urie Bronfenbrenner's theory of human development: Its evolution from ecology to bioecology. *Journal of Family Theory & Review, 5*(4), 243–258. https://doi.org/10.1111/jftr.12022

Shin, E., Choi, K., Resor, J., & Smith, C. L. (2021). Why do parents use screen media with toddlers? The role of child temperament and parenting stress in early screen use. *Infant Behavior and Development, 64*, 101595. https://doi.org/10.1016/j.infbeh.2021.101595

Srivastava, K., Chaudhury, S., Bhat, P. S., & Mujawar, S. (2018). Media and mental health. *Industrial Psychiatry Journal, 27*(1), 1–5. https://doi.org/10.4103/ipj.ipj_73_18

Stainback, K., Hearne, B. N., & Trieu, M. M. (2020). COVID-19 and the 24/7 news cycle: Does COVID-19 news exposure affect mental health? *Socius, 6*. https://doi.org/10.1177/2378023120969339

Sultana, A., Tasnim, S., Bhattacharya, S., Hossain, M. M., & Purohit, N. (2020). Digital screen time during COVID-19 pandemic: A public health concern. *F1000Research, 10*(81). https://doi.org/10.12688/f1000research.50880.1

Sween, J., Wallington, S. F., Sheppard, V., Taylor, T., Llanos, A. A., & Adams-Campbell, L. L. (2014). The role of exergaming in improving physical activity: A review. *Journal of Physical Activity & Health, 11*(4), 864–870. https://doi.org/10.1123/jpah.2011-0425

Takahashi, N., Tsuchiya, K. J., Okumura, A., Harada, T., Iwabuchi, T., Rahman, M. S., Kuwabara, H., Nomura, Y., & Nishimura, T. (2023). The association between screen time and genetic risks for neurodevelopmental disorders in children. *Psychiatry Research, 115395*. https://doi.org/10.1016/j.psychres.2023.115395

Thompson, R. A. (2016). What more has been learned? The science of early childhood development 15 years after neurons to neighborhoods. *Zero to Three Journal, 36*(3), 18–24.

Twenge, J. M., & Campbell, W. K. (2018). Associations between screen time and lower psychological Well-being among children and adolescents: Evidence from a population-based study. *Preventive Medicine Reports, 12*, 271–283. https://doi.org/10.1016/j.pmedr.2018.10.003

Twenge, J. M., & Campbell, W. K. (2019). Media use is linked to lower psychological Well-being: Evidence from three datasets. *Psychiatric Quarterly, 90*(2), 311–331. https://doi.org/10.1007/s11126-019-09630-7

Valkenburg, P. M., & Peter, J. (2013). The differential susceptibility to media effects model. *Journal of Communication, 63*(2), 221–243. https://doi.org/10.1111/jcom.12024

Wang, X. C., Berson, I. R., Jaruszewicz, C., Hartle, L., & Rosen, D. (2010). Young children's technology experiences in multiple contexts: Bronfenbrenner's ecological theory reconsidered. In I. R. Berson & M. J. Berson (Eds.), *High-tech tots: Childhood in a digital world*. IAP.

Williams, A. L., & Merten, M. J. (2011). iFamily: Internet and social media technology in the family context. *Family and Consumer Sciences Research Journal, 40*(2), 150–170. https://doi.org/10.1111/j.1552-3934.2011.02101.x

World Health Organization. (2019, April 24). *To grow up healthy, children need to sit less and play more*. https://www.who.int/news/item/24-04-2019-to-grow-up-healthy-children-need-to-sit-less-and-play-more

Xia, M., Li, X., & Tudge, J. R. H. (2020). Operationalizing Urie Bronfenbrenner's process-person-context-time model. *Human Development, 64*(1), 10–20. https://doi.org/10.1159/000507958

Zendle, D., & Bowden-Jones, H. (2019). Loot boxes and the convergence of video games and gambling. *The Lancet Psychiatry, 6*(9), 724–725. https://doi.org/10.1016/S2215-0366(19)30285-8

Chapter 4
Digital Contexts: A Theoretical Model for Researching Children's Digital Development

Daniel Abs

We face significant challenges with the technological advancement of recent decades. The digital world has gone from a promise to a reality in homes and in the daily life of school and work. With this, new challenges have been presented, and new solutions are demanded by society. What knowledge remains useful and effective in this new world? What values remain relevant in education and child development? What protections should be implemented for a healthy childhood? These are some of the recurring questions in the scientific and academic sphere concerned with the advances of the digital world in society. However, the advance of capitalism over structures, monetizing many aspects that were once bets of free circulation and thought, produced a very desolate scenario. This new reality, more tangible in the last decade, is characterized by the emergence and strengthening of big techs in the field of social media and a reach beyond geographical and national limits (Lee, 2018). Their products and their platforms encompass today activities of entertainment, education, culture, income, and work and have significant impacts on politics, economy, and social relations. Despite the efforts of families and educators, children, in general, are exposed to these scenarios and experience their development together with the adult population, consuming videos, music, cartoons, and information, which are often false (Howard et al., 2021). TikTok, YouTube, and Twitch are some of the platforms that circulate among this audience and establish daily challenges to understand what this new childhood that presents itself is (Neumann & Herodotou, 2020).

Initially, there is a difficulty for scientists and educators in recognizing and delimiting the digital phenomenon (Abs, 2023). This has expanded from the common use of technological devices such as television, computer, or cell phone to culture, language, values, and life perspectives. We remain continuously connected,

D. Abs (✉)
Instituto de Psicologia, Universidade de São Paulo, São Paulo, Brazil
e-mail: daniel.abs@ufrgs.br

G. B. Frizzo (ed.), *Digital Media and Early Child Development*,
https://doi.org/10.1007/978-3-031-69224-6_4

and this makes it difficult to establish research based on the number of hours with the use of technologies. This broader dimension of the digital, more complex, which involves beyond the PC and the smartphone and social, cultural, economic, and political factors we call digital contexts (Abs, 2022).

The Model of Digital Contexts

The central question refers to why the emphasis is on "digital contexts" instead of simply "digital technologies." The proposal of a theoretical model for digital contexts seeks to understand the inherent to the digital. When addressing this theme, it is essential to avoid frequent problems in research related to digital technologies. The first of these problems is the attribution of neutrality to technologies, considering them mere tools. Another issue is the linearity often established in relation to the causality of technologies. This linear approach often fails to capture the complexity of the phenomenon under study. In addition, it is fundamental to overcome the dichotomy established between human beings and machines. This simplistic separation hinders the understanding of digital relationships and processes mediated by digital technologies in human experience (see Simondon, 2020).

Given these challenges, establishing a theoretical model becomes an arduous task. The term "model" has been used in various areas, but its definition often proves ambiguous. A model indicates the highlight of the relationships between the main elements that constitute a certain structure (Guarany & Bentz, 1974). Proposing a model for digital contexts means identifying the structural articulations of the digital, highlighting its most relevant aspects. The goal is to gain a deeper understanding of the digital reality and, eventually, develop intervention strategies.

The proposed model is theoretical and analytical, serving as a tool for reflection. It adopts a systemic approach, suggesting the premise that everything functions as a system. Within this context, the psychological is also understood as a system, aligned with an ontology that defines phenomena and processes based on the idea of systems. In other words, from this perspective, the human being is understood as a complex system, interacting with various other systems. The psychological system, in turn, can be essentially described as symbolic and based on interactions.

It is important to note that, within the systemic paradigm, there is the understanding that reality can be known. This view is a legacy of modernity, which proposed that reality is not mysterious and can be discovered. In the Middle Ages, for example, the view prevailed that certain aspects of reality were unreachable or mysterious. However, with the emergence of modern science, there was an evolution in the understanding that nature and reality are susceptible to understanding. In the systemic context, it is understood that reality has a structure and this can be known and studied (Vieira & Santaella, 2008).

Understanding reality, from this thought, requires the recognition of the general laws that underpin it (Bunge, 2017). Many of these laws are still unknown to science. Reality, in this context, serves as a starting point to identify the transformations and changes that are occurring. Since the nineteenth century, we have observed the emergence and consolidation of the digital world in altering the relationships and interactions that exist in the world.

To carry out this analysis, we turn to Vieira and Santaella (2008) when they point out reality as systemic, complex, and legaliform. These are the fundamental principles of the model we propose. When we refer to child development in the context of digital technologies, we are doing so from the understanding that it is something that is systemic, complex, and legaliform; that is, it is based fundamentally on interactions, does not lend itself to linear responses, and has general laws to be recognized.

Another important concept is the environment. A system always exists in relation to other systems, forming an interconnected network. The environment of a system is, essentially, the set of external systems to it. There are no isolated systems. The idea of environment refers to the system that is external to the system in focus (Vieira & Santaella, 2008). What interests us in the model proposal and aligns with the understanding already widely developed by Bronfenbrenner (2005) and his collaborators is the understanding of the child as a complex system in relation to the digital environment. In other words, children and digital environments are both systems in interaction. It is up to us to describe, analyze, and understand the nature of these interactions and how they occur.

In this way, digital contexts are multiple systems in relation, which constitute the complex environment of human development characterized by mutual and inseparable interactions of machines. Digital, from computers to wearable peripherals, from the different languages involved, from programming to culture, and from the human body in interaction (Abs, 2022). This definition is inspired by the understanding of development contexts as already signaled by Bronfenbrenner (2005) in his work.

The study of certain contexts requires identifying what differentiates it from other development contexts, such as educational contexts or family contexts. This specificity refers us to the task of highlighting in the model those elements without which it is not possible to establish what a digital context is. This model should contemplate at the same time a reasonable diversity of permutations that allow recognizing in it the reality of human development. When doing this exercise, three elements are identified that are present in all digital systems and contexts and that distinguish them from other contexts of human development:

1. The machine: it is essential to understand the technological infrastructure that supports and enables the digital context. This is all the hardware developed in recent decades, which has advanced from the large computers of the 1940s to today's nanoprocessors. Future prospects point to major transformations in data processing, mainly with the advancement of supercomputers, cloud computing, quantum computers, and also peripherals such as virtual reality (VR) glasses and wearable devices, which will popularize what we today call the metaverse. Access to the most physical devices and their infrastructure networks is also a relevant element for the analysis of social inequalities and the sociopolitical impacts of technologies and for understanding access to rights and citizenship.

2. The language: digital language represents the symbolic aspect of this context. Without understanding the linguistic and symbolic component, the understanding of the digital context is incomplete. This is not only all the software developed, but also the strategies for translating reality and the decomposition of images, sounds, videos, and memories into storable and potentially marketable data. The aspects of language also involve the strategies for controlling and using these symbolic aspects, which is pointed out in studies on algorithmization. The most intense implications of these symbolic aspects are recognizable, more broadly, in culture itself, which goes beyond the idea of a digital culture that is restricted to social networks.
3. The body: it refers to the human interactions that occur within this context. For this, we resort to classic studies, such as those by McLuhan in the 1960s, which discuss how technologies act as extensions of the human body: the mouth and ears expand and amplify with the emergence of the telephone, the eyes do so on television, and the legs in the car (McLuhan, 2011). This notion of bodily expansion in the virtual is essential to understand how childhood interacts with different digital media, such as social networks and digital games.

Digital contexts, therefore, are made up of processes of interaction of these elements—machines, languages, and bodies—in constant development today. There is intense investment by large corporations for the development of technologies that expand access, use, and resources available in the digital world. With the accelerated development we have, we identify some central processes currently, for the analysis of digital contexts.

Characterization of Analysis Processes

The Convergence of Technologies

Digital machines, during their historical development process, have been showing a characteristic of convergence in their technologies. Current devices integrate into their organization and process previous technologies. Smartphones today present previous generations of media: we have in them the newspaper, television, cinema, radio, VCR, telephone, modem, camcorder, the computer itself, and the Internet. All these technologies are today in convergence in current smartphones. Others, in development, promise new more powerful devices with greater appeals to interaction and immersion (Santaella, 2010).

Machine Intelligence

In the process of developing more complex digital machines with greater processing power, new programming strategies have been added. Artificial intelligence (AI) is an important and disruptive advancement at the moment (Gabriel, 2022). Despite being a mid-century theme, it has been developing at an accelerated pace in the last decade and is fully integrated into the operation of our smartphones. When using an Uber, the route is plotted by an artificial intelligence algorithm. Today, debates are intense on the uses and ethical repercussions of artificial intelligences (Sijing & Lan, 2018; Owe & Baum, 2021) and especially of generative artificial intelligences, such as Midjourney, ChatGPT, and other Large Language Models (LLMs) (Klimova et al., 2023), which process a massive amount of data through statistics and probabilities to generate new and plausible results in image, sound, video, or text. We also have significant challenges in education to incorporate these technologies into educational processes in the face of sometimes problematic use by teachers and students in everyday school life (Ifenthaler & Schumacher, 2023).

Human Hybridization with Technologies

Machines do not constitute a possible space for interaction if they do not have powerful peripherals in their architecture that allow the input and output of their data to humans. The mouse, keyboards, monitors, and smartwatches are examples of this type of peripherals. The current goal is greater interaction and immersion of users, with ease of use. Virtual reality glasses are receiving heavy investments from big techs in the promise of increasing user immersion in so-called persistent worlds (Ball, 2022). We already have a significant contingent of children using virtual worlds and a set of games already designed for use in VR. The current use of peripherals, from smartphones to the glasses we will have in the future, supports the assertion that we are today in an intense process of hybridization, in which our cognitive, social, and emotional abilities are shared between experiences that are and are not mediated by digital technologies (Santaella, 2021). This is a significant challenge in the analysis of childhood, considering the relations already widely pointed out by Bronfenbrenner between child development and the environment that surrounds it. This environment, today, is hybrid (Santaella, 2021).

Reality Translated into Codes

The improvement of programs and applications today implies that they increasingly simulate environments and processes and expand possibilities for interaction. In an application, there is a set of languages in interaction, from the binary code necessary for the processing of information by the powerful current processors to the icons and indicators used by the design to establish an optimal user experience (UX). The complexity of the relationships of these languages is increasing as they incorporate into digital language materials that have historically been analog. Cinema, dance, music, theater, and touch and emotional experiences are translated into digital languages to be processed and interact with users. The translation processes have been widely studied by authors of the semiotics of culture and allow a deeper analysis of the relationships of meaning and significance that are constituted on these platforms.

The Control and Automation of Algorithms

Applications have been increasingly incorporated into everyday life, with systems adapted to view images, take photos, make videos, transmit in real time, generate knowledge, play simultaneously, write and dictate materials, locate maps, find a ride, and call an Uber. These applications exist today in a relationship that breaks with the utopian ideals of the 1990s for the Internet. They are directed by algorithms to amplify data capture, which is a relevant capital in the current world, and to make the user experience a fundamental marketing and sales strategy today. Algorithmization implies this direction and management of the experience and use no longer by the user, but by the corporations that order and organize specialized algorithms for this. When it comes to childhood, the challenge is gigantic, in terms of directing content to this audience, both for sales marketing and for informational content. These materials exist not only on social networks, but on games aimed at the child audience, and it is a current feature of digital contexts.

The Characteristics of a Digital Culture

In a broader aspect, the use of platforms and applications for access to entertainment and information has created a new culture (Santaella, 2007a). There are social, political, and economic aspects that involve the use of social networks. In Brazil and the world, currently, politicians use their social networks to make statements, do political campaigns, and, not infrequently, disseminate fake news. Large corporations and also professionals seeking visibility use social networks to publicize their work. The use of digital media has become a relevant learning for professions and for career development. Emotional support and the intensity of networks, the famous "hate," translate the intense exchanges and the exposure lived today daily mainly by teenagers. A set of new meanings are built daily in the production of memes, and new values are shared. There is a great challenge in digital culture to understand what is forming a new childhood, which will lead to another society that is certainly different from the one we are experiencing today.

The Expansion of Bodies in Machines

There is an intense experience of transformation of the understanding of the body with the use of digital machines. McLuhan (2011) already pointed to the transformation that the emergence of technologies produces in the human body. This experience of virtual bodies and of mediated experiences outside the organic body, on screens and peripherals, expands the understanding of the borders of the body. If we understand that the human being is also a complex system, the relationship of this same system with increasingly powerful machines amplifies its perception and action, causing emotions and learning to happen between people and environments that are distant from each other and often at different times. The immersion of the human being in virtual environments characterizes very well the concept of extension that McLuhan (2011) produced to explain this process. The body extends in machines and amplifies its existence in avatars and profiles on social networks (Santaella, 2007b). There are direct implications when it is the child who experiences this process. The amplitude of relationships is much greater than the traditionally recognized limits of the body.

The Construction of Multiple Identities on Networks

This process becomes complex with the emergence of social networks and of interaction platforms, like Instagram and TikTok. In child development, the construction of the self has been the object of different theories, which diverge on many points, but recognize that at some point there are interactions that forge a certain understanding of the self. There is a field still unexplored of research on this theme in the constitution of the current subject when considered that from a very young age children already use screens, have user profiles, and interact many times. Even with parental supervision, the effects are still unknown. As adults, we establish different profiles and relationships, depending on the platform and the application that welcomes us. We are constituting a relationship of multiple insertions in the digital that determine important processes of life, such as affective, social, and work relationships.

Social, Economic, and Geopolitical Implications in the Digital

Networks were fundamental in the social transformations that the digital produced in the last 20 years. In the 1990s, it was still very optimistically expected that the emergence of networks, the Internet, and more democratic possibilities of participation in the media would be a promising future for humanity. From 2010 onwards, a certain pessimism coined the term post-digital, which signaled that dangers existed, that optimism had failed, and that more extreme care was necessary (Santaella, 2016), including more direct government regulations to prevent abuses from big techs that today dominate the digital scene. Networks have become an arena for political, social, and economic decisions in which children, teenagers, adults, thinkers, politicians, influencers, and lobbyists coexist. The interests in these arenas are of economic order and also geopolitical in the dissemination of ideas and information, constituting a certain biopolitics of the digital. Childhood is immersed in this same space and suggests the need to expand our education strategies for the digital. However, other movements also took place present. On the networks, movements for more citizen rights and for the fight against racism, fascism, transphobia, and homophobia have found space to be seen and heard. Digital has entered slums and indigenous villages and has also made the struggles of these communities visible. These resistance movements coexist with more reactionary movements in society. The tensions produced today establish an environment that deserves our attention.

Suggestions for Use

We consider these different processes as initial indicators for the study of digital currently, which can be revised as new technologies are developed and other relationships are established.

The first step would be to establish some questions guided by these processes: (1) What technologies converge in this device and are involved in the object I am analyzing? (2) How do the involved software effectively operate? (3) What hybridization effects do they produce on the user? (4) How is reality being translated in this digital object? (5) Which and how are the control operations by the algorithms acting on this digital object? (6) What aspects of digital culture are being created by this digital object? (7) How does the user perceive their body expanding in this digital territory? (8) What possibilities of different identities and experiences are produced in this new digital space? (9) What biopolitical aspects are involved in this new space?

A second step, in search of a certain synthesis of this context in analysis, we propose that readings of the relationships between these elements be made. For example: At a first level of analysis, we can highlight the relationships that exist between the convergence of technologies, the translation of different languages, and their effects on the production of the expansion of bodies in the digital in this digital object. At a second level of analysis, we can highlight the relationship between the operation of the software, the processes of control and algorithmization, and their effects on the creation of new "selves" for the human being. And at a third and last level, we can have the effects of this digital object in the amplification of a hybridization between human and machine, reverberating in transformations of digital culture, with implications and reflections proper to biopolitics in its critical dimension to the power arrangements established by technologies.

A Brief Example of Analysis

If we take the entertainment platform TikTok, which, according to the survey on Internet use by children in Brazil (2023), represents 60% of the profiles of users aged 9–17, we will find an application focused on short videos, with a diversity of content, strong engagement, and interactivity with children and adults. With a brief analysis, understanding TikTok as a context to be analyzed, we have as a convergence of the technologies involved the processing of video, machine learning algorithms for content recommendation, facial recognition, augmented reality, and many interaction strategies already developed by previous platforms such as Facebook, Instagram, and YouTube. This operating mechanism, despite not indicating a direct effect on childhood, will support the understanding of the platform's operation. In relation to artificial intelligences, it is possible to observe that they assist in the creation, editing, and sharing of short videos. The platform uses algorithms that analyze user behavior to suggest personalized content, with the intention of retaining more users. The affective exchanges, expressed in comments, shares, and likes, favor the user's blend of reality with digital elements. There are filters, music, and special effects. Regarding the process of translating reality, short videos stand out, which narrate everyday life, actions, dances, and music through the lens of the platform's resources. This can sometimes distort reality to fit the trends and desires of the audience. The TikTok algorithm strongly influences what users see, based on their behavior, interests, and previous interactions. The most explicit effect would be the creation of bubbles of content, where children are repeatedly exposed to similar types of interactions. Regarding culture, the most striking feature is instantaneity, where the content is brief, but highly engaging. The affective and social relationships shared by TikTok expand the child's interaction space, which can experience a sense of omnipresence, as their videos can be viewed globally. Finally, there is a brief analysis that should be made about the way other children are exposed in the videos, their uses, and commercializations. A very relevant aspect currently is how the platform collects data and user privacy. These would be basic and initial aspects that would be under analysis using the proposed model. Certainly, it is a small example; however, it already provides small clues about the complexity of the phenomenon and alternative ways it can be analyzed.

Limits and Final Considerations

The proposal of an analysis model based on a robust theory like that of Bronfenbrenner (2005) requires the researcher to consider what limits this relationship can be made. There is an intense concern about the interference of big techs in the ethical development of artificial intelligences and in the provision of information and fake news (Prado, 2022). The complexity of this exposure, which expands without a defined geographical territory, is a challenge for a theory that in its proposition constituted the microsystem as the child's closest environment. This environment today is populated by interactive screens, with individuals and corporations establishing ideas and affections, from their room. In the current processes of discussion of regulation of these technologies, which are still in the beginning, a very absent theme is the impact on childhood.

Another aspect of Bronfenbrenner's theory (2005) that deserves better development in digital contexts is the chronosystem. The passage of time is a differential of the theory presented by him. However, the chronosystem thought by the author was modified with the different synchronous and asynchronous processes of the digital. Responses and interactions and the fear of not following them and being left out (FOMO) characterize much of the current child and adolescent development.

The way security policies, data monitoring, and content moderation are carried out today constitutes a significant challenge to parents and childhood researchers. Each large corporation, often operating within the limits that the law allows, allows or ceases contents that exploit various forms of violence. This control is deposited in the judgment of these corporations, without major interferences from society, parents, or educators.

Another aspect to be highlighted is the potential use of the model to expand discussions about family and educational contexts in the relationships they establish with children and technologies. Schools and family units, concerned with the constant use of children, can expand the digital issue beyond the use of a particular device and complexify this understanding.

What other challenges will we still find? There are serious political implications in the contributions that research should make, directed not only to the regulation of digital technologies but also to the performance of big techs with childhood. We still have for the next few years the convergence of technologies indicating the establishment of metaverses and the expansion of generative technologies (see ChatGPT and similar). The generations born now will live with personal assistants generated by AI and will have to learn to live with such dilemmas.

Acknowledgments The original version of this chapter was written in Portuguese and translated into English with the help of artificial intelligence. A subsequent human revision was done primarily in terms of content.

References

Abs, D. (2022). Contextos Digitais de Desenvolvimento Humano. In D. Abs (Org.), *Contextos Digitais: encontros, pesquisas e práticas* (pp. 8–21). UFRGS.

Abs, D. (2023). A pesquisa sobre o digital: expansões, dispersões e convergências. In D. Abs (Org.), *Inscrições Digitais: encontros entre linguagens, trabalho e tecnologias* (pp. 166–181). UFRGS.

Ball, M. (2022). *The Metaverse*. Liveright.

Bronfenbrenner, U. (2005). The bioecological theory of human development. In U. Bronfenbrenner (Org.), *Making human beings human: Bioecological perspectives on human development* (pp. 3–15). Sage.

Bunge, M. (2017). *Teoria e Realidade*. Perspectiva.
Gabriel, M. (2022). *Inteligência Artificial: do zero ao metaverso*. Atlas.
Guarany, W. C., & Bentz, I. M. G. (1974). *Metacomunicação*. FERVI.
Howard, P. H., Neudert, L. M., & Prakash, N. (2021). *Digital misinfor-mation/disinformation and children*. Unicef.
Ifenthaler, D., & Schumacher, C. (2023). Reciprocal issues of artificial and hu-man intelligence in education. *Journal of Research on Technology in Education, 55*, 1–6. https://doi.org/10.1080/15391523.2022.2154511
Klimova, B., Pikhart, M., & Kacetl, J. (2023). Ethical issues of the use of AI-driven mobile apps for education. *Frontiers in Public Health, 10*. https://doi.org/10.3389/fpubh.2022.1118116
Lee, K. F. (2018). *AI super-powers: China, silicon valley and the new world order*. Houghton Mfflin Harcourt.
McLuhan, M. (2011). *Os meios de comunicação como extensões do homem*. Cultrix.
Neumann, M. M., & Herodotou, C. (2020). Young Children and YouTube: A global phenomenon. *Childhood Education, 96*(4), 72–77. https://doi.org/10.1080/00094056.2020.1796459
Owe, A., & Baum, S. (2021). Consideração moral dos não-humanos na ética da inteligência artificial. *IA e Ética, 1*, 517–528. https://doi.org/10.1007/s43681-021-00065-0
Prado, M. (2022). *Fake News e Inteligência Artificial: o Poder dos Algoritmos na Guerra da Desinformação*. Edições 70.
Santaella, L. (2007a). *Linguagens líquidas na era da mobilidade*. Paulus.
Santaella, L. (2007b). Figurações do corpo biológico ao virtual. *Revista Interin, 4*(2), 1–12.
Santaella, L., & Vieira, J.A. (2008). *Metaciência como guia de pesquisa: uma proposta semiótica e sistêmica*. São Paulo: Mérito.
Santaella, L. (2010). *A ecologia pluralista da comunicação: conectividade, mobi-lidade, ubiquidade*. Paulus.
Santaella, L. (2016). *Temas e dilemas do pós-digital: a voz da política*. Paulus.
Santaella, L. (2021). *Humanos hiper-híbridos: linguagens e cultura na segunda era da internet*. Paulus.
Sijing, L., & Lan, W. (2018). Artificial intelligence education ethical problems and solutions. In *2018 13th international conference on Computer Science & Edu-cation (ICCSE)* (pp. 1–5). https://doi.org/10.1109/ICCSE.2018.8468773
Simondon, G. (2020). *Do modo de existência dos objetos técnicos*. Contraponto.

Chapter 5
Digital Media Use During Children's Sleeping and Eating Routines

Sofia Sebben, Fernanda Martins Marques, Gabriela Vescovi, Indianara Sehaparini, and Giana Bitencourt Frizzo

Introduction

In the age of digitalization, children[1] are immersed in daily life filled with digital media. Recent data shows that children have been using digital media in a variety of places, such as in schools, restaurants, parks, and museums (Kabali et al., 2015). Nevertheless, routines at home such as bedtime and mealtime are among the moments children have been using media the most. A study by our research group (Azevedo et al., 2022) found that the use of screens during routine activities increased according to the child's age, especially from 13 months of age onwards. The majority of mothers of babies aged 0–12 months (82.5%) reported not using screens during routine moments. This proportion decreased to 61.8% among children aged 13–24 months, remaining stable among children aged 25–36 months. In line with these findings, research shows that exposure to digital devices increases with children's age (Bellagamba et al., 2021; Rideout & Robb, 2020).

Parents have been using digital media such as TV, videos, smartphones, and tablets to calm down their kids and make eating and sleeping routines less rowdy (Zimmerman, 2008). Many parents think of digital media as a strategy to get their children to cooperate during routine moments believing that the child becomes more receptive when using digital media. During feeding times, parents tend to find

[1] In the chapter, we discuss various developmental stages, including infants, preschoolers, and school-aged children. Therefore, we decided to standardize and employ the term "child" in a broad and inclusive manner to encompass the different ages and developmental periods covered.

S. Sebben · F. M. Marques · G. Vescovi · I. Sehaparini · G. B. Frizzo (✉)
Universidade Federal do Rio Grande do Sul (UFRGS), Porto Alegre, Brazil
e-mail: sofia.colognese@ufrgs.br; martins.marques@ufrgs.br;
gabriela-vescovi@saude.rs.gov.br; indianara.sehaparini@ufrgs.br; giana.frizzo@ufrgs.br

G. B. Frizzo (ed.), *Digital Media and Early Child Development*,
https://doi.org/10.1007/978-3-031-69224-6_5

it easier to introduce different foods to the child in the presence of media (Teekavanich et al., 2022). During sleeping routines, digital media is used to distract the child until they fall asleep (Bellagamba et al., 2021). However, this particular use during eating and sleeping routines may be detrimental to a child's well-being and development.

Despite the considerable pervasiveness of digital media in children's routines, there has been a common concern among scholars and healthcare professionals regarding the possible negative effects of this use during routine moments. Indeed, the World Health Organization (World Health Organization (WHO), 2019) established that digital media should not interfere with activities that are essential for child development, that is, during eating and sleeping routines and during movement and human interaction. Many pediatric societies around the world, such as the American Academy of Paediatrics (2016), the Royal College of Pediatrics and Child Health (2019), the Brazilian Society of Paediatrics (2019), the Canadian Paediatric Society (2022), and the American Academy of Child and Adolescent Psychiatry (2020), also recommend that digital media should be limited or avoided during daily routines, especially oversleep and meal routines. The current literature in the area also shows supporting evidence for these recommendations. Children who spend more time in front of screens during routine activities such as feeding, bathing, changing diapers, and bedtime are at greater risk of socioemotional delay (Raman et al., 2017; Wan et al., 2021). Indeed, a meta-analysis of 23 studies showed strong associations between excessive use of digital media at bedtime and mealtime and detrimental outcomes for children's sleep quality and quantity and also nutritional health (Li et al., 2020).

It is important to highlight that the pandemic of COVID-19 was a landmark responsible for the increased use of digital media in the family environment. Due to the need for social distance, digital media has become one of the main resources for communication, work, and distraction for families. Children's exposure to screens has also become more recurrent due to parents' need to carry out different work activities and domestic chores. However, using screens during feeding times and bedtimes is associated with more negative indicators of physical and mental health in children (Francisco et al., 2020).

Following evidence, in the past few years, there has been an ongoing trend recommending parents to keep children's bedtime and mealtime screen-free. Given this, in the next sections, we will review current evidence regarding the ways digital media has been used during children's sleeping and eating routines, respectively, and the possible relations of such use with their sleeping and eating lifestyles.

Media and Sleep: Digital Media Impact on Sleep Quality and Child Behavior

A quality sleep time is vital for physical and mental health. While the child sleeps, several processes occur in the brain, such as the consolidation of memories and learning carried out during the day and the production of defense cells that constitute the human immune system (Zimmerman, 2008). Sleep is crucial for infants and young children as it supports the development of the brain and cognitive functions, such as memory and attention (Tham et al., 2017). The decrease in the duration and quality of sleep, in the long term, has an impact on the reduction of hormones that are important for child growth and development, such as melatonin (which prepares the body for sleep), cortisol (related to stress, emotional regulation, and inflammation control), and somatotropin (responsible for regulating growth) (Tham et al., 2017). When sleep is insufficient or of poor quality, negative effects on the development of brain functions can occur, facilitating the onset of health problems such as obesity. If not properly addressed, sleeping problems may have lifelong impacts (Garrison et al., 2011; Magee et al., 2014).

The WHO (2019) makes recommendations on the daily amount of sleep needed in each age group during the first years of life, as seen in Table 5.1. Any sleep pattern that makes it troublesome for the child to get the necessary amount for her or his normal growth and development is considered a sleep problem. About 20–30% of young children have difficulty sleeping, with different causes that can overlap such as biological (mouth breathing), emotional (psychosomatic), and behavioral (related to habits and routines close to bedtime) symptoms (Blackham et al., 2019).

In addition to the total hours, sleep quality is analyzed by different criteria, such as the amount of time the child takes from going to bed to falling asleep (called latency time), the number of times the child wakes up during the night, consolidation sleep duration (number of hours of sleep that occur at night), sleepiness during the day (measured by the number and duration of naps), and parent's perception of the existence, or not, of sleep problems (Blackham et al., 2019). In contemporary society, the pervasiveness of screens in families' routines is a factor that can impair the quality of children's sleep, with negative consequences for their health and development (Cheung et al., 2017; Domingues-Montanari, 2017; Staples et al., 2021).

To understand the relationship between screens and infant sleep, it is important to consider the concept of circadian rhythms, also called circadian clock. This is a natural internal process repeated every 24 hours that regulates sleep–wake cycles. It is influenced by genetic aspects and by environmental factors, such as sunlight and routine schedules. This process has the important function of signaling that we are

Table 5.1 WHO recommendations on sleep hours during the first years of life[a]

Age group	Daily amount of sleep recommended (hours) including naps
First 3 months	14–17
Up to 1 year	12–16
Between 1 and 2 years	11–14
Between 3 and 4 years	10–13

[a]Source: World Health Organization (2019)

sleepy and should go to bed and also when we have got enough sleep and can wake up (Walker et al., 2020). Because infants and young children are learning to regulate their sleep–wake cycle, bedtime can turn into a challenging moment for many families. Going to sleep can be facilitated or hindered, according to the family's sleep hygiene habits (Blackham et al., 2019).

Sleep hygiene refers to habits and routines that occur close to bedtime. Stimulating activities at night, such as using the bed to play, eat, and watch TV; a room with too much light, noise, cold, or heat; taking many naps during the day; and irregular sleep and wake times are examples of inadequate sleep hygiene habits (Zimmerman, 2008). In turn, good sleep hygiene for children is linked to stability in the bedtime routine. For the child, the family must have habits that signal the approach of bedtime because they help children get organized and regulate their circadian clock. Studies have indicated that one of the behaviors that hinder this preparation, constituting an inadequate sleep hygiene habit, is the excessive use of screens, especially close to bedtime. Prolonged or frequent use of screens during sleep routines can alter sleep-related habits due to the hyperstimulus that the blue light of the screen can emit, in addition to the type of content watched by the child (e.g., aggressive content can make the child agitated and difficult to calm down). Therefore, this practice can affect the quantity and quality of sleep, as well as increase daytime sleepiness, which tends to deregulate the child's circadian clock (LeBourgeois et al., 2023; Wong et al., 2022).

The use of media at bedtime has been associated with decreased sleep quality (Nathanson & Beyens, 2018). For instance, television use has been associated with sleeping problems, such as shorter duration and irregular sleep or nap schedules. A study found that each additional hour of television use during evening time was associated with greater odds of parents reporting sleep problems in their 3- to 5-year-old children (Garrison et al., 2011). In another study carried out in the United Kingdom (Cheung et al., 2017), researchers found that each additional hour of touchscreen media use was associated with 15.6 minutes less sleep in children aged 6 months to 3 years.

Screens can interfere with children's sleep in multiple ways, both directly and indirectly. The literature points to four hypotheses that seek to explain the interference of screens in children's sleep. The first hypothesis is related to the physiological arousal caused by the content that the child watches. If violent, impactful, or frightening, it can cause agitation at bedtime. As a consequence, there may be an increase in the sleep latency time and induction of nightmares, leading the child to wake up more often during the night. If the state of greater alertness and activity at bedtime is maintained over time, changes in the circadian clock may occur due to the activation of the cortisol hormone (Tham et al., 2017). The second hypothesis states that the blue light emitted by electronic devices would decrease the production of melatonin in the brain, the hormone responsible for inducing sleep. In this way, the child would need longer to feel sleepy, go to bed later than usual, increase the latency time, or decrease the total number of hours of sleep (Higuchi et al., 2014). The third explanation is that using screens at night delays bedtime, causing the child to sleep later. As the family routine is usually maintained, the child wakes up at the usual time, resulting in fewer hours of sleep (Hale et al., 2018). The fourth and final hypothesis proposes that the use of digital media close to bedtime may increase the chances of the child going to bed later and waking up later the next morning. Although the child may have the same amount of sleep hours, the shift in the sleep schedule may increase the amount of daytime sleep and interfere with sleep consolidation (Blackham et al., 2019).

In addition to these direct mechanisms, screens can impact child sleep indirectly. When using electronic devices during the day, the child reduces the time devoted to other activities that are important for their development and to energy expenditure, such as physical and outdoor activities, running, jumping, and playing (Janssen et al., 2020). All these direct and indirect impacts could create a vicious cycle, such as the child, when excessively exposed to screens, could have worse sleep quality, resulting in more tiredness during the day, which impacts the disposition and energy for active behaviors creating a sedentary routine. When a child is tired, there is an increased chance that he may spend more time on screens, which in turn negatively impacts his sleep, forming a feedback cycle (Lin et al., 2022).

Despite these impacts, many parents use screens as a resource to make their child sleep. Parents want to help their children sleep better, but many of them are unaware of the risks associated with this behavior and use screens as a way to calm the children down or keep them quiet in bed (Radesky et al., 2016). In our research group (Azevedo et al., 2022), we found that the use of screens at bedtime by Brazilian children remained relatively stable up to 24 months, with an increase among children aged 25–36 months. Among mothers of infants and toddlers, about 8% reported using screens at bedtime. In children aged 25–36 months, this proportion increased to 16.4%. This suggests that there are factors related to child development associated with the practice of offering screens at bedtime, which still need to be further investigated. It should be noted that the sample of this study was composed of Brazilian mothers living in urban areas and with high levels of education, who generally have easier access to information about the potentially harm caused by screen use in childhood. These numbers may be different in studies made with samples of other sociodemographic profiles.

Sleep has been impacted by the COVID-19 pandemic, and screen time, which influences sleep, has increased during this period (Drumheller & Fan, 2022). In a study carried out in Canada during the COVID-19 pandemic, Fitzpatrick et al. (2022) found that most preschool children in the sample (56%) were habitually exposed to screens within the hour before bedtime (4–7 times/week). Additionally, 27% were exposed moderately (1–3 times/week), and only 17% were never or rarely exposed to screens before bedtime (less than 1 time/week). The researchers also found that certain child and family characteristics contributed to the risk of media use before bedtime during the pandemic. Regarding the child, those who had better ability to regulate their emotions, attention, and movement were less likely to use media before bedtime. Concerning the family, parents who used more digital media themselves and those accustomed to the practice of co-viewing and instructive approaches exposed their children to bedtime media more often. On the other hand, parents who had a restrictive style exposed their children to bedtime media less frequently. These results indicate the relevance of considering the family context in interventions aimed at reducing screen use at bedtime in childhood. They also point to the importance of taking into account the long-term effects of the pandemic on children's screen use and sleep.

Besides sleep, nutrition is another essential component in a child's optimal development. Food is not only beneficial for a child's physical growth but also for establishing affection and bonding with caregivers. We now turn to explore the relationship between digital media use and eating habits.

Media Use and Nutrition: Digital Media Impact on Eating Habits and Child Development

In the early years, through breastfeeding, whether directly from the breast or a bottle, infants start to engage with the world and familiarize themselves with it. The period of food introduction reinforces the bond with caregivers, also providing the child the possibility to learn about food flavors, colors, smells, temperature, textures, consistencies, and preferences (Brazilian Society of Paediatric, 2022). Furthermore, mealtime is a rich moment for children to learn about their culture and their family's habits. All these experiences help to shape identity, build a relationship with food, and establish healthy habits for life (WHO, 2020).

Hunger and satiety are two of the main mechanisms linked to the nutrition process, and so is physical growth. These two mechanisms work through a complex neurophysiological process, in which the brain sends signals to the human body for food intake. Food then provides the body with energy and allows for adjusted bodily functions. The hypothalamus is the portion in the brain that stimulates the feeling of hunger, through the ghrelin hormone. This mechanism can be characterized as the stimulus expected to lead to the beginning of the meal. When one is eating, their stomach naturally expands, and at some point, this signal notifies the brain that it is time to stop eating, reducing the ghrelin hormone (Sarma et al., 2020). In turn, the fat tissue releases the hormone leptin, which is responsible to signal and regulate satiation to an individual after they have eaten enough. Therefore, a good balance between these hormones is key to healthy development, appropriate food intake, and energy storage (Kharbanda et al., 2022), especially during childhood. A well-nourished child is capable of favorable physical, cognitive, and social development (WHO, 2020), increasing the chances of being a healthy adult. Hence, a child's attention should be focused on the experiences of eating during meals, without the presence of distractions which may take the child's attention away (Silva et al., 2016).

Nowadays, it is well-reported that the children's use of digital media during mealtime occurs in many families (Bahadur et al., 2021). In this view, a child who is distracted by screens during meals and whose main focus is not on the experience of eating could be missing out on the experience of meals and important information for their healthy development. This, in turn, can lead to a series of behavioral and developmental changes in the child.

Children who use digital media during mealtime often lose interest in eating which hinders their understanding of food. Those who watch more TV can increase their intake of desserts and sweets (Jensen et al., 2022). Eating without paying attention to food may also affect vital functions, like loss of reduced awareness over hunger and satiety, with a consequent increase in food intake (Robinson et al., 2017; Tabares-Tabares et al., 2022) and, in the long term, excessive weight gain. This can bring greater impairment for young children, as they gradually learn to regulate their hunger and satiety system in the early years of life (Brazilian Society of Paediatric, 2022).

In this sense, it is relevant to question the use of screens during meals. It can contribute to the child remaining oblivious to eating experiences, mostly submitting her body to the mechanical performance of this activity. In this way, the child may not actively participate in the meal. He is often only passively involved, being fed by adults, without engaging in this experience, learning from it, or being aware of his physiological signals. Research in the area found some variables to be associated with higher children's exposure to screens while feeding in the first years of life: parents' lower educational level, having a television in the child's bedroom, infant's higher activity level, and more child negative affectivity (Cost et al., 2020; Domoff et al., 2017; Thimmig et al., 2017; Thompson et al., 2013). Despite that, all these associations need to be deeply investigated in future studies.

Besides this active use of digital media, children can also employ a passive use of digital media during mealtime, like through background TV (BTV). BTV is a term used to characterize a situation in which a TV is turned on in the background while a child is in the room performing another activity (Lapierre et al., 2012). The child could be by himself doing a parallel activity, for instance, eating while the TV is turned on in the room. Or the caregiver could be watching something on the TV, while the child is in the same room but engaged in another task.

Passive screen use, like BTV, may seem less harmful than active screen use during eating routines, since the child may not be directly visually watching TV or interacting with it. However, recent research shows a relevant perspective on the relations between BTV and child nutrition and behavior. Children often exposed to BTV can increase junk food intake, lower fruit and vegetable consumption, and have higher active digital media use during meals (Jusienė et al., 2019). Parents of children who live in environments with frequent BTV exposure and increased use of digital media during meals also report a higher incidence of challenging behavior in their children (Munzer et al., 2018). However, most of these studies are cross-sectional, so these hypotheses need to be tested in future longitudinal research to find causal relations.

When adults are the ones who use screens during child feeding times, they can decrease their attention and sensitivity to the child's needs and signals. In these circumstances, adults can respond with a repressive tone or even physically, giving orders mechanically, without eye contact or appropriate voice intonation. Consequently, the child may react by showing difficulty accepting new foods or testing limits with oppositional behaviors (Radesky et al., 2014). All these negative interactive dynamics can impair the development of taste and eating habits, affecting the emotional connection between caregiver and child. In that way, a great opportunity for parents to interact and stimulate child development during family meals is potentially lost.

It is also important to consider why adults appeal to screens when feeding the child. Often due to difficulties in managing the toddler's refusal to eat and try new foods or out of concern about the amount of food the child eats, caregivers end up using electronic devices to make children eat more, faster, or with fewer interruptions. In these cases, parents must receive guidance from doctors, nutritionists, or other healthcare providers. As for sleep, there is evidence that the practice of offering screens at mealtime changes according to the child's age. In a study by our research group, screen use at feeding times increased from 5.6% among infants to over 20% among children aged 13–36 months (Azevedo et al., 2022). Cost et al. (2020) also found that children from 13 to 18 months were more likely to have screen exposure combined with feeding compared with younger children.

Apart from that, digital media use in childhood can also target youngsters to food or beverage advertisements (Delgado et al., 2022). In the next topic, we will approach current legislation and existing empirical evidence regarding this phenomenon.

Food and Beverage Advertisements to Children

Food and beverage advertisement is a marketing strategy for selling many types of healthy and unhealthy products to customers through a variety of forms and channels. The food industry targets the population in general, but especially children, with marketing in a variety of media types, such as television and, in the last few years, on digital media, through the Internet, online games, social media, and other apps (WHO, 2023). Although advertising to children is common in many countries, some legislation sees this practice through another lens. Up to the present, the United Kingdom, Greece, Denmark, and Belgium restrict advertising to children. In other countries like Norway, Brazil, Sweden, and some provinces of Canada, like Quebec, advertising to children under the age of 12 is illegal. Concerning this, it is important to point out that most legislation refers to restricting television and other printed media of food and beverage advertisements for children (Tatlow-Golden & Garde, 2020).

On the other hand, many countries lack government laws that aim to regulate and restrict advertisements on digital media. Children are smartphone and tablet "owners" from an early age, meaning they can have firsthand and broader access to propaganda materials with potentially less adult supervision. These digital platforms are also fertile grounds for targeted advertising since advertisers can collect data on children's browsing habits, preferences, and demographics, allowing them to tailor their ads specifically to their target audience, increasing the effectiveness of these advertisements (Van Reijmersdal et al., 2016). Furthermore, the widespread use of digital media exposes children to advertisements during TV commercial breaks and through various platforms and devices, particularly while playing games or watching videos online. This almost constant exposure can make it challenging for children to escape the influence of these persuasive messages, pointing to the importance of discussing these issues in our times. Indeed, access to specific advertisements can impact aspects that range from children's relation to the consumption of certain types of food, consumerism, to weight gain and contribute to higher rates of childhood obesity (Delgado et al., 2022; Von Nordheim et al., 2022; Russell et al., 2019).

Research on the area has shown that children can have different eating patterns depending on the content of the advertisements they access. Advertisement exposure in childhood, which influences children to eat more unhealthy food, may create a behavior trend that tends to last into adulthood (Norman et al., 2020) because children normally have access to advertisements that show ultra-processed and junk food content. These materials also promote the consumption of unhealthy foods (high in saturated fat, salt, and sugar) or immediate calorie consumption by children (Russell et al., 2019). Moreover, foods high in saturated fat, salt, and sugar can impair good sleep quality, leading to weight gain and obesity over time (Delgado et al., 2022; van Meer et al., 2015).

On the other hand, children who commonly watch healthy food advertisements are more likely to reach the daily recommended vegetable and fruit intake (Von Nordheim et al., 2022). Nevertheless, children can easily mix up reality with the fiction of advertising content. Until the age of 7–8, they are not fully capable of perceiving persuasive intents of marketing advertisements, because they are still developing parts of the brain related to judgment and decision-making skills (Delgado et al., 2022).

Even on channels considered appropriate for children, food or beverage advertisements in TV programs or games have been linked to encouraging consumerism in children (Delgado et al., 2022). The presence of toys and characters in the advertisements can further increase the consumption of these foods. The association of the product (food or toy) with pleasant feelings (such as being strong, being cool, being joyful) can lead to the false notion of problem-solving through consumption, since the advertisements show happy individuals spending money, buying things, or consuming a certain food or drink (Dixon et al., 2017). Furthermore, many videos sponsored by food and beverage companies and made by channels or people linked to children's audiences can encourage food waste.

Another topic that needs to be considered is that many food and beverage advertisements to children are also directed to parents. As we stated earlier on, it is likely that eating behaviors are promoted by parents from children's early age. Therefore, a child will probably follow and get used to the parents' diet, which entails a need for parents to acknowledge the importance of introducing healthy food into children's, but also their own diet. However, there seems to be an interplay between the child–parent relationship and diet that needs to be considered. Although young children may not yet have the autonomy to purchase their own food, they can affect their parents' buying decisions (Baldassarre et al., 2016). According to Baldassarre et al. (2016), this influence may decrease when caregivers have more awareness of the importance of a quality-based diet. Therefore, children's food and diet preferences may shape and influence the whole family's consumption patterns from the advertising content they have access to, and this is exploited by marketing. Thus, parents need to be informed about the importance of offering children a more balanced diet and how this can affect their health and the family's eating behaviors. Having a better comprehension about how advertisements foster consumption of certain types of foods and beverages can help parents choose healthier options (Peters et al., 2014, Sina et al., 2022).

In sum, current evidence shows that children may be influenced by food and beverage advertisements, which could impact their eating habits, weight gain, sleep patterns, and risk of obesity. Especially in digital resources, there may be an even higher consumption to this type of propaganda, in which contents are available during other contexts beside commercial breaks, like during children's leisure time. But evidence on this topic is relatively recent and limited, being that most literature still focuses on advertisements on television (Boyland et al., 2022). There is still a need for more research to investigate this phenomenon on digital media in order to provide scientifically informed interventions for families with children and to encourage review of current policies that include regulations on advertisements available on digital media.

Practical Implications

In this chapter, we reviewed evidence on the possible developmental impacts of children's digital media use during sleeping and eating routines, as well as childhood exposure to food and beverage advertisements. Media use during sleep and meals can be detrimental to their sleeping and eating routines, potentially having long lasting effects on their development. It can also disrupt the rich social interactions between children and their caregivers during those moments. Access to food and beverage advertisements in digital media can also impair their eating experiences and prospectively lead to unhealthy food intake and risk of obesity. In the face of this scientific knowledge, we now conclude with practical implications for parents, educators, health professionals, and policymakers.

First, it is important for parents to receive guidelines on how to manage their children's sleep routine, in order to protect them from the potentially harmful effects of screen use at bedtime. As young children are still regulating their circadian clock, it is important that they have a consistent bedtime routine, without distraction from screens. Pediatricians' guidelines recommend to stop using screens at least 1 hour before bedtime and avoid having television or cell phones available in the bedroom. It is also essential that the child has a regular bedtime routine, with clear rules about using screens late in the day and close to bedtime. Sleep moments can be a great opportunity for parents to strengthen the bond with the child, reading stories, listening to calm music, and creating a cozy and silent environment, without interference from lights and strong noises. If the whole family follows these rules, it will be easier for the child to understand and respect them. Children learn a lot about habits, routines, and how to behave by observing their parents and engaging in daily activities with them (Rosa & Tudge, 2013). Therefore, recommendations such as the guidelines from the Royal College of Pediatrics and Child Health (2019) that go beyond children's screen time are important, which focus on the whole family's media use and propose critical reflection on the whole family media habits and needs.

Health professionals and educators should raise awareness with caregivers about what it means for a child to eat well, going beyond the focus on the amount of food ingested. Promoting an active engagement of the child with the food and creating a safe and warm environment while eating is essential. It is needed that mothers and fathers understand the importance of children being aware of their bodily cues to identify when they are hungry or satiated and to allow healthy food choices based on their own preferences. Irritation, rushing, and blackmailing the child to eat, in turn, are behaviors to be avoided, as well as the incentive to "nibble" on sweets and snacking while using screens. Caregivers should also be encouraged to reflect on their own use of digital media during meals, as their behavior serves as an example to their child's. There should also be orientation towards BTV during meals, as many families are unaware of the potential harmful impacts of this passive practice on their child's food-related behaviors and overall physiological development.

As the child gets older and his autonomy behaviors and unwanted tantrums begin to emerge, it seems like digital media is more often used to calm them down. An important consideration to be made is at what cost this happens, because the use of digital media as a way of managing the child can lead to several dysfunctional behaviors. Distraction by digital media in order to avoid such behaviors can prevent children from starting to express their emotions, like discontent, to pay attention to their satiety and hunger, and to recognize signs of sleepiness and tiredness. To always expect passive and obedient behavior from children in this age group is to disregard the importance of this early acquisition of their autonomy. Caregivers should be instructed on developmental marks and how important autonomy is to be developed at a young age. Furthermore, they ought to receive recommendations on how to manage children's difficult behaviors, so that screens are not the only or first choice when it comes to helping children to regulate their emotions or when parents feel the need to distract the child.

In order to address these issues during a health appointment or in an educational setting, professionals should be up to date with scientific evidence. As making way throughout scientific knowledge may be overwhelming to clinicians and educators, initiatives aiming at science dissemination regarding media use are essential. Models of such initiatives are shared in Chap. 6. Besides, brief interventions regarding family's sleep hygiene, eating habits and the development of a family media plan can be performed by different professionals such as nurses, pediatricians, family doctors, and psychologists.

On a macrolevel, governments should consider the elaboration of evidence-based policies to regulate and restrict unhealthy food and beverage advertising that are screened on digital media. Researchers are also encouraged to keep studying the possible associations between different types of food and beverage advertisements, the relations to unhealthier or healthier drinking eating habits, and impacts on child development. These actions should be implemented in order to help improve children's healthy nutrition and minimize junk food intake, consumerism, and risk of weight gain in childhood. Also, evidence of the relations between watching unhealthy food and drink advertisements and negative outcomes in children's nutrition and behaviors should be better disseminated to the community. This way, caregivers, teachers, and other adults responsible for children can be attentive and protect them from consuming this type of marketing. For example, Canada has a program called Stop Marketing to Kids Coalition (Stop Marketing to Kids Coalition, n.d.) which aims to bring awareness about food and beverage advertisements. They offer diverse content (videos and webinars) for adults and children to access. They are also encouraging adults to use social media as a strategy to support the restriction of marketing to kids, through the use of hashtags and slogans to reach more members of the community. Through evidence-based policies, they encourage governments to have strict regulations on marketing to preserve children's health.

Final Considerations

Many habits are built during early childhood, and the relationship with sleep and food is among them. Developing preferences for foods and flavors, the ritual of sitting down at the table to share a meal with others, enjoying the end of the day routine, and having good quality sleep are healthy habits that every child should have the chance to develop. However, these processes take time and require support, attention, affection, and patience from the people responsible for taking care of the child. Children need encouragement and caregivers are a source of example for healthy behaviors like trying new foods or having a healthy diet and engaging in the family bedtime routine.

Finally, societal norms and values may put unrealistic expectations on families regarding child development. Once again, we emphasize the value of proper guidance by health and education professionals for caregivers to provide quality family moments, with or without the presence of digital media. It is essential to help families find possible solutions for children's routines that are so challenging, especially sleeping and eating time.

References

American Academy of Child and Adolescent Psychiatry. (2020). *Screen Time and Children*. https://www.aacap.org/AACAP/Families_and_Youth/Facts_for_Families/FFF-Guide/Children-And-Watching-TV-054.aspx#:~:text=For%20children%202%2D5%2C%20limit,during%20family%20meals%20and%20outings

American Academy of Paediatrics. (2016). Media and young minds. *Pediatrics, 138*(5), e20162591. https://doi.org/10.1542/peds.2016-2591
Azevedo, E. C., Riter, H. S., Pieta, M. A. M., & Frizzo, G. B. (2022). Digital media use on interactions between mother and child: Differences in infants' early years. *Paidéia, 32*. https://doi.org/10.1590/1982-4327e321
Bahadur, E. İ., Akkuş, P. Z., Yoldaş, T. Ç., & Özmert, E. N. (2021). How effective is family counselling on screen exposure of pre-school children?. *The Turkish Journal of Pediatrics, 63*(2), 282–290. https://doi.org/10.24953/turkjped.2021.02.012
Baldassarre, F., Campo, R., & Falcone, A. (2016). Food for kids: How children influence their parents purchasing decisions. *Journal of Food Products Marketing, 22*(5), 596–609. https://doi.org/10.1080/10454446.2016.1141143
Bellagamba, F., Presaghi, F., Di Marco, M., D'Abundo, E., Blanchfield, O., & Barr, R. (2021). How infant and toddlers' media use is related to sleeping habits in everyday life in Italy. *Frontiers in Psychology, 12*. https://doi.org/10.3389/fpsyg.2021.589664
Blackham, A., McDaniel, J. R., Chauvin, I. A., Nelson, K. L., & Buboltz, W. C. (2019). Sleep disruptions and disorders in children and adolescents: A review of the impact of parents and family on sleeping behaviors. *Annals of. Sleep Medicine, 2*(1), 10.36959/532/321.
Boyland, E., McGale, L., Maden, M., Hounsome, J., Boland, A., Angus, K., & Jones, A. (2022). Association of Food and Nonalcoholic Beverage Marketing with Children and Adolescents' eating behaviors and health: A systematic review and meta-analysis. *JAMA Pediatrics, 176*(7), e221037. https://doi.org/10.1001/jamapediatrics.2022.1037
Brazilian Society of Paediatric. (2019). #MENOS TELAS #MAIS SAÚDE. https://www.sbp.com.br/fileadmin/user_upload/_22246c-ManOrient_-__MenosTelas__MaisSaude.pdf
Brazilian Society of Paediatric. (2022). *Guia prático de alimentação. Crianças de 0 a 5 anos*. https://www.sbp.com.br/fileadmin/user_upload/Guia_de_alimentac__a__o_e_nutric__a__o_-_versa__o_fami__lias_compressed.pdf
Canadian Paediatric Society. (2022). *Screen time and preschool children: Promoting health and development in a digital world*. https://cps.ca/en/documents/position/screen-time-and-preschool-children#:~:text=For%20children%202%20to%205,children%20younger%20than%205%20year
Cheung, C. H. M., Bedford, R., Saez de Urabain, I. R., Karmiloff-Smith, A., & Smith, T. J. (2017). Daily touchscreen use in infants and toddlers is associated with reduced sleep and delayed sleep onset. *Scientific Reports, 7*(46104), 1–7. https://doi.org/10.1038/srep46104
Cost, K. T., Korczak, D., Charach, A., Birken, C., Maguire, J. L., Parkin, P. C., & Szatmari, P. (2020). Association of parental and contextual stressors with child screen exposure and child screen exposure combined with feeding. *JAMA Network Open, 3*(2). https://doi.org/10.1001/jamanetworkopen.2019.20557
Delgado, J.R., Campoy, C., Galera Martínez, R., Gallego Mayo, E., Gil-Campos, M., González Jiménez, D., Redecillas Ferreiro, S., Sáenz de Pipaón, M., & Leis, R. (2022). Publicidad de alimentos no saludables. Posicionamiento del Comité de Nutrición y Lactancia Materna de la Asociación Española de Pediatría. *Anales de Pediatría, 97*(3), 206.e1–206.e9. https://doi.org/10.1016/j.anpedi.2022.07.004
Dixon, H., Niven, P., Scully, M., & Wakefield, M. (2017). Food marketing with movie character toys: Effects on young children's preferences for unhealthy and healthier fast food meals. *Appetite, 117*, 342–350. https://doi.org/10.1016/j.appet.2017.07.014
Domingues-Montanari, S. (2017). Clinical and psychological effects of excessive screen time on children. Journal of Paediatrics and Child Health, 53, 333–338. http://doi.org/https://doi.org/10.1111/jpc.13462
Domoff, S. E., Lumeng, J. C., Kaciroti, N., & Miller, A. L. (2017). Early childhood risk factors for mealtime TV exposure and engagement in low-income families. *Academic Pediatrics, 17*(4), 411–415. https://doi.org/10.1016/j.acap.2016.12.003

Drumheller, K., & Fan, C. W. (2022). Unprecedented times and uncertain connections: A systematic review examining sleep problems and screentime during the COVID-19 pandemic. *Sleep Epidemiology, 2*. https://doi.org/10.1016/j.sleepe.2022.100029

Fitzpatrick, C., Almeida, M. L., Harvey, E., Garon-Carrier, G., Berrigan, F., & Asbridge, M. (2022). An examination of bedtime media and excessive screen time by Canadian preschoolers during the COVID-19 pandemic. *BMC Pediatrics, 22*. https://doi.org/10.1186/s12887-022-03280-8

Francisco, R., Pedro, M., Delvecchio, E., Espada, J. P., Morales, A., Mazzeschi, C., & Orgilés, M. (2020). Psychological symptoms and behavioral changes in children and adolescents during the early phase of COVID-19 quarantine in three European countries. *Frontiers in Psychiatry, 11*. https://doi.org/10.3389/fpsyt.2020.570164

Garrison, M. M., Liekweg, K., & Christakis, D. A. (2011). Media use and child sleep: The impact of content, timing, and environment. *Pediatrics, 128*(1), 29–35. https://doi.org/10.1542/peds.2010-3304

Hale, L., Kirschen, G. W., LeBourgeois, M. K., Gradisar, M., Garrison, M. M., Montgomery-Downs, H., Kirschen, H., McHale, S. M., Chang, A. M., & Buxton, O. M. (2018). Youth screen media habits and sleep: Sleep-friendly screen behavior recommendations for clinicians, educators, and parents. *Child and Adolescent Psychiatric Clinics of North America, 27*(2), 229–245. https://doi.org/10.1016/j.chc.2017.11.014

Higuchi, S., Nagafuchi, Y., Lee, S. I., & Harada, T. (2014). Influence of light at night on melatonin suppression in children. *The Journal of Clinical Endocrinology and Metabolism, 99*(9), 3298–3303. https://doi.org/10.1210/jc.2014-1629

Janssen, X., Martin, A., Hughes, A. R., Hill, C. M., Kotronoulas, G., & Hesketh, K. R. (2020). Associations of screen time, sedentary time and physical activity with sleep in under 5s: A systematic review and meta-analysis. *Sleep Medicine Reviews, 49*, 101226. https://doi.org/10.1016/j.smrv.2019.101226

Jensen, M. L., Dillman Carpentier, F. R., Corvalán, C., Popkin, B. M., Evenson, K. R., Adair, L., & Taillie, L. S. (2022). Television viewing and using screens while eating: Associations with dietary intake in children and adolescents. *Appetite, 168*, 105670. https://doi.org/10.1016/j.appet.2021.105670

Jusienė, R., Urbonas, V., Laurinaitytė, I., Rakickienė, L., Breidokienė, R., Kuzminskaitė, M., & Praninskienė, R. (2019). Screen use during meals among young children: Exploration of associated variables. *Medicina, 55*(10), 688. MDPI AG. https://doi.org/10.3390/medicina55100688

Kabali, H. K., Irigoyen, M. M., Nunez-Davis, R., Budacki, J. G., Mohanty, S. H., Leister, K. P., & Bonner, R. L., Jr. (2015). Exposure and use of Mobile media devices by young children. *Pediatrics, 136*(6), 1044–1050. https://doi.org/10.1542/peds.2015-2151

Kharbanda, C., Bansal, S., & Aneja, P. (2022). Role and significance of ghrelin and leptin in hunger, satiety, and energy homeostasis. *Journal of the Scientific Society, 49*(1), 12. https://doi.org/10.4103/jss.jss_126_21

Lapierre, M. A., Piotrowski, J. T., & Linebarger, D. L. (2012). Background television in the homes of US children. *Pediatrics, 130*(5), 839–846. https://doi.org/10.1542/peds.2011-2581

LeBourgeois, M. K., Hartstein, L. E., Wong, S. D., & Ricker, A. A. (2023). Optimal sleep and circadian habits in infants and children. In *Encyclopedia of sleep and circadian rhythms* (pp. 102–109). Elsevier. https://doi.org/10.1016/B978-0-12-822963-7.00020-7

Li, C., Cheng, G., Sha, T., Cheng, W., & Yan, Y. (2020). The relationships between screen use and health indicators among infants, toddlers, and preschoolers: A meta-analysis and systematic review. *International Journal of Environmental Research and Public Health, 17*(19), 7324. MDPI AG. https://doi.org/10.3390/ijerph17197324

Lin, Y., Zhang, X., Huang, Y., Jia, Z., Chen, J., Hou, W., Zhao, L., Wang, G., & Zhu, J. (2022). Relationships between screen viewing and sleep quality for infants and toddlers in China: A cross-sectional study. *Frontiers in Pediatrics, 10*, 987523. https://doi.org/10.3389/fped.2022.987523

Magee, C. A., Lee, J. K., & Vella, S. A. (2014). Bidirectional relationships between sleep duration and screen time in early childhood. *JAMA Pediatrics, 168*(5), 465–470. https://doi.org/10.1001/jamapediatrics.2013.4183

Munzer, T. G., Miller, A. L., Peterson, K. E., Brophy-Herb, H. E., Horodynski, M. A., Contreras, D., et al. (2018). Media exposure in low-income preschool-aged children is associated with multiple measures of self-regulatory behavior. *Journal of developmental and behavioral pediatrics: JDBP, 39*(4), 303–309. https://doi.org/10.1097/DBP.0000000000000560

Nathanson, A. I., & Beyens, I. (2018). The role of sleep in the relation between young children's mobile media use and effortful control. *British Journal of Developmental Psychology, 36*, 1–21. https://doi.org/10.1111/bjdp.12196

Norman, J., Kelly, B., McMahon, A.-T., Boyland, E., Chapman, K., & King, L. (2020). Remember me? Exposure to unfamiliar food brands in television advertising and online advergames drives children's brand recognition, attitudes, and desire to eat foods: A secondary analysis from a crossover experimental-control study with randomization at. *Journal of the Academy of Nutrition and Dietetics, 120*(1), 120–129. https://doi.org/10.1016/j.jand.2019.05.006

Peters, J., Parletta, N., Lynch, J., & Campbell, K. (2014). A comparison of parental views of their pre-school children's 'healthy' versus 'unhealthy' diets. A qualitative study. *Appetite, 76*, 129–136. https://doi.org/10.1016/j.appet.2014.02.001

Radesky, J. S., Kistin, C. J., Zuckerman, B., Nitzberg, K., Gross, J., Kaplan-Sanoff, M., et al. (2014). Patterns of mobile device use by caregivers and children during meals in fast food restaurants. *Pediatrics, 133*(4), 843–849. https://doi.org/10.1542/peds.2013-3703

Radesky, J. S., Peacock-Chambers, E., Zuckerman, B., & Silverstein, M. (2016). Use of mobile technology to calm upset children: Associations with social-emotional development. *JAMA Pediatrics, 170*(4), 397–399. https://doi.org/10.1001/jamapediatrics.2015.4260

Raman, S., Guerrero-Duby, S., McCullough, J. L., Brown, M., Ostrowski-Delahanty, S., Langkamp, D., & Duby, J. C. (2017). Screen exposure during daily routines and a young child's risk for having social-emotional delay. *Clinical Pediatrics, 56*(13), 1244–1253. https://doi.org/10.1177/0009922816684

Rideout, V., & Robb, M. B. (2020). *The common sense census: Media use by kids age zero to eight, 2020*. Common Sense Media.

Robinson, T. N., Banda, J. A., Hale, L., Lu, A. S., Fleming-Milici, F., Calvert, S. L., & Wartella, E. (2017). Screen media exposure and obesity in children and adolescents. *Pediatrics, 140*(Suppl 2), S97–S101. https://doi.org/10.1542/peds.2016-1758K

Rosa, E. M., & Tudge, J. (2013). Urie Bronfenbrenner's theory of human development: Its evolution from ecology to bioecology. *Journal of Family Theory & Review, 5*, 243–258. https://doi.org/10.1111/jftr.12022

Royal College of Pediatric and Child Health. (2019). *The health impacts of screen time: A guide for clinicians and parents*. https://www.rcpch.ac.uk/sites/default/files/2018-12/rcpch_screen_time_guide_-_final.pdf

Russell, S. J., Croker, H., & Viner, R. M. (2019). The effect of screen advertising on children's dietary intake: A systematic review and meta-analysis. *Obesity Reviews: An Official Journal of the International Association for the Study of Obesity, 20*(4), 554–568. https://doi.org/10.1111/obr.12812

Sarma, R., Krishnamoorthy, C., & Chidambaram, R. (2020). Child appetite. In T. Gutiérrez (Ed.), *Food science, technology and nutrition for babies and children*. Springer. https://doi.org/10.1007/978-3-030-35997-3_9

Silva, G. A. P., Costa, K. A. O., & Giugliani, E. R. J. (2016). Infant feeding: Beyond the nutritional aspects. *Jornal de Pediatria, 92*(3), 2–7. https://doi.org/10.1016/j.jped.2016.02.006

Sina, E., Boakye, D., Christianson, L., Ahrens, W., & Hebestreit, A. (2022). Social media and children's and adolescents' diets: A systematic review of the underlying social and physiological mechanisms. *Advances in Nutrition, 13*(3), 913–937. https://doi.org/10.1093/advances/nmac018

Staples, A. D., Hoyniak, C., McQuillan, M. E., Molfese, V., & Bates, J. E. (2021). Screen use before bedtime: Consequences for nighttime sleep in young children. *Infant Behavior & Development, 62*. https://doi.org/10.1016/j.infbeh.2020.101522

Stop Marketing to Kids Coalition. (n.d.). *Stop Marketing to Kids*. https://stopmarketingtokids.ca/

Tabares-Tabares, M., Moreno Aznar, L. A., Aguilera-Cervantes, V. G., León-Landa, E., & López-Espinoza, A. (2022). Screen use during food consumption: Does it cause increased food intake? A systematic review. *Appetite, 171*, 105928. https://doi.org/10.1016/j.appet.2022.105928

Tatlow-Golden, M., & Garde, A. (2020). Digital food marketing to children: Exploitation, surveillance and rights violations. *Global Food Security, 27*, 100423. https://doi.org/10.1016/j.gfs.2020.100423

Teekavanich, S., Rukprayoon, H., Sutchritpongsa, S., & Rojmahamongkol, P. (2022). Electronic media use and food intake in Thai toddlers. *Appetite, 176*, 106121. https://doi.org/10.1016/j.appet.2022.106121

Tham, E. K., Schneider, N., & Broekman, B. F. (2017). Infant sleep and its relation with cognition and growth: A narrative review. *Nature and Science of Sleep, 9*, 135–149. https://doi.org/10.2147/NSS.S125992

Thimmig, L. M., Cabana, M. D., Bentz, M. G., Potocka, K., Beck, A., Fong, L., Chao, C., Caughey, A. B., Wong, A., & McKean, M. (2017). Television during meals in the first 4 years of life. *Clinical Pediatrics, 56*(7), 659–666. https://doi.org/10.1177/0009922816678585

Thompson, A. L., Adair, L. S., & Bentley, M. E. (2013). Maternal characteristics and perception of temperament associated with infant TV exposure. *Pediatrics, 131*(2). https://doi.org/10.1542/peds.2012-1224

Van Meer, F., van der Laan, L. N., Adan, R. A., Viergever, M. A., & Smeets, P. A. (2015). What you see is what you eat: An ALE meta-analysis of the neural correlates of food viewing in children and adolescents. *NeuroImage, 104*, 35–43. https://doi.org/10.1016/j.neuroimage.2014.09.069

Van Reijmersdal, E. A., Rozendaal, E., Smink, N., van Noort, G., & Buijzen, M. (2016). Processes and effects of targeted online advertising among children. *International Journal of Advertising, 36*(3), 396–414. https://doi.org/10.1080/02650487.2016.1196904

Von Nordheim, L., Blades, M., Oates, C., & Buckland, N. J. (2022). Manipulated exposure to television-style healthy food advertising and children's healthy food intake in nurseries. *Appetite, 168*, 105791. https://doi.org/10.1016/j.appet.2021.105791

Walker, W. H., Walton, J. C., DeVries, A. C., et al. (2020). Circadian rhythm disruption and mental health. *Translational Psychiatry, 10*(28). https://doi.org/10.1038/s41398-020-0694-0

Wan, M. W., Fitch-Bunce, C., Heron, K., & Lester, E. (2021). Infant screen media usage and social-emotional functioning. *Infant Behavior & Development, 62*. https://doi.org/10.1016/j.infbeh.2020.101509

Wong, S. D., Wright, K. P., Jr., Spencer, R. L., Vetter, C., Hicks, L. M., Jenni, O. G., & LeBourgeois, M. K. (2022). Development of the circadian system in early life: Maternal and environmental factors. *Journal of Physiological Anthropology, 41*(1), 22. https://doi.org/10.1186/s40101-022-00294-0

World Health Organization. (2019). *Guidelines on physical activity, sedentary behaviour and sleep for children under 5 years of age*. World Health Organization. https://apps.who.int/iris/handle/10665/311664

World Health Organization. (2020). *Healthy diet*. https://www.who.int/news-room/fact-sheets/detail/healthy-diet

World Health Organization. (2023). *New WHO tool aim to protect children from unhealthy food marketing*. https://www.who.int/europe/news/item/14-03-2023-new-who-guidelines-aim-to-protect-children-from-unhealthy-food-marketing

Zimmerman, F. J. (2008). *Children's media use and sleep problems: Issues and unanswered questions*. Kaiser Family Foundation. https://files.eric.ed.gov/fulltext/ED527857.pdf

Chapter 6
Perspectives on Preschooler Screen Time and Global Development

Marie-Andrée Binet, Mélanie Couture, Maíra Lopes Almeida, Mathieu Bégin, and Caroline Fitzpatrick

Preschoolers' Digital Landscape

The digital landscape in which families grow and interact has undergone vast transformations across the last two decades. Notably, newer mobile screen-based devices offer multiplied viewing opportunities as they are now portable and connected to the Internet. Furthermore, their increased affordability has made it easier for families to own more than one device. Preschoolers' access to mobile devices has almost doubled from 2011 to 2020, going from 52% to 98%, with about half of children aged 2–4 owning their own tablet or smartphone (Rideout & Robb, 2020). Moreover, children today are exposed to screens for longer periods of time and at earlier development stages (McArthur et al., 2022; Reid Chassiakos et al., 2016).

M.-A. Binet (✉) · M. Couture
Faculty of Medicine and Health Sciences, Université de Sherbrooke, Sherbrooke, QC, Canada
e-mail: marie-andree.binet@usherbrooke.ca; melanie.m.couture@usherbrooke.ca

M. L. Almeida
Faculty of Education, Universidade Federal de Goiás, Goiânia, Brazil

M. Bégin
Department of Preschool and Primary Education, Université de Sherbrooke, Sherbrooke, QC, Canada
e-mail: mathieu.begin3@usherbrooke.ca

C. Fitzpatrick
Department of Preschool and Primary Education, Université de Sherbrooke, Sherbrooke, QC, Canada

Department of Childhood Education, University of Johannesburg, Johannesburg, South Africa
e-mail: caroline.fitzpatrick@usherbrooke.ca

G. B. Frizzo (ed.), *Digital Media and Early Child Development*,
https://doi.org/10.1007/978-3-031-69224-6_6

Importance of Global Development for Future Outcomes

Young children develop within the context of relationships and interactions. From research on early brain development, it is known that early experiences have a great influence on a child's brain development (Shonkoff, 2016). If these experiences provide emotional support and favorable conditions for development, children are also provided with strong bases for resilience across their lifespan (Shonkoff, 2016). In that sense, it becomes important to better understand how their interactions with screens may be contributing to their acquisition of foundational skills and development. Child global development refers to skills acquired across cognitive/language, physical/motor, and social/emotional domains (World Health Organization, 2007). Achieving autonomy and maturity in these areas of development is then a key determinant of child readiness to learn when entering kindergarten (Williams et al., 2019). Furthermore, the set of skills acquired by children when transitioning to formal schooling seem to forecast long-term achievement by the end of high school (Fitzpatrick et al., 2020). Academic success is also related to better life outcomes (Heckman, 2007). Early vulnerabilities in global development can increase risks for many aspects of adolescent and adult well-being, including obesity, mental health, and employability (Hertzman, 2010). Unfortunately, many children enter school with insufficient skills, either in social, emotional, physical, or cognitive/language domains, putting at risk their ability to benefit from schooling experiences (Browne et al., 2018).

In order to maximize children's opportunities for growth and learning, many pediatric organizations recommend limiting 2- to 5-year-olds' screen time to 1 h daily (Hill et al., 2016). Adherence to these guidelines is rather low in families with preschoolers, with studies reporting averages of 1.5–2.5 h of daily screen time (Carson et al., 2019; Madigan et al., 2020b). A recent meta-analysis of 63 studies revealed a rate of adherence of about 36% among 2–5-year-old children (McArthur et al., 2022). The COVID-19 crisis is likely to have favored an increase in preschoolers' screen time, which could represent an additional 60 minutes daily (Madigan et al., 2022).

From Child Screen Time to Child Media Diets

Research on screen use and child global development has been overwhelmingly focused on screen use or screen time duration. However, other features of children's media diets also merit investigation as they are susceptible to having a wide range of effects. For instance, media content and contexts in which screens are being used are important aspects of a child's media diet. All three dimensions of the media diet—duration, contents, and contexts—will be examined in the next sections.

Duration of Screen Use

The length and frequency of preschoolers' screen exposure have been linked to negative developmental outcomes. This is likely to be the case because screen time can displace time available for other activities, like child–caregiver interactions or unstructured play (Kirkorian et al., 2009; Putnick et al., 2022; Radesky et al., 2015). Studies vary in how they have conceptualized screen time. For instance, many have considered TV only, while others examine aggregate time across multiple devices. Studies have also differed in how they have assessed child developmental outcomes. Most have focused on one domain of development, either cognitive, language, socio-emotional, or motor, whereas only a few have examined an integrated measure of global development. In the present section, we review evidence linking screen time to preschoolers' developmental outcomes.

Overall, most studies indicate negative associations between preschoolers' screen time and cognitive development, including executive functions, general intellectual abilities, and pre-academic skills (Almeida et al., 2023; Munzer et al., 2018; Nathanson & Beyens, 2018; Pagani et al., 2013; Ribner et al., 2017; Zhao et al., 2022). For instance, one study following Chinese preschoolers over the first 6 years of life found that children whose screen use trajectories featured more screen time and earlier exposure onset reported weaker cognitive abilities including intellectual quotient and working memory (Zhao et al., 2022). These associations were found while taking into account risk factors such as maternal education and family income, as well as maternal mental health and child difficult temperament. Research also indicates negative effects of screen time on preschoolers' language development, including expressive and receptive language and vocabulary and communication skills (Byeon & Hong, 2015; Duch et al., 2013; Dynia et al., 2021; Gialamas et al., 2020; Kühhirt & Klein, 2020). Also, studies on socio-emotional development tend to find deleterious effects of screen time, namely on internalized and externalized behaviors, self-regulation skills, and social skills (Eirich et al., 2022; Fitzpatrick et al., 2023; McDaniel & Radesky, 2020; Neville et al., 2021a, b; Pagani et al., 2013; Tamana et al., 2019; Zhao et al., 2022).

Although very few studies on screen use have looked at motor development in preschoolers, they suggest that increased screen time may negatively affect fine motor skills, especially manual dexterity, and gross motor development, including ball skills and locomotion (Felix et al., 2020; Lin et al., 2015; Pagani et al., 2013; Webster et al., 2019). In one Canadian study of 1314 children followed longitudinally, authors found that each additional hour spent watching television at 2.5 years was associated with a decrease in a standing long jump performance, an indicator of physical fitness, at 4.5 years (Fitzpatrick et al., 2012a, b). Increased television exposure also predicted higher odds of at-risk status in this performance (Fitzpatrick et al., 2012a, b).

Most studies looking at preschooler development globally find that global development indices are lower when screen use increases (Kim & Chung, 2021; Madigan et al., 2019; McArthur et al., 2020; Vanderloo et al., 2022). Additionally, among all developmental domains, at least two or three are affected by screen use, primarily language, followed by cognitive and socio-emotional skills (Kerai et al., 2022; Rocha et al., 2021; Vanderloo et al., 2022; Yu et al., 2022).

Few studies have investigated the risks of delays, although these risks have great implications for clinicians and parents (Duch et al., 2013; Felix et al., 2020; Lin et al., 2015; McArthur et al., 2021a, b; Tamana et al., 2019; Vanderloo et al., 2022). Duch et al. (2013) observed that 21-month-old children were more likely to present with language delays when they exceeded 2 h of daily screen time. These risks were also present at follow-up when children were 33 months of age. Risks of global delays were also found to be higher in a Canadian cohort when screen time exceeded 1 hour per day, even when taking into account confounding factors like child age and sex, parent education and stress, and family income (McArthur et al., 2021a, b).

Research using a threshold approach categorizes screen use based on varying doses to verify if being under or over a certain threshold relates to different levels of developmental risks. Research using the threshold approach suggests that exceeding the 1 hour limit is associated with negative developmental effects across developmental domains and that risks increase as the threshold increases (Duch et al., 2013; McArthur et al., 2021a, b; McNeill et al., 2020; Plancoulaine et al., 2017; Yu et al., 2022). For instance, Yu et al. (2022) observed that, compared to children who stayed within the 0–1 h range, exposure to 2–3 h was associated with increased risks of developmental delays across cognitive, expressive language, and social adaptation domains. Furthermore, children exposed to over 3 h of screen time per day had even higher risks of delays, and more developmental domains were affected, such as receptive language, fine and gross motor, and social emotion. As such, children who stay within a 0–1 h range appear to be facing little risks, whereas harm appears to increase for children beyond that range.

Studies on the effect of screen time are limited by the use of correlational designs, which do not allow researchers to reach a cause-and-effect conclusion. In addition, they usually find small effect sizes, meaning that screen time contributes little to outcomes. However, when many people are exposed to the same risk factor over many consecutive years, even small effects can accumulate and become important health risks (Huesmann & Taylor, 2006).

Content and Nature of Use

Content

In order to more fully understand the impact of digital media on young children, it is also essential to consider media *content*. The most studied feature of media content has been the presence of violence. Many studies have revealed associations between preschooler exposure to violent shows and movies and increased risk of later aggression, behavioral and emotional problems, decreased empathy, and poorer sleep and cognitive development (Anderson et al., 2010; Christakis et al.,

2013; Fitzpatrick et al., 2012a; Garrison et al., 2011; Pagani et al., 2023). Zimmerman and Christakis (2007) observed that children under 3 years old exposed to violent entertainment television had increased risks of attentional difficulties 5 years later, in comparison to those who were exposed to nonviolent content.

In addition to violent content, fast-paced (i.e., featuring rapid scene changes) or fantastical programming may also foster risks for cognitive development (Christakis, 2011; Lillard et al., 2015). Using an experimental design, Lillard and Peterson (2011) showed that 4-year-olds who watched a fast-paced television cartoon (e.g., *SpongeBob*) had worse performance on an assessment of executive functioning immediately after viewing in comparison to children who had viewed an educational program (e.g. *Arthur*).

In contrast, exposure to high-quality and age-appropriate prosocial or educational content may be related to more neutral or even positive consequences (Christakis et al., 2013; Coyne et al., 2018; Huber et al., 2018). Indeed, educational TV programs like *Sesame Street* or *Daniel Tiger's Neighborhood* can offer cognitive and psychosocial benefits for preschoolers (Mares & Pan, 2013; Rasmussen et al., 2019). For example, in an experimental study, 121 children aged 3 and 4 were either assigned to an experimental or a control condition. The experimental group used the *Daniel Tiger's Neighborhood* app and watched the homologous TV program for at least 10 min per day for 2 weeks. The control group watched a popular program broadcast on Nick Jr. and played its assigned app at the same frequency. Children in the experimental group had increased emotional knowledge and were using emotion regulation strategies depicted in the media more frequently after 1 month (Rasmussen et al., 2019). Similarly, using a longitudinal design, Anderson et al. (2001) found that preschoolers who viewed more educational content had higher academic success, read more, and were less aggressive by adolescence.

Nature of Use

Interactive video chat technology may provide preschoolers with contexts more favorable for learning as it allows for contingent and sensitive back-and-forth interactions (Gaudreau et al., 2020; Myers et al., 2019). Gaudreau et al. (2020) observed that children who participated in a book-reading activity with a live or a video chat partner had similar performance in vocabulary and comprehension after the activity. Myers et al. (2019) observed that 2- and 3-year-olds who interacted with live or video chat adult partners imitated and responded to the partner's bids in a similar fashion, allowing them to learn new words (Gaudreau et al., 2020; Myers et al., 2019).

Research on newer screen devices such as smartphones or tablets, which require tactile input from the user and which are designed for individual use, has been scarcer. One study has linked mobile device use to negative effects on socio-cognitive development in 4- to 6-year-olds, more precisely on the child's theory of mind, an ability allowing the child to view the world from someone else's perspective (Konok et al., 2021). Studies have found effects of touchscreen use on poorer executive functioning, lower sleep consolidation, and disrupted sleep routines.

Notably, mobile use negatively affects executive functioning through lower sleep quality (Beyens & Nathanson, 2019; Nathanson & Beyens, 2018). Finally, using a case-control design, Lin et al. (2017) observed that preschoolers who spent 20 min per day using an app designed to improve fine motor skills performed *worse* on an assessment of fine motor skills than children from the control group who practiced more traditional fine motor activities (e.g., using scissors, drawing, etc.).

Context of Use

Exposure to screens before bedtime has been linked with lower cognitive functioning, notably through reduced sleep quality (Beyens & Nathanson, 2019; Nathanson & Fries, 2014; Staples et al., 2021). One Canadian study with over 1800 children found that having a television in the bedroom at age 4 was related to higher body mass index, less healthy eating habits, and lower social-emotional well-being at 12, adjusting for confounding individual and family risk factors (Pagani et al., 2019).

Similarly, exposure to screens in the background, notably during mealtimes, is associated with unhealthy eating habits, poorer cardiometabolic outcomes, lower cognitive and self-regulation development, as well as more difficult parent-reported child temperament (Alroqi et al., 2022; Carson & Kuzik, 2021; Corkin et al., 2021; Jamnik et al., 2022; Martinot et al., 2021; Munzer et al., 2018; Parkes et al., 2013; Schlesinger et al., 2019; Wenhold & Harrison, 2018).

Although these contexts are more detrimental to child development, others might be more favorable. In contrast, children may benefit from screen use when a caregiver co-views content with them. Active co-viewing by parents involves shared viewing between the child and an adult. Contrary to solitary screen use, co-viewing may favor bidirectional interactions and lead to improved learning outcomes (Barr, 2019). Indeed, according to one study with 127 preschoolers aged 2–6, psychosocial outcomes such as empathy are improved when children frequently co-viewed an educational program (*Daniel Tiger's Neighborhood*) with a parent (Rasmussen et al., 2016). Furthermore, a Korean study found that when children aged 0–5 years engaged more frequently in reading, physical activity, and screen-based activities with caregivers, they were more likely to be in the highest-performing quartile for cognitive and linguistic development (Lee et al., 2017).

Mechanisms

Understanding the mechanisms linking preschoolers' media diet to positive and negative developmental outcomes remains relevant to developing effective interventions.

Duration-Related Hypotheses

Children aged 2–5 years old are awake between 11 and 14 hours per day (World Health Organization, 2019), and they have much to do and learn during those precious hours. Time spent in front of screens is thus likely to displace time for other more enriching and social activities (Neville et al., 2021b; Radesky et al., 2015). When they are in front of a screen, they are not climbing, building, exploring their environment, or having rich back-and-forth interactions with caregivers. Screen use could displace sleep, play time with peers, and reading activities (Downing et al., 2017; McArthur et al., 2021a; Putnick et al., 2022). To date, few studies have directly examined how screen time may displace developmentally important activities. As an exception, Putnick et al. (2022) observed that preschoolers who accumulated more screen time between 12 and 36 months were at higher risk for developmental delays at 36 months across cognitive, motor, and social–emotional domains through the decreased time spent playing with peers.

Time displacement hypotheses are embedded in neurodevelopment principles, where screen time is viewed as a *lower-quality* activity. Early brain development is highly environment-dependent. As such, developing brains undergo structural changes as a function of experience and stimulation (Shonkoff, 2016). This characteristic, known as neuroplasticity, makes preschoolers particularly disposed to make significant learnings and developmental progress through the repeated establishment of neural connections. However, neuroplasticity is maximal in the early years and declines over time, resulting in a gradual loss of unused neural connections and an increased effort required to make such progress later in life (National Council on the Developing Child, 2007). Recent studies using brain imagery support these hypotheses by revealing a possible relationship between high screen time and less-than-optimal brain development in regions supporting literacy and cognitive development (Hutton et al., 2020b). In contrast, reading activities may stimulate brain tracts supporting language skills (Hutton et al., 2020a). In a longitudinal study also using brain imagery (Law et al., 2023), physical brain alterations mediated the association between screen time at 12 months and executive functioning at 8 years old.

In other words, how children spend their time matters. Screen time may displace time spent engaged in imaginary play, sleeping, doing physical activity, interacting with peers, or practicing language. These missed opportunities may have deleterious effects on sleep and physical/motor, cognitive, and social development.

Content and Nature of Use-Related Hypotheses

Disruption of Attentional and Physiological Systems

Certain types of content may present specific risks to children's cognitive development. For instance, certain contents may be disruptive to children's attentional and physiological systems. Many shows and movies directed at children contain fast-paced and fantastical content, including perceptually salient visual cues such as rapid changes of scenes, camera cuts, and zoom in (Goodrich et al., 2009). These features may be overstimulating for young children's brains, meaning the visual and auditory sensory stimulation provided by media might be excessive (Christakis et al., 2018). In addition, these features are also effective at sustaining child attention to media content without requiring cognitive effort. Over time, this is believed to undermine the development of sustained attention and the ability to inhibit distractors (Christakis et al., 2018). Many television programs capture child attention through sensory stimulation, through a *bottom–up* process, rather than engaging effortful attention directed by the prefrontal cortex in a *top–down* manner (Buschman & Miller, 2007). In addition, watching a rapid-paced succession of stimuli, especially when they are unrealistic or impossible (e.g., fantastical events, a human transforming into a piece of candy), might deplete attentional resources (Lillard & Peterson, 2011). Children may not be able to encode fantastical events the same way as more realistic events, because they are new or rare or in contradiction with their internal understanding of the world. As such, fantastical contents are more difficult to reconcile and may require heavy cognitive resources (Smith, 2020).

Child screen use habits may also have an impact on dopaminergic responses in the brain. Dopamine plays a major role in reward, motivation, pleasure, and addictive behaviors. Some characteristics of media use, such as intermittent positive reinforcement found in video games, may involve immediate rewards and strong incentives to stay engaged in the screen-based activity. The amount of dopamine secreted during video game play may be similar to that of alcohol or psychostimulant drug consumption in humans (Boileau et al., 2003; Cox et al., 2009; Koepp et al., 1998). Thus, rewards obtained in the context of gaming could be associated with increased dopamine secretion in the brain, although we know much less on the impacts of screen exposure on dopamine secretion in young children (Lissak, 2018).

Nature of Use

Touchscreen technologies have a higher potential for interactivity compared to passive television viewing, so they may be associated with different, even positive, effects on child learning. However, compared to manipulating objects or drawing, which require coordination and dexterity, they require simpler motor skills, such as tapping, pressing, or sliding fingers across the screen (Price et al., 2015). Additionally, their omni-availability and portability make them more susceptible to displace time for other activities (Christakis, 2014).

Social Learning Mechanism

As previously noted, the quality of the content children are exposed to matters. Children learn a tremendous amount from observing and imitating models that surround them. Parents and close family members represent important models for children (Bandura, 1977). However, children may also choose to imitate their favorite character from a television show, movie, or game (Greitemeyer & Osswald, 2010). In a classic aggression study, kindergarteners were exposed to an aggressive act by an adult toward a *Bobo* clown doll. Children then had the opportunity to play with the doll after experiencing a frustrating situation. Results indicated that children who had been previously exposed to an aggressive act, either in real life or through a cartoon on TV, were more likely to behave aggressively toward the doll. In comparison, children from the control group who did not witness the aggressive act did not behave aggressively toward the doll (Bandura et al., 1963). Children committed more aggressive behaviors when they had seen the model get rewarded for their actions and less when the model was punished (Bandura, 1965; Bandura & Kupers, 1964). Learning may also occur through simple repeated exposure to stimuli. Repeated exposure to media violence can increase perceived familiarity and normality, leading to habituation and adoption of more aggressive internal cognitive "scripts" or schemas (Bushman & Huesmann, 2012). A study conducted by Gentile et al. (2014) followed 3000 children aged 8–17 years over a 2-year span and observed that exposure to media violence could foster the development of aggressive thoughts or attitudes (e.g., daydreaming or imagining hitting somebody or attributing a hostile intention to someone in an ambiguous situation), which were associated with aggressive behaviors (e.g., hitting someone).

Exposure to prosocial content may similarly lead to more prosocial or altruistic behavior, through similar social learning mechanisms (Coyne et al., 2018). In addition, slow-paced television shows that include familiar situations (e.g., other preschoolers in the context of home) and lots of repetitions, such as *Sesame Street*, facilitate learning by allowing them to relate content to prior experience and information (Mares & Pan, 2013; Valkenburg & Piotrowski, 2017). In coherence with these findings, reducing exposure to violent content and increasing exposure to educational content has been found to benefit preschoolers' social–emotional outcomes (Christakis et al., 2013).

Context-Related Mechanisms

The timing and location of child screen use may influence its consequences on development. When screens disrupt routines, family interactions, or play, they most likely pose developmental risks. Because young children are largely sensory-oriented, sounds and movements have the potential to disrupt them from their ongoing activities (ex., during mealtime) by soliciting attentional resources (Gillioz et al., 2022; Kirkorian et al., 2009). For example, research has shown that when screens are being used during a child's playtime, the child experiences disruption in their playtime behaviors, meaning play episode lengths are reduced and their attention is less focused (Schmidt et al., 2008; Setliff & Courage, 2011). In addition, watching television during mealtimes may distract the child from their satiety cues or expose them to food and beverage advertising, leading to increased amount of calorie intake (Robinson et al., 2017; Robinson & Matheson, 2015). As another example, the psychological and physiological stimulation provided by exposure to screens at night, before bedtime, may contribute to sleep problems in preschoolers (Staples et al., 2021). This disruption in preschooler sleep could notably be due to decreased melatonin secretion, a hormone involved in the circadian rhythm, following exposure to the blue light emitted by electronic devices (Chang et al., 2015; Cheung et al., 2017; LeBourgeois et al., 2017; Salti et al., 2006).

Individual and Family Characteristics

Differential susceptibility and stress–diathesis models (Valkenburg & Peter, 2013) stipulate that sensitivity to environmental influences varies based on individual characteristics. In the present section, we will present the different variables responsible for individual differences in susceptibility to screen influences: age, sex, temperament, and family context.

Although some studies have found no sex differences in the associations between screen time and outcomes (Cliff et al., 2018; Neville et al., 2021a, b; Vanderloo et al., 2022), other research observed that boys may be more vulnerable to screen effects on externalized problems and language skills (Gentile et al., 2017; MacGowan & Schmidt, 2021; Pagani et al., 2023). Experimental research has notably shown increased cardiovascular arousal in boys after playing a violent video game (Gentile et al., 2017). Moreover, a meta-analysis suggests that the protective effects of co-viewing may be especially true in boys (Madigan et al., 2020a, b).

Children with more challenging behaviors and temperament may also be exposed to higher amounts of screen time and show higher sensitivity to the negative impact of screens. For example, children expressing more difficult temperamental characteristics may be exposed to more media, possibly as a parental emotional regulation strategy (Radesky et al., 2016). However, this strategy seems to backfire, leading to increased subsequent emotional reactivity in the child, notably extreme emotions when the screen is removed (Coyne et al., 2021; Radesky et al., 2023). Additionally, children who are described as difficult eaters by their parents are more likely to be exposed to screens during mealtimes, which can lead to further behavioral difficulties (Teekavanich et al., 2022).

The impacts of preschoolers' screen use may also be influenced by the family context. For example, when parents are heavier screen users, their children have higher levels of screen exposure (Lauricella et al., 2015; Madigan et al., 2020a, b). Moreover, lower socioeconomic status (SES) families tend to accumulate more screen time (Rideout & Robb, 2020), and the deleterious effects of screen time on child mathematic skills and executive functioning were found to be increased in lower-income families (Ribner et al., 2017).

Discussion

Young children are exposed to various media diets that differ in amount, content, and context. Briefer screen use duration of high-quality educational content in the presence of an interacting parent appears to facilitate learning and may provide benefits to children. In contrast, media diets characterized by prolonged periods of time, exposure to violent content, and during specific contexts like family meals could lead to decrements in global development. Time displacement, disruption of attentional processes, social learning, and disruption of family interactions are proposed as explanations for these effects. It is also important to consider child and family characteristics, such as child behavioral and temperament profiles, as protective or risk factors moderating the impact of screen use on child development.

Clinical Implications

The Canadian Pediatric Society recommends certain practices to maximize the benefits and reduce the risks associated with screen use by young children. These practices notably include a family media plan that establishes time limits, moments, rooms, and contexts where screen use is allowed or not, prioritizes co-viewing and educational content rather than individual use, and turns off devices that are not being used (Ponti, 2022).

The present review can inform clinical interventions. First, interventions are likely to be successful when beginning in early childhood (Wahi et al., 2011). Second, interventions targeting parents need to be prolonged over time. A recent meta-analysis of 21 clinical trials aimed at reducing time spent in front of screens in children 0–18 also supports the benefits of screen time reduction interventions (including home- or school-based health promotion curriculum, family counseling, etc.), with stronger effects when interventions lasted for at least 7 months (Akçay & Barış, 2021). Third, content can also be targeted as a way to increase the quality of media diets in preschoolers. As an example of content intervention, a randomized controlled trial aiming at modifying media content but not screen time in preschoolers observed that assisting parents in replacing violent content by prosocial and educational programming had positive effects on social competence and reduction of externalizing behaviors and sleep problems (Christakis et al., 2013; Garrison & Christakis, 2012). This study supports the importance of considering media content in the context of early intervention in order to foster developmental benefits. Fourth, interventions could benefit from including parental screen time as it strongly predicts the child's own use (Lauricella et al., 2015).

Research Implications

Although research on preschooler screen use and development has increased in the past decade, there is still much to be learned. Notably, most existing research focuses on screen time rather than content and context of use. Further investigation is needed regarding the mechanisms behind screen use effects, notably how the displacement of sleep or physical activity may indirectly influence global development or how blue light may disrupt circadian cycles. Finally, a great number of studies do not include important child and family characteristics that are susceptible to help identify individuals who are more at risk to the effects of screens (Kostyrka-Allchorne et al., 2017).

References

Akçay, D., & Barış, N. (2021). Evaluating the effectiveness of interventions to reducing screen time in children : Meta-analysis of randomized controlled trials. *Journal of Public Mental Health, 21*, 179–196. https://doi.org/10.1108/JPMH-03-2021-0039

Almeida, M. L., Garon-Carrier, G., Cinar, E., Frizzo, G. B., & Fitzpatrick, C. (2023). Prospective associations between child screen time and parenting stress and later inattention symptoms in preschoolers during the COVID-19 pandemic. *Frontiers in Psychology, 14*, 1053146. https://doi.org/10.3389/fpsyg.2023.1053146

Alroqi, H., Serratrice, L., & Cameron-Faulkner, T. (2022). The association between screen media quantity, content, and context and language development. *Journal of Child Language, 50*, 1155–1183. https://doi.org/10.1017/S0305000922000265

Anderson, D. R., Huston, A. C., Schmitt, K. L., Linebarger, D. L., Wright, J. C., & Larson, R. (2001). Early childhood television viewing and adolescent behavior: The Recontact study. *Monographs of the Society for Research in Child Development, 66*, i–154.

Anderson, C. A., Shibuya, A., Ihori, N., Swing, E. L., Bushman, B. J., Sakamoto, A., Rothstein, H. R., & Saleem, M. (2010). Violent video game effects on aggression, empathy, and prosocial behavior in eastern and Western countries: A meta-analytic review. *Psychological Bulletin, 136*, 151–173. https://doi.org/10.1037/a0018251

Bandura, A. (1965). Influence of models' reinforcement contingencies on the acquisition of imitative responses. *Journal of Personality and Social Psychology, 1*, 589–595. https://doi.org/10.1037/h0022070

Bandura, A. (1977). *Social learning theory*. Prentice-Hall.

Bandura, A., & Kupers, C. J. (1964). Transmission of patterns of self-reinforcement through modeling. *The Journal of Abnormal and Social Psychology, 69*, 1–9. https://doi.org/10.1037/h0041187

Bandura, A., Ross, D., & Ross, S. A. (1963). Imitation of film-mediated aggressive models. *The Journal of Abnormal and Social Psychology, 66*, 3–11. https://doi.org/10.1037/h0048687

Barr, R. (2019). Growing up in the digital age: Early learning and family media ecology. *Current Directions in Psychological Science, 28*, 341–346. https://doi.org/10.1177/0963721419838245

Beyens, I., & Nathanson, A. I. (2019). Electronic media use and sleep among preschoolers: Evidence for time-shifted and less consolidated sleep. *Health Communication, 34*, 537–544. https://doi.org/10.1080/10410236.2017.1422102

Boileau, I., Assaad, J.-M., Pihl, R. O., Benkelfat, C., Leyton, M., Diksic, M., Tremblay, R. E., & Dagher, A. (2003). Alcohol promotes dopamine release in the human nucleus accumbens. *Synapse, 49*, 226–231. https://doi.org/10.1002/syn.10226

Browne, D. T., Wade, M., Prime, H., & Jenkins, J. M. (2018). School readiness amongst urban Canadian families: Risk profiles and family mediation. *Journal of Educational Psychology, 110*, 133–146. https://doi.org/10.1037/edu0000202

Buschman, T. J., & Miller, E. K. (2007). Top-down versus bottom-up control of attention in the prefrontal and posterior parietal cortices. *Science, 315*, 1860–1862. https://doi.org/10.1126/science.1138071

Bushman, B. J., & Huesmann, L. R. (2012). Effects of violent media on aggression. In D. G. Singer & J. L. Singer (Eds.), *Handbook of children and the media* (2nd ed., pp. 231–248). Sage Publications, Inc.

Byeon, H., & Hong, S. (2015). Relationship between television viewing and language delay in toddlers: Evidence from a Korea national cross-sectional survey. *PLoS One, 10*, e0120663. https://doi.org/10.1371/journal.pone.0120663

Carson, V., & Kuzik, N. (2021). The association between parent–child technology interference and cognitive and social–emotional development in preschool-aged children. *Child: Care, Health and Development, 47*, 477–483. https://doi.org/10.1111/cch.12859

Carson, V., Ezeugwu, V. E., Tamana, S. K., Chikuma, J., Lefebvre, D. L., Azad, M. B., Moraes, T. J., Subbarao, P., Becker, A. B., Turvey, S. E., Sears, M. R., & Mandhane, P. J. (2019). Associations between meeting the Canadian 24-hour movement guidelines for the early years and behavioral and emotional problems among 3-year-olds. *Journal of Science and Medicine in Sport, 22*, 797–802. https://doi.org/10.1016/j.jsams.2019.01.003

Chang, A.-M., Aeschbach, D., Duffy, J. F., & Czeisler, C. A. (2015). Evening use of light-emitting eReaders negatively affects sleep, circadian timing, and next-morning alertness. *Proceedings of the National Academy of Sciences of the United States of America, 112*, 1232–1237. https://doi.org/10.1073/pnas.1418490112

Cheung, C. H. M., Bedford, R., Saez De Urabain, I. R., Karmiloff-Smith, A., & Smith, T. J. (2017). Daily touchscreen use in infants and toddlers is associated with reduced sleep and delayed sleep onset. *Scientific Reports, 7*, 46104. https://doi.org/10.1038/srep46104

Christakis, D. A. (2011). The effects of fast-paced cartoons. *Pediatrics, 128*, 772–774. https://doi.org/10.1542/peds.2011-2071

Christakis, D. A. (2014). Interactive media use at younger than the age of 2 years: Time to rethink the American Academy of Pediatrics guideline? *JAMA Pediatrics, 168*, 399–400. https://doi.org/10.1001/jamapediatrics.2013.5081

Christakis, D. A., Garrison, M. M., Herrenkohl, T., Haggerty, K., Rivara, F. P., Zhou, C., & Liekweg, K. (2013). Modifying media content for preschool children: A randomized controlled trial. *Pediatrics, 131*, 431–438. https://doi.org/10.1542/peds.2012-1493

Christakis, D. A., Ramirez, J. S. B., Ferguson, S. M., Ravinder, S., & Ramirez, J.-M. (2018). How early media exposure may affect cognitive function: A review of results from observations in humans and experiments in mice. *Proceedings of the National Academy of Sciences of the United States of America, 115*, 9851–9858. https://doi.org/10.1073/pnas.1711548115

Cliff, D. P., Howard, S. J., Radesky, J. S., McNeill, J., & Vella, S. A. (2018). Early childhood media exposure and self-regulation: Bidirectional longitudinal associations. *Academic Pediatrics, 18*, 813–819. https://doi.org/10.1016/j.acap.2018.04.012

Corkin, M. T., Peterson, E. R., Henderson, A. M. E., Waldie, K. E., Reese, E., & Morton, S. M. B. (2021). Preschool screen media exposure, executive functions and symptoms of inattention/hyperactivity. *Journal of Applied Developmental Psychology, 73*, 101237. https://doi.org/10.1016/j.appdev.2020.101237

Cox, S. M. L., Benkelfat, C., Dagher, A., Delaney, J. S., Durand, F., McKenzie, S. A., Kolivakis, T., Casey, K. F., & Leyton, M. (2009). Striatal dopamine responses to intranasal cocaine self-administration in humans. *Biological Psychiatry, 65*, 846–850. https://doi.org/10.1016/j.biopsych.2009.01.021

Coyne, S. M., Padilla-Walker, L. M., Holmgren, H. G., Davis, E. J., Collier, K. M., Memmott-Elison, M. K., & Hawkins, A. J. (2018). A meta-analysis of prosocial media on prosocial behavior, aggression, and empathic concern: A multidimensional approach. *Developmental Psychology, 54*, 331–347. https://doi.org/10.1037/dev0000412

Coyne, S. M., Shawcroft, J., Gale, M., Gentile, D. A., Etherington, J. T., Holmgren, H., & Stockdale, L. (2021). Tantrums, toddlers and technology: Temperament, media emotion regulation, and problematic media use in early childhood. *Computers in Human Behavior, 120*, 106762. https://doi.org/10.1016/j.chb.2021.106762

Downing, K. L., Hinkley, T., Salmon, J., Hnatiuk, J. A., & Hesketh, K. D. (2017). Do the correlates of screen time and sedentary time differ in preschool children? *BMC Public Health, 17*, 285. https://doi.org/10.1186/s12889-017-4195-x

Duch, H., Fisher, E. M., Ensari, I., & Harrington, A. (2013). Screen time use in children under 3 years old: A systematic review of correlates. *The International Journal of Behavioral Nutrition and Physical Activity, 10*, 102. https://doi.org/10.1186/1479-5868-10-102

Dynia, J. M., Dore, R. A., Bates, R. A., & Justice, L. M. (2021). Media exposure and language for toddlers from low-income homes. *Infant Behavior & Development, 63*, 101542. https://doi.org/10.1016/j.infbeh.2021.101542

Eirich, R., McArthur, B. A., Anhorn, C., McGuinness, C., Christakis, D. A., & Madigan, S. (2022). Association of screen time with internalizing and externalizing behavior problems in children 12 years or younger: A systematic review and meta-analysis. *JAMA Psychiatry, 79*, 393–405. https://doi.org/10.1001/jamapsychiatry.2022.0155

Felix, E., Silva, V., Caetano, M., Ribeiro, M. V. V., Fidalgo, T. M., Rosa Neto, F., Sanchez, Z. M., Surkan, P. J., Martins, S. S., & Caetano, S. C. (2020). Excessive screen media use in preschoolers is associated with poor motor skills. *Cyberpsychology, Behavior, and Social Networking, 23*, 418–425. https://doi.org/10.1089/cyber.2019.0238

Fitzpatrick, C., Barnett, T., & Pagani, L. S. (2012a). Early exposure to media violence and later child adjustment. *Journal of Developmental and Behavioral Pediatrics, 33*, 291–297. https://doi.org/10.1097/DBP.0b013e31824eaab3

Fitzpatrick, C., Pagani, L. S., & Barnett, T. A. (2012b). Early childhood television viewing predicts explosive leg strength and waist circumference by middle childhood. *The International Journal of Behavioral Nutrition and Physical Activity, 9*, 87. https://doi.org/10.1186/1479-5868-9-87

Fitzpatrick, C., Boers, E., & Pagani, L. S. (2020). Kindergarten readiness, later health, and social costs. *Pediatrics, 146*, e20200978. https://doi.org/10.1542/peds.2020-0978

Fitzpatrick, C., Binet, M.-A., Harvey, E., Barr, R., Couture, M., & Garon-Carrier, G. (2023). Preschooler screen time and temperamental anger/frustration during the COVID-19 pandemic. *Pediatric Research, 94*, 820–825. https://doi.org/10.1038/s41390-023-02485-6

Garrison, M. M., & Christakis, D. A. (2012). The impact of a healthy media use intervention on sleep in preschool children. *Pediatrics, 130*, 492–499. https://doi.org/10.1542/peds.2011-3153

Garrison, M. M., Liekweg, K., & Christakis, D. A. (2011). Media use and child sleep: The impact of content, timing, and environment. *Pediatrics, 128*, 29–35. https://doi.org/10.1542/peds.2010-3304

Gaudreau, C., King, Y. A., Dore, R. A., Puttre, H., Nichols, D., Hirsh-Pasek, K., & Golinkoff, R. M. (2020). Preschoolers benefit equally from video chat, pseudo-contingent video, and live book reading: Implications for storytime during the coronavirus pandemic and beyond. *Frontiers in Psychology, 11*, 2158. https://doi.org/10.3389/fpsyg.2020.02158

Gentile, D. A., Li, D., Khoo, A., Prot, S., & Anderson, C. A. (2014). Mediators and moderators of long-term effects of violent video games on aggressive behavior: Practice, thinking, and action. *JAMA Pediatrics, 168*, 450–457. https://doi.org/10.1001/jamapediatrics.2014.63

Gentile, D. A., Bender, P. K., & Anderson, C. A. (2017). Violent video game effects on salivary cortisol, arousal, and aggressive thoughts in children. *Computers in Human Behavior, 70*, 39–43. https://doi.org/10.1016/j.chb.2016.12.045

Gialamas, A., Haag, D. G., Mittinty, M. N., & Lynch, J. (2020). Which time investments in the first 5 years of life matter most for children's language and behavioural outcomes at school entry? *International Journal of Epidemiology, 49*, 548–558. https://doi.org/10.1093/ije/dyz192

Gillioz, E., Bellucci, T., Borghini, A., Gentaz, É., & Lejeune, F. (2022). Les écrans et les jeunes enfants (0-3 ans) dans un contexte de pandémie de COVID-19: une enquête en ligne conduite auprès de 486 parents. *A.N.A.E., 178*, 321–331.

Goodrich, S. A., Pempek, T. A., & Calvert, S. L. (2009). Formal production features of infant and toddler DVDs. *Archives of Pediatrics & Adolescent Medicine, 163*, 1151–1156. https://doi.org/10.1001/archpediatrics.2009.201

Greitemeyer, T., & Osswald, S. (2010). Effects of prosocial video games on prosocial behavior. *Journal of Personality & Social Psychology, 98*, 211–221. https://doi.org/10.1037/a0016997

Heckman, J. J. (2007). The economics, technology, and neuroscience of human capability formation. *Proceedings of the National Academy of Sciences, 104*, 13250–13255. https://doi.org/10.1073/pnas.0701362104

Hertzman, C. (2010). Social geography of developmental health in the early years. *Healthcare Quarterly, 14*, 32–40. https://doi.org/10.12927/hcq.2010.21981

Hill, D., Ameenuddin, N., Chassiakos, Y. R., Cross, C., Radesky, J., Hutchinson, J., Boyd, R., Mendelson, R., Moreno, M. A., Smith, J., Swanson, W. S., & Council on Communications and Media. (2016). Media and young minds. *Pediatrics, 138*, e20162591. https://doi.org/10.1542/peds.2016-2591

Huber, B., Yeates, M., Meyer, D., Fleckhammer, L., & Kaufman, J. (2018). The effects of screen media content on young children's executive functioning. *Journal of Experimental Child Psychology, 170*, 72–85. https://doi.org/10.1016/j.jecp.2018.01.006

Huesmann, L. R., & Taylor, L. D. (2006). The role of media violence in violent behavior. *Annual Review of Public Health, 27*, 393–415. https://doi.org/10.1146/annurev.publhealth.26.021304.144640

Hutton, J. S., Dudley, J., Horowitz-Kraus, T., DeWitt, T., & Holland, S. K. (2020a). Associations between home literacy environment, brain white matter integrity and cognitive abilities in preschool-age children. *Acta Paediatrica, 109*, 1376–1386. https://doi.org/10.1111/apa.15124

Hutton, J. S., Dudley, J., Horowitz-Kraus, T., DeWitt, T., & Holland, S. K. (2020b). Associations between screen-based media use and brain white matter integrity in preschool-aged children. *JAMA Pediatrics, 174*, e193869. https://doi.org/10.1001/jamapediatrics.2019.3869

Jamnik, J., Keown-Stoneman, C., Eny, K. M., Maguire, J. L., & Birken, C. S. (2022). Mealtime media use and cardiometabolic risk in children. *Public Health Nutrition, 25*, 670–679. https://doi.org/10.1017/S1368980020003821

Kerai, S., Almas, A., Guhn, M., Forer, B., & Oberle, E. (2022). Screen time and developmental health: Results from an early childhood study in Canada. *BMC Public Health, 22*, 310. https://doi.org/10.1186/s12889-022-12701-3

Kim, K. M., & Chung, U. S. (2021). Associations among exposure to television or video, language development, and school achievement in childhood: A prospective birth cohort study. *Social Psychiatry and Psychiatric Epidemiology, 56*, 847–856. https://doi.org/10.1007/s00127-020-01967-w

Kirkorian, H. L., Pempek, T. A., Murphy, L. A., Schmidt, M. E., & Anderson, D. R. (2009). The impact of background television on parent-child interaction. *Child Development, 80*, 1350–1359. https://doi.org/10.1111/cdev.2009.80.issue-510.1111/j.1467-8624.2009.01337.x

Koepp, M. J., Gunn, R. N., Lawrence, A. D., Cunningham, V. J., Dagher, A., Jones, T., Brooks, D. J., Bench, C. J., & Grasby, P. M. (1998). Evidence for striatal dopamine release during a video game. *Nature, 393*, 266–268. https://doi.org/10.1038/30498

Konok, V., Liszkai-Peres, K., Bunford, N., Ferdinandy, B., Jurányi, Z., Ujfalussy, D. J., Réti, Z., Pogány, Á., Kampis, G., & Miklósi, Á. (2021). Mobile use induces local attentional precedence and is associated with limited socio-cognitive skills in preschoolers. *Computers in Human Behavior, 120*, 106758. https://doi.org/10.1016/j.chb.2021.106758

Kostyrka-Allchorne, K., Cooper, N. R., & Simpson, A. (2017). The relationship between television exposure and children's cognition and behaviour: A systematic review. *Developmental Review, 44*, 19–58. https://doi.org/10.1016/j.dr.2016.12.002

Kühhirt, M., & Klein, M. (2020). Parental education, television exposure, and children's early cognitive, language and behavioral development. *Social Science Research, 86*, 102391. https://doi.org/10.1016/j.ssresearch.2019.102391

Lauricella, A. R., Wartella, E., & Rideout, V. J. (2015). Young children's screen time: The complex role of parent and child factors. *Journal of Applied Developmental Psychology, 36*, 11–17. https://doi.org/10.1016/j.appdev.2014.12.001

Law, E. C., Han, M. X., Lai, Z., Lim, S., Ong, Z. Y., Ng, V., Gabard-Durnam, L. J., Wilkinson, C. L., Levin, A. R., Rifkin-Graboi, A., Daniel, L. M., Gluckman, P. D., Chong, Y. S., Meaney, M. J., & Nelson, C. A. (2023). Associations between infant screen use, electroencephalography markers, and cognitive outcomes. *JAMA Pediatrics, 177*, 311–318. https://doi.org/10.1001/jamapediatrics.2022.5674

LeBourgeois, M. K., Hale, L., Chang, A.-M., Akacem, L. D., Montgomery-Downs, H. E., & Buxton, O. M. (2017). Digital media and sleep in childhood and adolescence. *Pediatrics, 140*, S92–S96. https://doi.org/10.1542/peds.2016-1758J

Lee, E.-Y., Spence, J. C., & Carson, V. (2017). Television viewing, reading, physical activity and brain development among young south Korean children. *Journal of Science and Medicine in Sport, 20*, 672–677. https://doi.org/10.1016/j.jsams.2016.11.014

Lillard, A., & Peterson, J. (2011). The immediate impact of different types of television on young children's executive function. *Pediatrics, 128*, 644–649. https://doi.org/10.1542/peds.2010-1919

Lillard, A. S., Li, H., & Boguszewski, K. (2015). Television and children's executive function. *Advances in Child Development and Behavior, 48*, 219–248. https://doi.org/10.1016/bs.acdb.2014.11.006

Lin, L.-Y., Cherng, R.-J., Chen, Y.-J., Chen, Y.-J., & Yang, H.-M. (2015). Effects of television exposure on developmental skills among young children. *Infant Behavior & Development, 38*, 20–26. https://doi.org/10.1016/j.infbeh.2014.12.005

Lin, L.-Y., Cherng, R.-J., & Chen, Y.-J. (2017). Effect of touch screen tablet use on fine motor development of young children. *Physical & Occupational Therapy in Pediatrics, 37*, 457–467. https://doi.org/10.1080/01942638.2016.1255290

Lissak, G. (2018). Adverse physiological and psychological effects of screen time on children and adolescents: Literature review and case study. *Environmental Research, 164*, 149–157. https://doi.org/10.1016/j.envres.2018.01.015

MacGowan, T. L., & Schmidt, L. A. (2021). Preschoolers' social cognitive development in the age of screen time ubiquity. *Cyberpsychology, Behavior and Social Networking, 24*, 141–144. https://doi.org/10.1089/cyber.2020.0093

Madigan, S., Browne, D., Racine, N., Mori, C., & Tough, S. (2019). Association between screen time and children's performance on a developmental screening test. *JAMA Pediatrics, 173*, 244–250. https://doi.org/10.1001/jamapediatrics.2018.5056

Madigan, S., McArthur, B. A., Anhorn, C., Eirich, R., & Christakis, D. A. (2020a). Associations between screen use and child language skills: A systematic review and meta-analysis. *JAMA Pediatrics, 174*, 665–675. https://doi.org/10.1001/jamapediatrics.2020.0327

Madigan, S., Racine, N., & Tough, S. (2020b). Prevalence of preschoolers meeting vs exceeding screen time guidelines. *JAMA Pediatrics, 174*, 93–95. https://doi.org/10.1001/jamapediatrics.2019.4495

Madigan, S., Eirich, R., Pador, P., McArthur, B. A., & Neville, R. D. (2022). Assessment of changes in child and adolescent screen time during the covid-19 pandemic: A systematic review and meta-analysis. *JAMA Pediatrics, 176*, 1188–1198. https://doi.org/10.1001/jamapediatrics.2022.4116

Mares, M.-L., & Pan, Z. (2013). Effects of sesame street: A meta-analysis of children's learning in 15 countries. *Journal of Applied Developmental Psychology, 34*, 140–151. https://doi.org/10.1016/j.appdev.2013.01.001

Martinot, P., Bernard, J. Y., Peyre, H., De Agostini, M., Forhan, A., Charles, M.-A., Plancoulaine, S., & Heude, B. (2021). Exposure to screens and children's language development in the EDEN mother-child cohort. *Scientific Reports, 11*, 11863. https://doi.org/10.1038/s41598-021-90867-3

McArthur, B. A., Browne, D., Tough, S., & Madigan, S. (2020). Trajectories of screen use during early childhood: Predictors and associated behavior and learning outcomes. *Computers in Human Behavior, 113*, 106501. https://doi.org/10.1016/j.chb.2020.106501

McArthur, B. A., Browne, D., McDonald, S., Tough, S., & Madigan, S. (2021a). Longitudinal associations between screen use and reading in preschool-aged children. *Pediatrics, 147*, e2020011429. https://doi.org/10.1542/peds.2020-011429

McArthur, B. A., Tough, S., & Madigan, S. (2021b). Screen time and developmental and behavioral outcomes for preschool children. *Pediatric Research, 91*, 1616–1621. https://doi.org/10.1038/s41390-021-01572-w

McArthur, B. A., Volkova, V., Tomopoulos, S., & Madigan, S. (2022). Global prevalence of meeting screen time guidelines among children 5 years and younger: A systematic review and meta-analysis. *JAMA Pediatrics, 176*, 373–383. https://doi.org/10.1001/jamapediatrics.2021.6386

McDaniel, B. T., & Radesky, J. S. (2020). Longitudinal associations between early childhood externalizing behavior, parenting stress, and child media use. *Cyberpsychology, Behavior and Social Networking, 23*, 384–391. https://doi.org/10.1089/cyber.2019.0478

McNeill, J., Howard, S. J., Vella, S. A., & Cliff, D. P. (2020). Compliance with the 24-hour movement guidelines for the early years: Cross-sectional and longitudinal associations with executive function and psychosocial health in preschool children. *Journal of Science and Medicine in Sport, 23*, 846–853. https://doi.org/10.1016/j.jsams.2020.02.011

Munzer, T. G., Miller, A. L., Peterson, K. E., Brophy-Herb, H. E., Horodynski, M. A., Contreras, D., Sturza, J., Lumeng, J. C., & Radesky, J. (2018). Media exposure in low-income preschool-aged children is associated with multiple measures of self-regulatory behavior. *Journal of Developmental and Behavioral Pediatrics, 39*, 303–309. https://doi.org/10.1097/DBP.0000000000000560

Myers, L. J., Keyser, H., & Cors, M. (2019). Co-viewers support participation in video chat interactions, but live experiences promote richer word learning for 24- to 36-month-olds in the USA. *Journal of Children and Media, 13*, 415–432. https://doi.org/10.1080/17482798.2019.1646294

Nathanson, A. I., & Beyens, I. (2018). The role of sleep in the relation between young children's mobile media use and effortful control. *British Journal of Developmental Psychology, 36*, 1–21. https://doi.org/10.1111/bjdp.12196

Nathanson, A. I., & Fries, P. T. (2014). Television exposure, sleep time, and neuropsychological function among preschoolers. *Media Psychology, 17*, 237–261. https://doi.org/10.1080/15213269.2014.915197

National Scientific Council on the Developing Child. (2007). *The timing and quality of early experiences combine to shape brain architecture: Working Paper #5*. http://www.developingchild.net

Neville, R. D., McArthur, B. A., Eirich, R., Lakes, K. D., & Madigan, S. (2021a). Bidirectional associations between screen time and children's externalizing and internalizing behaviors. *Journal of Child Psychology and Psychiatry, 62*, 1475–1484. https://doi.org/10.1111/jcpp.13425

Neville, R. D., Nelson, M. A., Madigan, S., Browne, D. T., & Lakes, K. D. (2021b). Does physical activity moderate the association between screen time and psychosocial development in early childhood? Analysis of a longitudinal infant cohort study in Ireland. *European Journal of Pediatrics, 180*, 2199–2211. https://doi.org/10.1007/s00431-021-04008-z

Pagani, L. S., Fitzpatrick, C., & Barnett, T. A. (2013). Early childhood television viewing and kindergarten entry readiness. *Pediatric Research, 74*, 350–355. https://doi.org/10.1038/pr.2013.105

Pagani, L. S., Harbec, M. J., & Barnett, T. A. (2019). Prospective associations between television in the preschool bedroom and later bio-psycho-social risks. *Pediatric Research, 85*, 967–973. https://doi.org/10.1038/s41390-018-0265-8

Pagani, L. S., Bernard, J., & Fitzpatrick, C. (2023). Prospective associations between preschool exposure to violent televiewing and psychosocial and academic risks in early adolescent boys and girls. *Journal of Developmental and Behavioral Pediatrics, 44*, e1–e11. https://doi.org/10.1097/DBP.0000000000001135

Parkes, A., Sweeting, H., Wight, D., & Henderson, M. (2013). Do television and electronic games predict children's psychosocial adjustment? Longitudinal research using the UK millennium cohort study. *Archives of Disease in Childhood, 98*, 341–348. https://doi.org/10.1136/archdischild-2011-301508

Plancoulaine, S., Stagnara, C., Flori, S., Bat-Pitault, F., Lin, J.-S., Patural, H., & Franco, P. (2017). Early features associated with the neurocognitive development at 36 months of age: The AuBE study. *Sleep Medicine, 30*, 222–228. https://doi.org/10.1016/j.sleep.2016.10.015

Ponti, M. (2022). Screen time and preschool children: Promoting health and development in a digital world. *Paediatrics & Child Health, 28*, 184–202. https://doi.org/10.1093/pch/pxac125

Price, S., Jewitt, C., & Crescenzi, L. (2015). The role of iPads in pre-school children's mark making development. *Computers & Education, 87*, 131–141. https://doi.org/10.1016/j.compedu.2015.04.003

Putnick, D. L., Trinh, M.-H., Sundaram, R., Bell, E. M., Ghassabian, A., Robinson, S. L., & Yeung, E. (2022). Displacement of peer play by screen time: Associations with toddler development. *Pediatric Research, 93*, 1425–1431. https://doi.org/10.1038/s41390-022-02261-y

Radesky, J. S., Schumacher, J., & Zuckerman, B. (2015). Mobile and interactive media use by young children: The good, the bad, and the unknown. *Pediatrics, 135*, 1–3. https://doi.org/10.1542/peds.2014-2251

Radesky, J. S., Peacock-Chambers, E., Zuckerman, B., & Silverstein, M. (2016). Use of Mobile technology to calm upset children: Associations with social-emotional development. *JAMA Pediatrics, 170*, 397–399. https://doi.org/10.1001/jamapediatrics.2015.4260

Radesky, J. S., Kaciroti, N., Weeks, H. M., Schaller, A., & Miller, A. L. (2023). Longitudinal associations between use of mobile devices for calming and emotional reactivity and executive functioning in children aged 3 to 5 years. *JAMA Pediatrics, 177*, 62–70. https://doi.org/10.1001/jamapediatrics.2022.4793

Rasmussen, E. E., Shafer, A., Colwell, M. J., White, S., Punyanunt-Carter, N., Densley, R. L., & Wright, H. (2016). Relation between active mediation, exposure to Daniel Tiger's neighborhood, and US preschoolers' social and emotional development. *Journal of Children and Media, 10*, 443–461. https://doi.org/10.1080/17482798.2016.1203806

Rasmussen, E. E., Strouse, G. A., Colwell, M. J., Johnson, C. R., Holiday, S., Brady, K., Flores, I., Troseth, G., Wright, H. D., Densley, R. L., & Norman, M. S. (2019). Promoting preschoolers' emotional competence through prosocial TV and mobile app use. *Media Psychology, 22*, 1–22. https://doi.org/10.1080/15213269.2018.1476890

Reid Chassiakos, Y. (Linda), Radesky, J., Christakis, D., Moreno, M. A., & Cross, C. (2016). Children and adolescents and digital media. *Pediatrics, 138*, e1–e18.

Ribner, A., Fitzpatrick, C., & Blair, C. (2017). Family socioeconomic status moderates associations between television viewing and school readiness skills. *Journal of Developmental & Behavioral Pediatrics, 38*, 233–239. https://doi.org/10.1097/DBP.0000000000000425

Rideout, V., & Robb, M. B. (2020). *The common sense census: Media use by kids age zero to eight, 2020*. Common Sense Media.

Robinson, T. N., & Matheson, D. M. (2015). Environmental strategies for portion control in children. *Appetite, 88*, 33–38. https://doi.org/10.1016/j.appet.2014.12.001

Robinson, T. N., Banda, J. A., Hale, L., Lu, A. S., Fleming-Milici, F., Calvert, S. L., & Wartella, E. (2017). Screen media exposure and obesity in children and adolescents. *Pediatrics, 140*, S97–S101. https://doi.org/10.1542/peds.2016-1758K

Rocha, H. A. L., Correia, L. L., Leite, Á. J. M., Machado, M. M. T., Lindsay, A. C., Rocha, S. G. M. O., Campos, J. S., Silva, C. E., & A., & Sudfeld, C. R. (2021). Screen time and early childhood development in Ceará, Brazil: A population-based study. *BMC Public Health, 21*, 2072. https://doi.org/10.1186/s12889-021-12136-2

Salti, R., Tarquini, R., Stagi, S., Perfetto, F., Cornélissen, G., Laffi, G., Mazzoccoli, G., & Halberg, F. (2006). Age-dependent association of exposure to television screen with children's urinary melatonin excretion? *Neuro Endocrinology Letters, 27*, 73–80.

Schlesinger, M. A., Flynn, R. M., & Richert, R. A. (2019). Do parents care about TV? How parent factors mediate us children's media exposure and receptive vocabulary. *Journal of Children and Media, 13*, 395–414. https://doi.org/10.1080/17482798.2019.1627227

Schmidt, M. E., Pempek, T. A., Kirkorian, H. L., Lund, A. F., & Anderson, D. R. (2008). The effects of background television on the toy play behavior of very young children. *Child Development, 79*, 1137–1151. https://doi.org/10.1111/j.1467-8624.2008.01180.x

Setliff, A. E., & Courage, M. L. (2011). Background television and infants' allocation of their attention during toy play. *Infancy: The Official Journal of the International Society on Infant Studies, 16*, 611–639. https://doi.org/10.1111/j.1532-7078.2011.00070.x

Shonkoff, J. P. (2016). Capitalizing on advances in science to reduce the health consequences of early childhood adversity. *JAMA Pediatrics, 170*, 1003–1007. https://doi.org/10.1001/jamapediatrics.2016.1559

Smith, H. (2020). *Children, executive functioning, and digital media: A review*. https://www.commonsensemedia.org/research/children-executive-functioning-and-digital-media-a-review-2020

Staples, A. D., Hoyniak, C., McQuillan, M. E., Molfese, V., & Bates, J. E. (2021). Screen use before bedtime: Consequences for nighttime sleep in young children. *Infant Behavior & Development, 62*, 101522. https://doi.org/10.1016/j.infbeh.2020.101522

Tamana, S. K., Ezeugwu, V., Chikuma, J., Lefebvre, D. L., Azad, M. B., Moraes, T. J., Subbarao, P., Becker, A. B., Turvey, S. E., Sears, M. R., Dick, B. D., Carson, V., Rasmussen, C., Pei, J., & Mandhane, P. J. (2019). Screen-time is associated with inattention problems in preschoolers: Results from the CHILD birth cohort study. *PLoS One, 14*, e0213995. https://doi.org/10.1371/journal.pone.0213995

Teekavanich, S., Rukprayoon, H., Sutchritpongsa, S., & Rojmahamongkol, P. (2022). Electronic media use and food intake in Thai toddlers. *Appetite, 176*, 106121. https://doi.org/10.1016/j.appet.2022.106121

Valkenburg, P. M., & Peter, J. (2013). The differential susceptibility to media effects model. *Journal of Communication, 63*, 221–243. https://doi.org/10.1111/jcom.12024

Valkenburg, P. M., & Piotrowski, J. T. (2017). *Plugged in*. Yale University Press; JSTOR. http://www.jstor.org/stable/j.ctt1n2tvjd

Vanderloo, L. M., Janus, M., Omand, J. A., Keown-Stoneman, C. D. G., Borkhoff, C. M., Duku, E., Mamdani, M., Lebovic, G., Parkin, P. C., Simpson, J. R., Tremblay, M. S., Maguire, J. L., & Birken, C. S. (2022). Children's screen use and school readiness at 4-6 years: Prospective cohort study. *BMC Public Health, 22*, 382. https://doi.org/10.1186/s12889-022-12629-8

Wahi, G., Parkin, P. C., Beyene, J., Uleryk, E. M., & Birken, C. S. (2011). Effectiveness of interventions aimed at reducing screen time in children: A systematic review and meta-analysis of randomized controlled trials. *Archives of Pediatrics & Adolescent Medicine, 165*, 979–986. https://doi.org/10.1001/archpediatrics.2011.122

Webster, E. K., Martin, C. K., & Staiano, A. E. (2019). Fundamental motor skills, screen-time, and physical activity in preschoolers. *Journal of Sport and Health Science, 8*, 114–121. https://doi.org/10.1016/j.jshs.2018.11.006

Wenhold, H., & Harrison, K. (2018). Television use and family mealtimes among a sample of US families with preschoolers. *Journal of Children and Media, 12*, 98–115. https://doi.org/10.1080/17482798.2017.1395751

Williams, P. G., Lerner, M. A., & Council on Early Childhood, Council on School Health, Sells, J., Alderman, S. L., Hashikawa, A., Mendelsohn, A., McFadden, T., Navsaria, D., Peacock, G., Scholer, S., Takagishi, J., Vanderbilt, D., De Pinto, C. L., Attisha, E., Beers, N., Gibson, E., Gorski, P., … Weiss-Harrison, A. (2019). School readiness. *Pediatrics, 144*, e20191766. https://doi.org/10.1542/peds.2019-1766

World Health Organization. (2007). *Early Child Development: A Powerful Equalizer*. https://www.who.int/publications-detail-redirect/early-child-development-a-powerful-equalizer-final-report-for-the-world-health-organization-s-commission-on-the-social-determinants-of-health
World Health Organization. (2019). *Guidelines on physical activity, sedentary behaviour and sleep for children under 5 years of age*. World Health Organization; 2019. Licence: CC BY-NC-SA 3.0 IGO.
Yu, Y.-T., Hsieh, T.-L., Lin, G.-H., Lee, S.-C., Huang, C.-Y., & Chen, K.-L. (2022). High levels of screen time were associated with increased probabilities of lagged development in 3-year-old children. *Acta Paediatrica, 111*, 1736–1742. https://doi.org/10.1111/apa.16373
Zhao, J., Yu, Z., Sun, X., Wu, S., Zhang, J., Zhang, D., Zhang, Y., & Jiang, F. (2022). Association between screen time trajectory and early childhood development in children in China. *JAMA Pediatrics, 176*, 768–775. https://doi.org/10.1001/jamapediatrics.2022.1630
Zimmerman, F. J., & Christakis, D. A. (2007). Associations between content types of early media exposure and subsequent attentional problems. *Pediatrics, 120*, 986–992. https://doi.org/10.1542/peds.2006-3322

Chapter 7
Parental Digital Media Usage During Caregiving: How Can Technology Reverberate in Parent–Infant Emotional Connection?

Débora Becker and Tagma Marina Schneider Donelli

Introduction

The technological revolution has generated global changes in different domains in the last decades. Digital devices—smaller, more compact, and with a broader range of multimedia tools—are available to make adults' lives easier, as they offer real-time access to information and the possibility of communicating with geographically distant people (Konok et al., 2016). Although these technologies, along with the advent of the Internet, have created a world without borders, on the other hand, they have also proven to be a disruptive element in social ties, impacting social relationships (McDaniel & Coyne, 2016).

From a human development perspective, the early relationships established between the infant and their parents play a fundamental role in a child's development, especially concerning socio-emotional development (Ainsworth, 1989; Bowlby, 1984, 1988; Tronick, 2007; Winnicott, 1965/2013). Winnicott (1965/2013), in his studies on the theory of emotional development, already stated that the environment where a child is sufficiently cared for is crucial for them to acquire trust and feel protected from external dangers. It is essential to highlight that, compared with other species, human infants require intensive care for a more extended period, and during the first 36 months of life, the constant presence of a sensitive caregiver becomes indispensable. Additionally, this same caregiver needs to create a nurturing and affectionate environment for the infant, where the initial emotional bonds will be established (Ainsworth, 1989; Brazelton, 1994; Bowlby, 1984; Tronick, 2007; Winnicott, 1983/2007).

D. Becker (✉) · T. M. Schneider Donelli
Psychology Graduate Program—Universidade do Vale do Rio dos Sinos—UNISINOS University, São Leopoldo, RS, Brazil
e-mail: debbecker@edu.unisinos.br; tagmad@unisinos.br

G. B. Frizzo (ed.), *Digital Media and Early Child Development*,
https://doi.org/10.1007/978-3-031-69224-6_7

In the contemporary era, however, due to the massive influx of digital technologies into households, parent/caregiver–infant interactions are sometimes interrupted by adults' usage of digital media, such as smartphones and other portable devices, being shaped by the digital world. Moreover, children are exposed to screens from the beginning of life, usually provided by their caregivers, aiming to stimulate or entertain them (Becker & Donelli, 2024; Lauricella et al., 2015).

Given the need to better understand the possible repercussions of an environment pervaded by digital media on parent–infant interactions, this chapter will discuss parental usage of screens during caregiving and its possible repercussions on parent–infant emotional connection. The research thus far justifies the importance of broadening investigations into early interactions in light of the advent of the Internet and digital media, which are increasingly prevalent in the lives of contemporary families, especially since the beginning of the COVID-19 pandemic. Moreover, as reported by Braune-Krikau et al. (2021) in a scope review, the research regarding parental usage of digital media in the family context is mainly focused on older children, having the necessity of broadening the discussion of the impacts on the early years.

Parent–Infant Interactions and the Importance of Sensitive Caregiving During Early Years

Children learn about their inner world by experiencing it. How infants experience the world through social interactions shapes their mental health, which refers to the ability to express, regulate, and experience emotions; form secure relationships; explore the environment; and learn from their experiences (Zeanah & Zeanah, 2019). To provide mental health in the early years, the infant's caregiver plays a vital role in providing a secure base, which is crucial for the child's sense of security and independence (Ainsworth, 1989; Bowlby, 1984, 1988; Brazelton, 1994; Tronick, 2007; Winnicott, 1965/2013).

The early interactions established between the infant and their caregiver influence different stages of child development (Biringen et al., 2014; Tronick, 2007; Wendland, 2001), impacting the physical, cognitive, and emotional health of the child, as well as contributing to the formation of secure attachment patterns that resonate throughout different stages of life (Ainsworth, 1989; Biringen et al., 2014; Bowlby, 1988). In the 1980s, Ainsworth (1989) and Bowlby (1988) pointed out that from birth, the infant presents an innate tendency to maintain proximity to their attachment figure, identified as the most capable of dealing with the world and, in addition to providing food and primary care, will provide security during the performance of these caregiving tasks. The formation of a dependency bond between the child and their caregiver is based on an emotional connection and part of a unidirectional process, starting from the infant's behavior directed toward the caregiver (Bowlby, 1988), called by Bowlby as attachment behaviors. Smiling, crying, clinging, maintaining eye contact, and following the attachment figure aim to capture the caregiver's attention to obtain a satisfactory response that meets the primary infant's needs. An infant's attempts are not enough to establish an emotional bond since the caregiver must be available and responsive to the infant's cues (Ainsworth, 1989; Bowlby, 1984, 1988; Brazelton, 1994; Tronick, 2007).

While interacting with the world during their first years, children build their internal working models, encompassing aspects of the experienced world. These models are formed based on the child's caregivers' responses, influencing their perceptions of themselves, others, and the world (Bowlby, 1988). According to Cooke et al. (2019), insecure attachment in children can lead to the internalization of maladaptive internal working models. On the other hand, children with a secure attachment pattern internalize adaptive internal working models, which are generated through sensitive caregiver responses. Maladaptive internal working models may contribute to developing internalizing and externalizing problems. In contrast, adaptive internal working models act as a protective factor. So, sensitive care is the substratum for a child's socio-emotional development (Winnicott, 1983/2007; Zeanah et al., 2019), having an essential role in a child's physiological regulation of stress and the reduction of the incidence of psychopathology in childhood, being a protective factor for child's mental health.

Caregiver's Skills

Child caregivers are expected to possess specific abilities necessary for establishing a dyadic interaction with emotional quality. Mary Ainsworth (Ainsworth et al., 1974), from the attachment framework, primarily defined maternal sensitivity as an expected maternal ability that encompasses noticing, interpreting, and responding to the child's signals appropriately and promptly. Later, Biringen et al., (2014) introduced the concept of emotional availability, which is also considered an essential piece in the foundation of healthy socio-emotional development. Emotional availability refers to the capacity of parents and infants to share an emotionally healthy relationship. It depends on characteristics displayed by adults in response to the infant's emotional cues, such as sensitivity, structuring, non-intrusiveness, responsiveness, and non-hostility, as well as the child's ability to respond to the adult and actively engage in emotional interactions with them (Biringen et al., 2014). The parents' intentions and the expression of emotions during interactions demonstrate a supportive parental attitude, indicating availability and emotional attunement with their infant, facilitating an emotionally stable relationship (Biringen et al., 2014). Stern (1974), in the 1970s, also emphasizes that the parent–child interaction aims to create a shared positive emotional state, nurturing mutual joy.

Following the attachment approach, studies conducted by Fonagy et al. (1991) expanded the view about the importance of sensitive care. They introduced the concept of reflective functioning, defined as the capacity to reflect one's own and other's internal states. In the domain of parent–child relationships, the concept of reflective functioning concerns being curious and interested in the child's mind, which is called parental reflective functioning (Slade, 2005). Parental reflective functioning is important to maintain healthy and mutually rewarding relationships and can contribute to a child's socio-emotional development and emotional self-regulation process. Moreover, parents with satisfactory reflective functioning may favor the development of the same ability in their child (Slade, 2005). In addition, according to Fonagy and Alisson (2012), a child who has not been understood and cared for by a sensitive caregiver during their early years may have those skills negatively affected. To foster the development of such skills, including reflective functioning, and facilitate a healthy mutual interaction, the care provided to the infant should be appropriate, affectionate, and sensitive in a nurturing environment. Also, the nurturing environment should be safe so that the child, always supervised by an adult, can play freely and do their explorations. An emotionally healthy caregiver, capable of meeting the child's physical and emotional needs, is necessary in the environment (Box 7.1).

Box 7.1: The nurturing environment

- The environment should provide love and security.
- The environment where the child is appropriately care for is essential for them to gain confidence, feel safe, and be protected from the dangers of the world.
- A healthy environment is the child's safe harbor.

Existing literature has indicated that inconsistent or inadequate responses to a child's needs, poor verbal communication, and less visual contact, usually observed when screens are involved, may result in difficulties establishing interaction (Becker, 2020; Robinson, 2013). A child waits for responses to their communication attempts, demanding an attuned caregiver (Box 7.2). Furthermore, parents with lower levels of parental reflective functioning or sensitivity can impact a child's emotional regulation and the development of a secure attachment (Schaefer et al., 2023; Slade, 2005).

Box 7.2: How Do We Know If the Parent–Infant Interaction Is of Quality?

- Parents are sensitive and emotionally attuned to their child's needs.
- Parents engage in conversations with the child using a soft voice, avoiding shouting.
- Parents allow space for the infant to respond.
- Parents try to interpret the signals emitted by the infant and meet their needs.

(Continued)

- Parents show the ability to think about infant's desires, behaviors, and intentions.
- Parents treat the child as a subject with a mind, considering the child's inner world.
- Parents hold the infant in a loving and comforting manner.
- Parents are not rough or harsh with the child.
- The child feels seen by the adult.
- The child responds to the adult and actively engage in the interactions.

The Presence of Digital Media During Parent–Infant Interactions

Nowadays, the family environment is trespassed by several media devices, and the parent–infant interaction has been experiencing these interferences (McDaniel & Radesky, 2018). The nurturing environment, which should offer love and security to the child, is inundated by different stimuli from the screens. Moreover, children become immersed in front of screens from a very early age, profoundly changing how they navigate the new world. In addition, how can the emotional bond be established between the child and their caregiver when parents, and sometimes, children, are engaging with electronic devices instead of being available for each other, communicating and responding with synchrony?

It is impossible to go back and change what is already done. However, it is relevant to consider this new scenario and rethink how to preserve love and security in the place where the child is doing their explorations, interacting, and learning about emotions. It is important to stress that adults are losing control when using screens, and these patterns of screen usage are shaping children's screen usage habits since parents act as role models for children, as stressed by some authors (Bergmann et al., 2022; Lauricella et al., 2015).

The literature has highlighted that digital media connection, despite having a positive impact in different domains of contemporary lives, may generate disconnections in face-to-face interactions, affecting the quality of human relationships negatively (Konok et al., 2016; McDaniel & Coyne, 2016; McDaniel & Radesky, 2018). The interference generated by technology in relationships is called technoference, and it is considered a contemporary phenomenon, first described by McDaniel and Coyne (2016), perceived in different contexts, including family surroundings. Technological interference in face-to-face interactions results in changes in family dynamics, impacting the quality of the relationships between family members, including the early interactions between the infant and their parents (Kildare & Middlemiss, 2017; Kushlev & Dunn, 2018).

During caregiving, parents engaged with digital devices, such as smartphones, tend to present a weaker emotional connection with the child. Despite physically being present and available to the child, they are often mentally absent while engaging with the screen, connected to another reality, which relates to the concept of absent presence (Aagaard, 2016). Parental technology usage may result in less sensitive parenting, as research indicates impairments in essential parental skills (Becker, 2020; Knitter & Zemp, 2020; McDaniel & Radesky, 2018; Wolfers et al., 2020). Due to parent's screen usage during the child's routine, they often become disconnected from the infant's needs, impacting the child's development.

Parental skills, such as sensitivity and responsiveness, may be significantly affected by technology. Once the usage of devices, such as smartphones, demands individual interaction, the user is isolated from the interactions that may occur in the real world outside of the screens, affecting parental awareness. The interaction established between the adult and the machine creates what has been defined by Mantere and Raudaskoski (2017) as a sticky media device. The parental connection with a screen in the domain of parent–child interactions may interfere with the parental ability to be there for the child, leading a child to compete or beg for the caregiver's attention, affecting the quality of interaction (Becker, 2020; Boles & Roberts, 2008; Hiniker et al., 2015; Moser et al., 2016; Radesky et al., 2014).

Studies suggest that parental engagement with mobile technologies may decrease parental responsiveness to the child, as these devices distract parents and other caregivers from supervising children, putting infants in high-risk situations and increasing child injuries (Boles & Roberts, 2008; Hiniker et al., 2015). Home accidents have also seen an exponential increase worldwide in recent years, caused mainly by the frequency of distractions generated by interaction with mobile technology (Palsson, 2017). Furthermore, sensitivity is also an affected aspect. It can be observed in various situations, such as playgrounds, restaurants, and other naturalistic settings, where parents are focused on their screens instead of the children. Usually, adults are connected through their smartphones while their children explore the environment, whether playing or eating. The studies that have focused on parent–child interactions in playgrounds (Abels et al., 2018; Elias et al., 2021; Hiniker et al., 2015; Lemish et al., 2020; Mangan et al., 2018; Vanden et al., 2020; Wolfers et al., 2020) highlighted impairments in attention-seeking behavior, higher hostility, lower parental responsiveness, lower maternal sensitivity, and weaker and delayed reactions to children's bids for attention. For example, Lemish et al. (2020) highlighted that parental smartphone engagement promotes parent–child disengagement, reverberating in a child's socio-emotional development and safety. Likewise, Elias et al. (2021) reported similar findings in a naturalistic study conducted in playgrounds and eateries in the USA and Israel.

According to the authors, parents tend to be less emotionally supportive when engaged with screens, reverberating in their children's reactions. Furthermore, parents miss potentially dangerous situations when engaged with their phones. On the other hand, research by Radesky et al. (2014) indicated the importance of considering what parents do with their phones. For example, parents who were less absorbed in their devices while talking on the phone appeared to present a better visual connection with the child compared to parents who were entirely captivated by the screen while typing and swiping on the screen. The findings of the study by Lemish et al. (2020) also stressed that the level of disengagement from their children depends on how parents use their phones during caregiving. From what was discussed in the studies until now, talking on the phone seems less deleterious for the quality of parent–infant interactions compared with other types of mobile interaction. The observational studies conducted in playgrounds and restaurants, previously reported, pointed out that parents are primarily unresponsive when using smartphones during caregiving. When parents pay attention to the phone screen, they reduce the possibility of relating to the child through gaze, affecting the development of language and the emotional bonding between the dyad (Morris et al., 2022; Radesky et al., 2016). Radesky et al. (2015), in a study that investigated associations of maternal smartphone use with the frequency of mother–child interactions during a laboratory task, highlighted that mothers connected through their devices during interactive tasks with their child presented fewer verbal and nonverbal interactions in comparison with mothers who were not connected through a mobile device during the experiment. This finding suggested that adults tend to interact less with their children when connected through their devices, impacting the quality of parent–child interactions (Box 7.3). In addition, Morris et al. (2022) pointed out that parental smartphone usage during parent–child interactions leads to reduced joint attention, which results in fewer opportunities for caregivers to interact verbally with their children, impacting the child's language acquisition.

Box 7.3: Aspects Which May Negatively Affect the Quality of Dyadic Social Interactions

- Smartphone absorption may lead to interactive rule-violating experiences.
- Parental smartphone engagement may lead to disruptions on dyadic communication, also affecting the child's language development.
- Parental smartphone usage during caregiving might be associated with impairments in parental responsiveness and sensitivity.
- Parental smartphone usage during caregiving might be associated with higher parental hostility.
- Parents lack of responsiveness impacts child's social engagement.
- The activities parents are engaged with their screens during caregiving matters. Typing, playing games, or scrolling social media seem to have a stronger impact on parental skills, such as sensitivity, than activities that require less screen absorption.

Why Do Parents Seek Technology During Caregiving?

The smartphone is the most accessed mobile device worldwide, and it is configured in contemporary cultures as a socially accepted habit (Beamish et al., 2019). Smartphones are also perceived as an extension of the human body since, for many people, it is impossible to exist without them (Konok et al., 2016; Lee et al., 2014). With parents, it is no different.

Technology has increased significantly in the last decades, and by offering devices with a range of possibilities, the multitasking behavior is reinforced. Nowadays, through a simple touch of the fingers on a sensitive screen or voice commands, it is possible to be everywhere and do everything, including babysitting a child. Mobile technology has changed how people live and interact since the advent of mobile technology. In parenting, technology has been used as a tool to relieve parental stress and help with babysitting.

Studies have pointed out that parents are using digital technologies, especially smartphones, to talk with family and friends, send and receive emails from work, relate to what is happening around them or follow the news, play games, watch movies, and access social media through different apps. Parents are using technology to get support in dealing with parenting and work demands. For parents, digital technologies are handling computers, which make possible interaction with the world, favoring access to updated information and helping to relate to other parents who are dealing with the same challenges. Parents have seen technology as a support network, helping them with parental demands (Becker, 2020; Wolfers et al., 2021). Studies also stressed that caregiving a child may be very exhaustive, especially for mothers, and technology can help in those moments, being used as an entertainment tool and helping relieve the feeling of loneliness and sadness (Becker, 2020; Radesky et al., 2016) (Box 7.4).

Box 7.4: The Reasons Most Frequently Reported by Parents in the Literature for Engaging with Screens, Even When They Are Caregiving the Child

- Searching for support
- Seeking information
- Relieving stress or scaping from stress
- Family entertainment
- Dealing with negative emotions and feeling overwhelmed
- As a habit (need of checking the device constantly)
- Babysitting the child (offering screens to the child)

During the COVID-19 pandemic, digital media was a way people found to make possible social interactions, being an essential tool for the maintenance of emotional support in many families. However, screen time has increased drastically during the pandemic years, affecting the patterns of usage among adults and children (Bergmann et al., 2022; Bergonsi et al., 2022; Hemsing et al., 2022; Trott et al., 2022). With the worldwide adoption of social isolation, screen usage patterns have changed in many families, aggravating problematic Internet-related behaviors. Fathers and mothers began to face new challenges that escape the daily life and family organization previously instituted, such as the home office and general care for the operation of the house (shopping, cooking, cleaning), exacerbating parental demands, especially for families who could not count on their social support network and, especially, for mothers. In this context, the intensification and dependence on the use of digital technologies have been perceived, which have been used as nannies, remote school, maintenance of contact with friends and family, for working proposes (home office), for calming down children, and for entertainment and stress relief for parents (Ponte & Neves, 2020; Portinho et al., 2023).

The reasons reported in the literature, before and during the pandemic, converge with what parents are experiencing nowadays: Parents are feeling overwhelmed! Overwhelmed by work and parenting, which can be exhausting, especially without a social support network. The excessive demands of contemporary lives require more support to manage different tasks and relieve stress. Moreover, social support predicts parental sensitivity (Shin et al., 2006). Considering that many families do not have a social support network, this support is mainly obtained from screens, once they may offer the possibility to remain in touch with a world mediated far away from real life, providing an experience of shutdown. So, technologies are pointed out by parents as a social support network (Becker, 2020; Gibson & Hanson, 2013; Radesky et al., 2016), being used to stay connected with people and a tool used to relieve stress (Becker, 2020; Wolfers, 2021), serving as an overflow container. However, problematic smartphone use, as mentioned in some studies (Elhai et al., 2019; Newsham et al., 2018), is associated with depression and anxiety. Corroborating this, McDaniel (2019) highlighted that parents who present less sensitivity and higher levels of depression and stress may be more likely to use their smartphones when caregiving for their children.

Conclusions

Early experiences are important for human development in different ways. A human baby requires the presence of a sensitive caregiver full-time during the first 3 years of life, and the quality of parental emotional presence in a child's explorations will shape the child's inner life. Infants are highly impacted by how their caregivers care for them and express their emotions since infants learn about emotions by experiencing them. Besides, it is known that an infant who was treated harshly during their early experiences will have their attachment relationships negatively impacted, leading to difficulties in the development of empathy, reflective functioning, and other important abilities for their healthy socio-emotional development. So, once a child acquires those skills through sensitive care, all the negative interactions between the child and their caregiver during the first years of life will resonate with the child's emotion regulation process and attachment patterns (Fonagy, 1991). Nowadays, with the omnipresence of technology in family surroundings, early childhood experiences are happening in an environment with more distractions, affecting how parents and their children interact and build the most important emotional bonds, which will reverberate throughout their whole lives.

In the last decade, studies that have explored parental usage of screens during caregiving increased. As presented before, some are observational studies investigating the impact of smartphones and other devices during parent–child interactions, primarily in naturalistic settings, such as playgrounds and restaurants. Using a qualitative approach, other studies tried to understand the main reasons that lead parents to stay connected, even with their children. The literature pointed out that parental engagement with screens has the potential to impact dyadic communication negatively, crucial to the establishment of interaction with synchrony, since the parental habit of staying connected with mobile devices while caregiving may result in impaired parental sensitivity and responsiveness, gazing decreased, still-faced effect, and impacts in child's behaviors. Related to parental screen engagement, the pressure generated by excessive work demands, which increased with remote work since the COVID-19 pandemic, also generated a necessity to remain connected to screens even when parents are at home with their children, being used to escape from the work and parenting demands.

Exploring this field is essential for considering how to guide parents in clinical and primary healthcare settings, contributing to the quality of parent–infant interactions and, consequently, the child's and family's psychological well-being. In summary, the research addressed thus far worldwide justifies the importance of expanding investigations into these early interactions in the face of the advent of the Internet and digital media, which are increasing rapidly, especially after the COVID-19 pandemic. The research about the topic underlines that parents are claiming support and orientation. More studies are needed and may contribute to improving public policy, the development of programs, and updated guidelines.

References

Aagaard, J. (2016). Mobile devices, interaction and distraction: A qualitative exploration of absent presence. *AI & Society, 31*, 223–231. https://doi.org/10.1007/s00146-015-0638-z

Abels, M., Vanden Abeele, M., Van Telgen, T., & Van Meijl, H. (2018). Nod, nod, ignore: An exploratory observational study on the relation between parental mobile media use and parental responsiveness towards young children. In E. M. Luef & M. M. Marin (Eds.), *The talking species: Perspectives on the evolutionary, neuronal, and cultural foundations of language* (pp. 195–228). Uni-press Verlag.

Ainsworth, M. D. (1989). Attachments beyond infancy. *American Psychologist, 44*, 709–716.

Ainsworth, M. D. S., Bell, S. M., & Stayton, D. F. (1974). Infant-mother attachment and social development: Socialization as a product of reciprocal responsiveness to signals. In M. P. M. Richards (Ed.), *The integration of a child into a social world* (pp. 99–135). Cambridge University Press.

Beamish, N., Fisher, J., & Rowe, H. (2019). Parents' use of mobile computing devices, caregiving and the social and emotional development of children: A systematic review of the evidence. *Australasian Psychiatry, 27*(2), 132–143. https://doi.org/10.1177/1039856218789764

Becker, D. (2020). *Digital technologies in the context of mother-baby and father-baby interactions: An exploratory approach.* Master's Thesis. Universidade do Vale do Rio dos Sinos, UNISINOS.

Becker, D., & Donelli, T. M. S. (2024). It doesn't always work, but it helps: Parental perceptions of baby's screen exposure. *Psicologia Em Estudo, 29*, 1. https://doi.org/10.4025/psicolestud.v29i1.54957

Bergmann, C., Dimitrova, N., Alaslani, K., Almohammadi, A., Alroqi, H., Aussems, S., Barokova, M., Davies, C., Gonzalez-Gomez, N., Gibson, S. P., Havron, N., Horowitz-Kraus, T., Kanero,

J., Kartushina, N., Keller, C., Mayor, J., Mundry, R., Shinskey, J., & Mani, N. (2022). Young children's screen time during the first COVID-19 lockdown in 12 countries. *Scientific Reports 2022, 12*(1), 1–15. https://doi.org/10.1038/s41598-022-05840-5

Bergonsi, F., Becker, D., Paiani, R. L., & Donelli, T. M. S. (2022). *O bebê em isolamento social e à exposição às mídias digitais: um estudo exploratório*. 29. Mostra de iniciação científica e tecnológica UNISINOS. http://www.guaritadigital.com.br/casaleiria/unisinos/eventos/mostra2022/234/index.html

Biringen, Z., Derscheid, D., Vliegen, N., Closson, L., & Easterbrooks, M. A. (2014). Emotional availability (EA): Theoretical background, empirical research using the EA Scales, and clinical applications. *Developmental Review, 34*(2), 114–167. https://doi.org/10.1016/j.dr.2014.01.002

Boles, R. E., & Roberts, M. C. (2008). Supervising children during parental distractions. *Journal of Pediatric Psychology, 33*(8), 833–841.

Bowlby, J. (1984). *Apego e perda: Apego*. (1), Martins Fontes. (Original publicado em 1969).

Bowlby, J. (1988). A secure base: Parent-child attachment and healthy human development. Basic Books.

Braune-Krickau, K., Schneebeli, L., Pehlke-Milde, J., Gemperle, M., Koch, R., & von Wyl, A. (2021). Smartphones in the nursery: Parental smartphone use and parental sensitivity and responsiveness within parent-child interaction in early childhood (0–5 years): A scoping review. *Infant Mental Health Journal, 42*(2), 161–175. https://doi.org/10.1002/imhj.21908. Epub 2021 Jan 15. PMID: 33452702; PMCID: PMC8048888.

Brazelton, T. B. (1994). *Momentos decisivos do desenvolvimento infantil*. Martins Fontes.

Cooke, J. E., Kochendorfer, L. B., Stuart-Parrigon, K. L., Koehn, A. J., & Kerns, K. A. (2019). Parent-child attachment and children's experience and regulation of emotion: A meta-analytic review. *Emotion, 19*(6), 1103–1126. https://doi.org/10.1037/emo0000504

Elhai, J. D., Levine, J. C., & Hall, B. J. (2019). The relationship between anxiety symptom severity and problematic smartphone use: A review of the literature and conceptual frameworks. *Journal of Anxiety Disorders, 62*, 45–52.

Elias, N., Lemish, D., Dalyot, S., & Floegel, D. (2021). "Where are you?" an observational exploration of parental technoference in public places in the US and Israel. *Journal of Children and Media*. https://doi.org/10.1080/17482798.2020.1815228

Fonagy, P., Steele, M., Steele, H., Moran, G. S., & Higgitt, A. C. (1991). The capacity for understanding mental states: The reflective self in parent and child and its significance for security of attachment. *Infant Mental Health Journal, 12*(3), 201–218.

Fonagy, P., & Allison, E. (2012). What is mentalization? The concept and its foundations in developmental research. In N. Midgley & I. Vrouva (Eds.), Minding the child: Mentalization-based interventions with children, young people and their families(p. 11–34). Routledge/Taylor & Francis Group.

Gibson, L., & Hanson, V. L. (2013). 'Digital motherhood': How does technology support new mothers. In *Proceedings of the SIGCHI Conference on Human Factors in Computing Systems* (pp. 313–322). Association for Computing Machinery. https://doi.org/10.1145/2470654.2470700

Hemsing, S., Becker, D., Stein, L., Paiani, R. L., & Donelli, T.M.S. (2022). *Maternidade e a pandemia de COVID-19: saúde mental e uso de mídias digitais de mães de bebês residentes no estado do Rio Grande do Sul*. 29. Mostra de iniciação científica e tecnológica UNISINOS. http://www.guaritadigital.com.br/casaleiria/unisinos/eventos/mostra2022/232/index.html

Hiniker, A., Sobel, K., Suh, H., Sung, Y. C., Lee, C. P., & Kientz, J. A. (2015). *Texting while parenting: How adults use mobile phones while caring for children at the parent distraction with phones at playground* (pp. 727–736). In Proceedings of the 33rd Annual ACM Conference on Human Factors in Computing Systems.

Kildare, C. A., & Middlemiss, W. (2017). Impact of parents mobile device use on parent-child interaction: A literature review. *Computers in Human Behavior, 75*, 579–593. https://doi.org/10.1016/j.chb.2017.06.003

Knitter, B., & Zemp, M. (2020). Digital family life: A systematic review of the impact of parental smartphone use on parent-child interactions. *Digital Psychology (InPress), 1*, 29.

Konok, V., Gigler, D., Bereczky, B. M., & Miklósi, A. (2016). Human's attachment to their mobile phones and its relationship with interpersonal attatchment style. *Computers in Human Behavior, 61*, 537–547. https://doi.org/10.1016/j.chb.2016.03.062

Kushlev, K., & Dunn, W. E. (2018). Smartphones distract parents from cultivating feelings of connection when spending time with their children. *Journal of Social and Personal Relationships, 36*, 1–21. https://doi.org/10.1177/0265407518769387

Lauricella, A. R., Wartella, E., & Rideout, V. J. (2015). Young children's screen time: The complex role of parent and child factors. *Journal of Applied Developmental Psychology, 36*, 11–17. https://doi.org/10.1016/J.APPDEV.2014.12.001

Lee, Y., Chang, C., Lin, Y., & Cheng, Z. (2014). The dark side of smartphone usage: Psychological traits, compulsive behavior and technostress. *Computers in Human Behavior, 31*, 373–383. https://doi.org/10.1016/j.chb.2013.10.047

Lemish, D., Elias, N., & Floegel, D. (2020). *"Look at me!" Parental use of mobile phones at the playground.* Mobile Media and Communication. https://doi.org/10.1177/2050157919846916

Mangan, E., Leavy, J. E., & Jancey, J. M. (2018). Mobile device use when caring for children 0-5 years: A naturalistic playground study. *Health Promot J.Austral., 29*, 337–343. https://doi.org/10.1002/hpja.38

Mantere, E., & Raudaskoski, S. (2017). The sticky media device. In A. R. Lahikainen, T. Mälkiä, & K. Repo (Eds.), *Media, family interaction and the digitalization of childhood* (pp. 173–184). Edward Elgar. https://doi.org/10.4337/9781785366673.0001

McDaniel, B. T. (2019). Parent distraction with phones, reasons for use, and impacts on parenting and child outcomes: A review of the emerging research. *Human Behavior and Emerging Technologies, 1*(2), 72–80.

McDaniel, B. T., & Coyne, S. M. (2016). Technology interference in the parenting of young children: Implications for mother's perceptions of coparenting. *The Social Science Journal, 53*, 435–443. https://doi.org/10.1016/j.soscij.2016.04.010

McDaniel, B. T., & Radesky, J. S. (2018). Technoference: Parents distraction with technology and association with child behavior problems. *Child Development, 89*, 100–109. https://doi.org/10.1111/cdev.12822

Morris, A. J., Filippetti, M. L., & Rigato, S. (2022). The impact of parents' smartphone use on language development in young children. *Child Development Perspectives, 16*, 103–109. https://doi.org/10.1111/cdep.12449

Moser, C., Schoenebeck, S. Y., & Reinecke, K. (2016). Technology at the table: Attitudes about mobile phone use at mealtimes. In: Proceedings of the conference on human factors in computer systems, 1881–1892. http://dx.doi.org/10.1145/2858036.2858357

Newsham, G., Drouin, M., & McDaniel, B. T. (2018). Problematic phone use, depression, and technology interference among mothers. *Psychology of Popular Media Culture, 9*(2), 117–124. https://doi.org/10.1037/ppm0000220

Palsson, C. (2017). Smartphones and child injuries. *Journal of Public Economics, 156*, 200–213.

Ponte, V., & Neves, F. (2020). Vírus, telas e crianças: entrelaçamentos em época de pandemia. *Simbiótica. Revista Eletrônica, 7*(1), 87–106. https://doi.org/10.47456/simbitica.v7i1.30984

Portinho, D. F., Becker, D., Schaefer, M. P., Paiani, R., & Donelli, T. M. S. (2023). A pandemia de COVID-19 e suas repercussões na rotina de famílias com bebês residentes no estado do Rio Grande do Sul: uso de telas e saúde mental. Congresso da Sociedade de Cardiologia do Estado do Rio Grande do Sul. *Resumo das Comunicações.* SOCERGS. chrome-extension://efaidnbmnnnibpcajpcglclefindmkaj/, https://abccardiol.org/wp-content/uploads/2023/07/SOCERGS_2023.x55156.pdf.

Radesky, J. S., Silverstein, M., Zuckerman, B., & Christakis, D. A. (2014). Infant self-regulation and early childhood media exposure. *Pediatrics, 133*(5), E1172–E1178. https://doi.org/10.1542/peds.2013-2367

Radesky, J., Miller, A. L., Rosenblum, K. L., Appugliese, D., Kaciroti, N., & Lumeng, J. C. (2015). Maternal mobile device use during a structured parent-child interaction task. *Academic Pediatrics, 15*(2), 238–244. https://doi.org/10.1016/j.acap.2014.10.001

Radesky, J. S., Kistin, C., Eisenberg, S., Gross, J., Block, G., Zuckerman, B., & Silverstein, M. (2016). Parent perspectives on their mobile technology use: The excitement and exhaustion of parenting while connected. *Journal of Developmental & Behavioral Pediatrics, 37*(9), 694–701.

Robinson, S. (2013). *The relationship between the quality of caregiver-child interaction and social-emotional problems in toddlers*. Southern Connecticut State University.

Schaefer, M. P., Becker, D., & Donelli, T. M. S. (2023). Interventions to improve mentalization and reflective functioning: a scoping review. *Ciencias psicológicas, 17*(1), e-2478.

Shin, H., Park, Y.-J., & Kim, M. J. (2006). Predictors of maternal sensitivity during the early postpartum period. *Journal of Advanced Nursing, 55*, 425–434. https://doi.org/10.1111/j.1365-2648.2006.03943.x

Slade, A. (2005). Parental reflective functioning: An introduction. *Attachment & Human Development, 7*(3), 269–281. https://doi.org/10.1080/14616730500245906

Stern, D.N. (1974). The Goal and Structure of Mother-Infant Play. *Journal of the American Academy of Child Psychiatry, 13*(3), 402–421.

Tronick, E. (2007). *The neurobehavioral and social-emotional development of infants and children*. Norton & Company.

Trott, M., Driscoll, R., Irlado, E., & Pardhan, S. (2022). Changes and correlates of screen time in adults and children during the COVID-19 pandemic: A systematic review and meta-analysis. *EClinicalMedicine, 48*, 101452. https://doi.org/10.1016/j.eclinm.2022.101452

Vanden Abeele, M. M. P., Abels, M., & Hendrickson, A. T. (2020). Are parents less responsive to young children when they are on their phones? A systematic naturalistic observation study. *Cyberpsychology, Behavior and Social Networking, 23*(6), 363–370. https://doi.org/10.1089/cyber.2019.0472

Wendland, J. (2001). A abordagem clínica das interações pais-bebê: perspectivas teóricas e metodológicas. *Psicologia Reflexão e Crítica, 14*(1), 45–46.

Winnicott, D. W. (2007). *O ambiente e os processos de maturação: estudos sobre a teoria do desenvolvimento emocional*. Artmed. (Original published in 1983).

Winnicott, D. W. (2013). *A família e o desenvolvimento individual*. Martins Fontes. (Original published in 1965).

Wolfers, L. N. (2021). Parental mobile media use for coping with stress: A focus groups study. *Human Behavior & Emerging Tech, 3*, 304–315.

Wolfers, L. N., Kitzmann, S., Sauer, S., & Sommer, N. (2020). Phone use while parenting: An observational study to assess the association of maternal sensitivity and smartphone use in a playground setting. *Computers in Human Behavior*. Advance Online Publication, *102*, 31. https://doi.org/10.1016/j.chb.2019.08.013

Zeanah, C. H., Jr., & Zeanah, P. D. (2019). Infant mental health: The clinical science of early experience. In C. H. Zeanah Jr. (Ed.), *Handbook of infant mental health* (4th ed., pp. 5–24). The Guilford Press.

Chapter 8
Digital Media and Language Development: The Role of Child-Directed Speech

Gabriela Vescovi, Lauren Schilling, and Meredith L. Rowe

Introduction

Language development is a multidetermined process (Rvachew, 2013), but social interaction with caregivers is one of the essential ingredients for the development of this ability (Tomasello, 2009; Vygotsky, 1984). From this perspective, language acquisition is a social phenomenon, hypothesized to be driven by the purpose of communicating (Tomasello, 2009). Because of the importance of social interaction in language learning, variability in linguistic environments produces individual and group differences in the course and pace of development (Hoff, 2006).

Recently, there has been a major increase in the use of digital media in early childhood (Kabali et al., 2015; Rocha et al., 2021), raising concerns about how this may alter social interactions within the family and, consequently, children's language acquisition and development. In this first section, we review the most recent evidence on the relationship between screen use and language development. Next, we highlight an environmental factor that can shed light on those studies' findings: the quantity and quality of speech adults direct to children. We also seek to understand how child-directed speech varies according to the type of digital media used. Finally, we discuss recent initiatives to use technology to promote rich verbal interactions between children and caregivers in ways that foster language development.

G. Vescovi (✉)
Universidade Federal do Rio Grande do Sul, Porto Alegre, RS, Brazil
e-mail: gabriela-vescovi@saude.rs.gov.br

L. Schilling · M. L. Rowe
Graduate School of Education, Harvard University, Cambridge, MA, USA
e-mail: lschilling@g.harvard.edu; meredith_rowe@gse.harvard.edu

G. B. Frizzo (ed.), *Digital Media and Early Child Development*,
https://doi.org/10.1007/978-3-031-69224-6_8

Digital Media and Children's Language Development

A large body of research has shown that more screen use is associated with lower language skills and developmental delays in language acquisition and communication from infancy to preschool years (Medawar et al., 2023; McArthur et al., 2022; Vanderloo et al., 2022; Varadarajan et al., 2021; Hutton et al., 2020; Duch et al., 2013a, b). For example, each additional 30-minute increase in daily mobile device use is associated with increased odds of parent-reported expressive speech delay in 18-month-old children (van den Heuvel et al., 2019). A systematic review and meta-analysis of 42 studies (totaling 18,905 participants) suggest that a greater quantity of screen use (i.e., hours per use of both screen time and background television) is associated with lower language skills (Madigan et al., 2020). This association appears to be unidirectional in that poor language skills does not predict screen time, but vice versa (Madigan et al., 2019).

One possible explanation for the association between screen use and lower language skills is the displacement hypothesis, which states that the more time children spend with media, the less time they must engage in other language-promoting activities and interactions (Hurwitz et al., 2020). Supporting this hypothesis, a study of Chinese children aged 3–6 years found that a high frequency of TV and tablet use was linked to fewer stimulating practices at home, such as interaction with educational books and toys or shared reading (Chen et al., 2020). Conversely, increased access to stimulation at home is negatively associated with screen media exposure among children under 3 (Duch et al., 2013a, b).

Importantly, some correlational studies do not find a relationship between television or touchscreen usage time and language delay (Lin et al., 2020; Ruangdaraganon et al., 2009; Schmidt et al., 2009). A meta-analysis by Jing et al. (2023) found no evidence of a negative association between screen media exposure and vocabulary. This is surprising given that screen media might be expected to displace valuable vocabulary learning activities. Rather, Jing and collaborators (2023) reported an overall positive relationship between screen media exposure and vocabulary in children aged 6 years and under. These findings suggest that screen time alone may not be the most relevant factor (Barr, 2019; Martinot et al., 2021) since it is not simply a displacement of time that is occurring but rather a complex interaction of family and child factors (Linebarger & Vaala, 2010; Radesky, 2021).

The relations between digital media use and language development are not straightforward and seem to rely on different factors. Researchers have postulated that any associations between screen media and language and literacy development may be explained not by the quantity of use only, but rather by a more comprehensive view of household media use including aspects such as the type of media available, content (e.g., educational), background TV exposure, age of first contact with media, co-viewing, and parents' media use and beliefs (Barr, 2019; Turco et al., 2023a; Karani et al., 2022; Çelen et al., 2021).

Depending on when and how it is used, digital media can have negative or positive impacts on language skills (Barr, 2019; Jing et al., 2023). Regarding when technology is used, delaying the age of first contact with digital media seems to be crucial for promoting language development, where later age at screen use onset is associated with stronger child language skills (Alroqi et al., 2022; Madigan et al., 2020). Furthermore, research suggests that children with language delay have often started using screen devices earlier than their typically developing peers and they have higher durations of TV viewing and background TV with less frequent exposition to co-viewing (Çelen et al., 2021). How screen media is used and the qualities of its content also impact children's language development. For example, exposure to television during family meals at age 2 years is consistently associated with lower language scores (Martinot et al., 2021). Additionally, while educational television or video, e-books, and interactive features are associated with higher vocabulary scores, Jing and collaborators (2023) found no evidence that naturalistic exposure to noneducational media has a positive effect on vocabulary.

Co-viewing is one way that parents can transform screen media experiences into an opportunity for language stimulation (Madigan et al., 2020; Medawar et al., 2023). Co-viewing, or *joint media engagement*, is a practice where a child and one or more adults actively and jointly engage with digital media, such as watching and talking about a TV show or playing and communicating around a digital game (Sundqvist et al., 2022). These joint media engagements have been associated with positive gains in infants' learning from touchscreens (Zack & Barr, 2016) and children's expressive and receptive vocabulary (Alroqi et al., 2022). On the other hand, increased screen use without the presence of an adult is associated with weaker lexical and general language abilities (Medawar et al., 2023; Mustonen et al., 2022).

One essential aspect of co-viewing is the language input parents offer to children referred to as child-directed speech (CDS). This communication is an important environmental factor that contributes to individual differences in early language development (Hart & Risley, 1995; Hoff, 2003; Rowe, 2012). One way to assess the quality of social interactions for language development is to evaluate the features of child-directed speech that occur during digital media use.

Child-Directed Speech and Its Relation with Media Use

CDS refers to the properties of speech adults use with infants and young children. The style of speech used with infants (also termed "parentese") is distinguished by long pauses, short sentences, acute intonation, and many intonation peaks (Hoff, 2009). The speech directed to young children is often measured as the quantity of words spoken during parent–child interactions. While the association between the number of words heard by the child and the size of their vocabulary seems robust (Cartmill, 2016; Hart & Risley, 1995), it is also known that the quantity of child-directed speech is not sufficient to explain differences in language acquisition and development (Hirsh-Pasek et al., 2015; Rowe, 2012). Other qualities of child-directed speech, such as lexical diversity (Weizman & Snow, 2001), question-asking (Rowe et al., 2016), and conversational turns (e.g., Romeo et al., 2018) among others also play an important role especially in the second and third years of life (Rowe, 2012). A study using computational modeling found that lexical diversity was more predictive than the quantity of speech for new word learning and performance on language tests (Jones & Rowland, 2017). A meta-analysis also showed that the pooled effect size on children's language was more robust for quality (i.e., vocabulary diversity and syntactic complexity) than for quantity features (i.e., number of words or utterances) of parental linguistic input (Anderson et al., 2021). Infant vocabulary also predicts maternal vocabulary at subsequent ages, suggesting a mutual influence between caregiver and child (Fusaroli et al., 2019).

Evidence has suggested that the presence of digital media use may negatively impact the speech adults address to the child, irrespective of socioeconomic status and child age (Kirkorian et al., 2009; Ramírez et al., 2021). Comparing moments of interaction with and without television, the presence of this device decreased the number, complexity, and diversity of parental utterances (Lavigne et al., 2015; Tanimura et al., 2007). Indeed, studies find that audible television is associated with decreased exposure to adult speech and decreased child vocalizations (Christakis et al., 2009). Even in the presence of background TV, the number of words and utterances spoken by the parent decreased as did the number of new words per minute (Pempek et al., 2014). However, this same research found that the mean length of utterance (a measure of language complexity) did not differ depending on background TV presence.

Besides television, some recent research has also investigated other types of devices such as mobile device use. The study by Ewin et al. (2021) found that parents spoke more and used more new words during shared toy play compared to shared mobile device use, but the quality and quantity of parent language did not differ during mobile device use compared to magazine use. Other studies have assessed media use in more comprehensive ways, including automatized measures of exposure time to all types of devices available in the child's home environment. They have also found negative associations between increased media exposure and conversational turns (Cycyk & De Anda, 2021; Ferjan et al., 2022). However, there is some evidence suggesting educational media use could predict small increases in verbal interactions (Choi et al., 2018; Pempek et al., 2011). Pempek et al. (2011) found that interactions increased in quantity and quality immediately after viewing an educational video, but not while it was playing, as parents used the video content as a basis for later interaction.

Additionally, other researchers have focused on comparing CDS between electronic and traditional (nonelectronic) versions of toys and books, in an attempt to determine if parental verbal input differs among these conditions. During play with electronic toys, Sosa (2016) found fewer adult words, conversational turns, parental responses, and content-specific words than during play with traditional toys or books. In the same study, children vocalized less during play with electronic toys. Parents playing with a traditional and electronic shape sorter toy did not differ in the total number of words, but parents playing with the traditional toy used more varied language and more spatial words (Zosh et al., 2015). Regarding differences in parents' verbal interactions across digital and print book reading, researchers found that e-books yielded less decontextualized talk (Korat & Or, 2010; Parish-Morris et al., 2013; Ozturk & Hill, 2020), fewer story-related utterances (Parish-Morris et al., 2013), less verbalization, and lower collaboration between parents and children (Munzer et al., 2019) but more discourse initiated by the child (Korat & Or, 2010) and more maternal support for child engagement with the e-book (Eggleston et al., 2022). On the other hand, some studies found similar interactions across the two conditions (Lauricella et al., 2014; Strouse et al., 2023). In this latter study, the only difference found was for parent engagement in favor of electronic storybooks (Lauricella et al., 2014). Overall, available evidence seems to point out mixed results (Strouse et al., 2023; Eggleston et al., 2022), suggesting that electronic books and toys are not necessarily detrimental to CDS compared to their traditional counterparts (Dore et al., 2017).

Given those results, the field has come to understand CDS not only as an aspect impacted by the media but as both a mediator and a moderator of the relation between digital media and child language outcomes (Sundqvist et al., 2022). That means the negative association between media and language development could be driven by a decrease in CDS (mediation), but higher levels of CDS during media use could possibly diminish or even eliminate the negative impacts on language (moderation). Empirical evidence supports this perspective. For instance, studies found that different features of CDS (such as the quantity of speech, lexical diversity, and turn-taking) mediate the negative association between media exposure and children's language skills (Ambrose et al., 2014; Masur et al., 2016; Sundqvist et al., 2022; Zimmerman et al., 2009). Another study (Mendelsohn et al., 2010) showed that verbal interactions during media use moderated adverse impacts of media exposure on language development at 14 months, with negative associations found only in the absence of these verbal interactions. The same research also suggests that the back-and-forth conversations during media use may even have direct positive impacts on language, in that verbal interactions during co-viewing of educational content (but not other content) were predictive of language outcomes. Those are promising findings as they suggest parents can prevent the negative effects of media exposure by talking with their children during its use.

However, it seems that verbal interactions during media use are not a straightforward practice among parents. Ambrose et al. (2014) found a decreased frequency of conversational turns in households with high rates of electronic media exposure. Even in the presence of the same electronic device, parents vary significantly in the quantity and features of child-directed speech (Turco et al., 2023a, b). Mendelsohn et al. (2008) found that verbal interactions during media exposure occurred in less than one-quarter of exposures and programs with educational content were not more likely to be co-viewed than other programs. The good news is parents can be taught how to increase verbal interactions during media use in a way that promotes child learning. For example, parents trained to use dialogic questioning techniques during educational television viewing had children who learned more vocabulary than those whose parents did not receive the training (Strouse et al., 2013).

These promising findings from training studies lead one to wonder whether the digital media itself could help parents enhance the quantity and quality of their

CDS. Given the available knowledge about media and language development and the rapid pace with which technology is advancing, we now turn to whether it is possible to use digital media to promote rich verbal interactions that support early language learning.

Can Digital Media Promote Child-Directed Speech and Language Development?

Most of the research on using digital media to promote child-directed speech has been focused on apps. This research suggests that to promote rich verbal interactions, apps and other media resources should present specific characteristics that align with what is already known about child language development. First, apps should offer meaningful and preferably contingent opportunities for participation by the child and caregiver (Tatar & Gerde, 2023; Okumura & Kobayashi, 2021; Dore et al., 2017), for instance, a character that asks questions and pauses for a response (Strouse et al., 2013; Troseth et al., 2020) or discussion prompts built in e-books (Korat & Shneor, 2019; Yang et al., 2022). Second, they should provide explicit and didactic instructions and feedback, preferably automatically adjusting the difficulty or task demands according to the user's skill level, being appropriate not only age-wise but also considering the user's cultural background (Tatar & Gerde, 2023; Dore et al., 2017).

As part of the Reach Every Reader project at the Harvard Graduate School of Education, we followed this advice and shared our knowledge of language development with experts in digital media (FableVision, Inc) to design some apps to elicit conversations between caregivers and young children (Rowe et al., 2021). For example, in one of the games "Animal Antics," the child and caregiver can each become one of the animal characters in a variety of scenes (doctor's office, library) by taking turns recording their own voices that are played back in an animal conversation through the app. The app also has a conversation-turn counter to encourage longer and longer conversations. We found that these apps did indeed elicit rich conversations between parents and their preschool-aged children and that families who used the apps more during a 3-week period also increased the diversity and complexity of the language they used while interacting with the apps. Thus, interactive digital media can promote conversations between parents and young children (Rowe et al., 2021).

Additionally, the use of an immersive digital app aimed at encouraging home literacy activities and how to embed learning into everyday home routines was associated with increased verbal communication between low- and middle-income parents and their 3-year-old children (Leech et al., 2022). Another initiative is *Háblame Bebé*, a phone application designed to support Hispanic infants and toddlers' early language environments and bilingualism through videos on how to provide language-rich interactions, conversation starter topics, sociolinguistic pride, and a milestone tracker (Baralt et al., 2020). The app was proven to increase mother–child verbal interactions, and mothers reported feeling prouder about speaking in Spanish with their children (Baralt et al., 2020).

Despite these successful initiatives led by developmental researchers, the same cannot be said about all commercial apps directed at infants and toddlers. In a series of analyses of infant-directed media, Linebarger and Vaala (2010) found that their audio and visual production features (like pace, cuts, and visual special effects) were heavily demanding for infants' cognitive skills and the embedded language support was mostly simple labeling. Higher-order language processing support, such as encouraging questions, was rarely used. According to those authors, this scenario is most likely difficult for language learning to occur. In the same direction, a recent analysis of the most popular educational apps targeting preschoolers by Kolak et al. (2022) found that the apps-embedded discourse contained rare words, but had lower lexical diversity compared to CDS and shorter utterances compared to books. Those apps thus do not expose children to a high proportion of questions and complex sentences (Kolak et al., 2022), both of which are crucial for language development.

Studies that analyzed parents' and children's co-use of commercial educational apps found that adults do not seem to exploit the app's language potential, rarely providing expanded or distanced talk (Griffith et al., 2023) due to their strong concentration on operative prompts and instructions (Müller-Brauers et al., 2020). Perhaps this happens with commercial apps because they are usually targeted at children using them alone. In that way, they do not always have conversation-eliciting features that consider the participation of an adult interacting with the child during its use, as did the interactional apps developed by researchers mentioned above. However, it is precisely the interactional quality between caregiver and infant that plays a crucial role in making digital media an effective teaching tool for young children's language learning (Myers et al., 2018; Strouse et al., 2018; Zack & Barr, 2016).

And what if the interaction happens through a screen? Research has examined whether young children can learn words from someone on a computer or television screen. For example, in a study with children aged 30–42 months, younger children only learned verbs from video when the interaction was live and synchronized (such as Skype or Zoom), whereas older children were able to learn verbs from pre-recorded video alone (Roseberry et al., 2009). Similar results were found in other studies (Kirkorian et al., 2016; Myers et al., 2017; Roseberry et al., 2014; Krcmar et al., 2007). Additionally, toddlers learn words better if their mother appears on the screen rather than an unknown experimenter (Krcmar, 2010). However, findings suggest that the best word-learning situation, especially for younger children, is the interaction condition where an offscreen person teaches the target word whether in the presence of media or not (Krcmar et al., 2007; DeLoache et al., 2010; Strouse et al., 2013; Myers et al., 2019). An interesting study suggests that not only the presence of an adult but also the live interaction with a peer child (as young as 9 months old) increased language learning from video (Lytle et al., 2018).

Taken together, digital media resources can stimulate CDS and early word learning if they are designed to do so, considering the principles of language development, and if they are used in the context of rich social interactions.

Implications for Research and Practice

This chapter aimed to review evidence on digital media use, CDS, and language development. First, we described studies that investigated the relationship between media use and child language development. Most studies found detrimental effects of media on language. However, those effects were not exclusively driven by the number of hours children use digital media, but by a complex interaction of multiple individual and contextual factors (such as content, how media is used, age of first contact with media, and child factors). Then, we focused on understanding how the family's use of digital media affects child-directed speech, a relevant environmental factor for language development. The reviewed studies highlight that CDS is both a moderator and a mediator of the connection between digital media and children's language, suggesting that the speech parents address to children during media exposure may be a relevant target to interventions aiming at reducing negative effects on language. Lastly, we discussed recent attempts to use media as a way to promote rich verbal interactions between children and caregivers. If media is designed to be interactive and contingent, it can create opportunities for parents and children to engage in rich conversations.

However, caregivers are not always available for high-quality interactions, whether in the presence of media or not. When not available, parents may use digital media to entertain their children expecting that they could be learning from that digital input (Rothstein et al., 2021). For that, parents should favor educational media and offer it sparsely in a way that other developmental-promoting activities are also available to the child. Nevertheless, it is important that parents understand that it is precisely their presence that seems to enhance on-screen language learning opportunities. Apps and media resources targeted at promoting rich verbal interactions should be disseminated and preferred over commercial apps. Still, the importance of playing with traditional toys and books, especially in the presence of an adult or peers, should not be underestimated for child development.

As we live in a digital society where technology is omnipresent, research should concentrate on uncovering specific and complex processes that happen in language development in the face of early media use, determining which features of digital technology may promote learning and which may detract from learning (Dore et al., 2017). Simply suggesting that early media use be avoided may not be a sufficient answer to society anymore. Therefore, more research is needed to understand the mediation/moderation effect of CDS leading to the development of interventions to increase parental verbal interaction in the presence of media. Additionally, research should investigate sources of variation in CDS among different types of media and their nonelectronic correlates. Researchers should consider including technology itself to collect more complex data on the use of digital media by families, moving away from only assessing the parent-reported time of use. Noteworthy, most of the research presented here was conducted in developed countries with white high-income populations. Research on digital media and language conducted with more diverse populations should be encouraged.

Besides investigations, it is critical that scientific knowledge be appropriately translated into practice. One way that this could be achieved is by including developmental researchers in technology companies that produce media resources targeting children's audiences. This would ensure that developmental principles be attended to when creating apps and other types of digital media. Another way is promoting a societal debate about what constitutes an "educational" product for children. By considering the views of different stakeholders, policymakers could create principles and regulations for digital products and services aimed at children, having their optimal development as a major and nonnegotiable goal.

References

Alroqi, H., Serratrice, L., & Cameron-Faulkner, T. (2022). The association between screen media quantity, content, and context and language development. *Journal of Child Language, 1-29*, 1155. https://doi.org/10.1017/S0305000922000265

Ambrose, S. E., VanDam, M., & Moeller, M. P. (2014). Linguistic input, electronic media, and communication outcomes of toddlers with hearing loss. *Ear and Hearing, 35*(2), 139–147. https://doi.org/10.1097/AUD.0b013e3182a76768

Anderson, N. J., Graham, S. A., Prime, H., Jenkins, J. M., & Madigan, S. (2021). Linking quality and quantity of parental linguistic input to child language skills: A meta-analysis. *Child Development, 92*(2), 484–501. https://doi.org/10.1111/cdev.13508

Baralt, M., Mahoney, A. D., & Brito, N. (2020). Háblame Bebé: A phone application intervention to support Hispanic children's early language environments and bilingualism. *Child Language Teaching & Therapy, 36*(1), 33–57. https://doi.org/10.1177/0265659020903779

Barr, R. (2019). Growing up in the digital age: Early learning and family media ecology. *Current Directions in Psychological Science, 28*(4), 341–346. https://doi.org/10.1177/0963721419838245

Cartmill, E. A. (2016). Mind the gap: Assessing and addressing the word gap in early education. *Policy Insights From the Behavioral and Brain Sciences, 3*(2), 185–193. https://doi.org/10.1177/2372732216657565

Çelen Yoldaş, T., & Özmert, E. N. (2021). Communicative environmental factors including maternal depression and media usage patterns on early language development. *Maternal and Child Health Journal, 25*, 900–908. https://doi.org/10.1007/s10995-021-03125-3

Chen, C., Chen, S., Wen, P., & Snow, C. E. (2020). Are screen devices soothing children or soothing parents? Investigating the relationships among children's exposure to different types of screen media, parental efficacy, and home literacy practices. *Computers in Human Behavior, 112*, 1–14. https://doi.org/10.1016/j.chb.2020.106462

Choi, J. H., Mendelsohn, A. L., Weisleder, A., Cates, C. B., Canfield, C., Seery, A., Dreyer, B. P., & Tomopoulos, S. (2018). Real-world usage of educational media does not promote parent–child cognitive stimulation activities. *Academic Pediatrics, 18*(2), 172–178. https://doi.org/10.1016/j.acap.2017.04.020

Christakis, D. A., Gilkerson, J., Richards, J. A., Zimmerman, F. J., Garrison, M. M., Xu, D., Gray, S., & Yapanel, U. (2009). Audible television and decreased adult words, infant vocalizations, and conversational turns: A population-based study. *Archives of Pediatrics & Adolescent Medicine, 163*(6), 554–558. https://doi.org/10.1001/archpediatrics.2009.61

Cycyk, L. M., & De Anda, S. (2021). Media exposure and language experience: Examining associations from home observations in Mexican immigrant families in the US. *Infant Behavior and Development, 63*, 101554. https://doi.org/10.1016/j.infbeh.2021.101554

DeLoache, J. S., Chiong, C., Sherman, K., Islam, N., Vanderborght, M., Troseth, G. L., Strouse, G. A., & O'Doherty, K. (2010). Do babies learn from baby media? *Psychological Science, 21*(11), 1570–1574. https://doi.org/10.1177/0956797610384145

Dore, R. A., Zosh, J. M., Hirsh-Pasek, K., & Golinkoff, R. M. (2017). Plugging into word learning: The role of electronic toys and digital media in language development. *Cognitive Development in Digital Contexts*, 75–91. https://doi.org/10.1016/B978-0-12-809481-5.00004-3

Duch, H., Fisher, E. M., Ensari, I., Font, M., Harrington, A., Taromino, C., Yip, J., & Rodriguez, C. (2013a). Association of screen time use and language development in Hispanic toddlers: A cross-sectional and longitudinal study. *Clinical Pediatrics, 52*(9), 857–865. https://doi.org/10.1177/0009922813492881

Duch, H., Fisher, E. M., Ensari, I., & Harrington, A. (2013b). Screen time use in children under 3 years old: A systematic review of correlates. *International Journal of Behavioral Nutrition and Physical Activity, 10*, 102. https://doi.org/10.1186/1479-5868-10-102

Eggleston, C., Wang, X. C., & Choi, Y. (2022). Mother-toddler shared Reading with electronic versus print books: Mothers' language use and perspectives. *Early Education and Development, 33*(7), 1152–1174. https://doi.org/10.1080/10409289.2021.1943638

Ewin, C. A., Reupert, A., McLean, L. A., & Ewin, C. J. (2021). Mobile devices compared to non-digital toy play: The impact of activity type on the quality and quantity of parent language. *Computers in Human Behavior, 118*, 106669. https://doi.org/10.1016/j.chb.2020.106669

Ferjan Ramírez, N., Hippe, D. S., & Lindekugel, K. (2022). Electronic media and social features of language input in bilingually-raised Latinx infants. *Infant Behavior and Development, 68*, 101740. https://doi.org/10.1016/j.infbeh.2022.101740

Fusaroli, R., Weed, E., Fein, D., & Naigles, L. (2019). Hearing me hearing you: Reciprocal effects between child and parent language in autism and typical development. *Cognition, 183*, 1–18. https://doi.org/10.1016/j.cognition.2018.10.022

Griffith, S. F., Casanova, S. M., & Delisle, J. H. (2023). Back-and-forth conversation during parent-child co-use of an educational app game. *Early Child Development and Care, 193*, 1007. https://doi.org/10.1080/03004430.2023.2199173

Hart, B., & Risley, T. R. (1995). *Meaningful differences in the everyday experience of young American children*. Brookes Publishing.

Hirsh-Pasek, K., Adamson, L. B., Bakeman, R., Owen, M. T., Golinkoff, R. M., Pace, A. S., Yust, P. K., & Suma, K. (2015). The contribution of early communication quality to low-income children's language success. *Psychological Science, 26*(7), 1071. https://doi.org/10.1177/0956797615581493

Hoff, E. (2003). The specificity of environmental influence: Socioeconomic status affects early vocabulary development via maternal speech. *Child Development, 74*(5), 1368–1378. https://doi.org/10.1111/1467-8624.00612

Hoff, E. (2006). How social contexts support and shape language development. *Developmental Review, 26*(1), 55–88. https://doi.org/10.1016/j.dr.2005.11.002

Hoff, E. (2009). *Language development* (4th ed.).

Hurwitz, L. B., Bickham, D. S., Moukalled, S. H., & Rich, M. (2020). Only so many hours in a day: Early childhood screen time in Boston and Mexico City. *International Journal of Communication, 14*, 4014–4034.

Hutton, J. S., Dudley, J., Horowitz-Kraus, T., DeWitt, T., & Holland, S. K. (2020). Associations between screen-based media use and brain white matter integrity in preschool-aged children. *Journal of the American Medical Association Pediatrics, 174*(1), 1–10. https://doi.org/10.1001/jamapediatrics.2019.3869

Jing, M., Ye, T., Kirkorian, H. L., & Mares, M.-L. (2023). Screen media exposure and young children's vocabulary learning and development: A meta-analysis. *Child Development, 10*, 1–21. https://doi.org/10.1111/cdev.13927

Jones, G., & Rowland, C. F. (2017). Diversity not quantity in caregiver speech: Using computational modeling to isolate the effects of the quantity and the diversity of the input on vocabulary growth. *Cognitive Psychology, 98*, 1–21. https://doi.org/10.1016/j.cogpsych.2017.07.002

Kabali, H. K., Irigoyen, M. M., Nunez-Davis, R., Budacki, J. G., Mohanty, S. H., Leister, K. P., & Bonner, R. L., Jr. (2015). Exposure and use of mobile media devices by young children. *Pediatrics, 136*(6), 1044–1050. https://doi.org/10.1542/peds.2015-2151

Karani, N. F., Sher, J., & Mophosho, M. (2022). The influence of screen time on children's language development: A scoping review. *South African Journal of Communication Disorders, 69*(1), 1–7. https://doi.org/10.4102/sajcd.v69i1.825

Kirkorian, H. L., Choi, K., & Pempek, T. A. (2016). Toddlers' word learning from contingent and noncontingent video on touch screens. *Child Development, 87*, 405–413. https://doi.org/10.1111/cdev.12508

Kirkorian, H. L., Pempek, T. A., Murphy, L. A., Schmidt, M. E., & Anderson, D. R. (2009). The impact of background television on parent–child interaction. *Child Development, 80*, 1350–1359. https://doi.org/10.1111/j.1467-8624.2009.01337.x

Kolak, J., Monaghan, P., & Taylor, G. (2022). Language in educational apps for pre-schoolers: A comparison of grammatical constructions and psycholinguistic features in apps, books, and child-directed speech. *Journal of Child Language, 1–27*, 895. https://doi.org/10.1017/S0305000922000198

Korat, O., & Or, T. (2010). How new technology influences parent-child interaction: The case of E-book Reading. *First Language, 30*(2), 139–154. https://doi.org/10.1177/0142723709359242

Korat, O., & Shneor, D. (2019). Can e-books support low SES parental mediation to enrich children's vocabulary? *First Language, 39*(3), 344–364. https://doi.org/10.1177/0142723718822443

Krcmar, M. (2010). Can social meaningfulness and repeat exposure help infants and toddlers overcome the video deficit? *Media Psychology, 13*(1), 31–53. https://doi.org/10.1080/15213260903562917

Krcmar, M., Grela, B., & Lin, K. (2007). Can Toddlers Learn Vocabulary from Television? An Experimental Approach. *Media Psychology, 10*(1), 41–63. https://doi.org/10.1080/15213260701300931

Lauricella, A. R., Barr, R., & Calvert, S. L. (2014). Parent-child interactions during traditional and computer storybook reading for children's comprehension: Implications for electronic storybook design. *International Journal of Child-Computer Interaction, 2*(1), 17–25. https://doi.org/10.1016/j.ijcci.2014.07.001

Lavigne, H. J., Hanson, K. G., & Anderson, D. R. (2015). The influence of television coviewing on parent language directed at toddlers. *Journal of Applied Developmental Psychology, 36*, 1–10. https://doi.org/10.1016/j.appdev.2014.11.004

Leech, K. A., Wheat, D., Rowe, M. L., Blatt, J., & Dede, C. (2022). "Literacy is everywhere!": Using digital technology to broaden how parents view the home literacy environment. *Applied Developmental Science*. https://doi.org/10.1080/10888691.2022.2125392

Lin, H., Chen, K., Chou, W., Yuan, K., Yen, S., Chen, Y., & Chow, J. C. (2020). Prolonged touch screen device usage is associated with emotional and behavioral problems, but not language delay, in toddlers. *Infant Behavior and Development, 58*, 1–10. https://doi.org/10.1016/j.infbeh.2020.101424

Linebarger, D. L., & Vaala, S. E. (2010). Screen media and language development in infants and toddlers: An ecological perspective. *Developmental Review, 30*(2), 176–202. https://doi.org/10.1016/j.dr.2010.03.006

Lytle, S. R., Garcia-Sierra, A., & Kuhl, P. K. (2018). Two are better than one: Infant language learning from video improves in the presence of peers. *Proceedings of the National Academy of Sciences, 115*(40), 9859–9866. https://doi.org/10.1073/pnas.1611621115

Madigan, S., Browne, D., Racine, N., Mori, C., & Tough, S. (2019). Association between screen time and children's performance on a developmental screening test. *Journal of the American Medical Association Pediatrics, 173*(3), 244–250. https://doi.org/10.1001/jamapediatrics.2018.5056

Madigan, S., McArthur, B. A., Anhorn, C., Eirich, R., & Christakis, D. A. (2020). Associations between screen use and child language skills: A systematic review and meta-analysis. *Journal of the American Medical Association Pediatrics, 174*(7), 665–675. https://doi.org/10.1001/jamapediatrics.2020.0327

Martinot, P., Bernard, J. Y., Peyre, H., De Agostini, M., Forhan, A., Charles, M., Plancoulaine, S., & Heude, B. (2021). Exposure to screens and children's language development in the EDEN mother–child cohort. *Scientific Reports, 11*, 11863. https://doi.org/10.1038/s41598-021-90867-3

Masur, E. F., Flynn, V., & Olson, J. (2016). Infants' background television exposure during play: Negative relations to the quantity and quality of mothers' speech and infants' vocabulary acquisition. *First Language, 36*(2), 109–123. https://doi.org/10.1177/0142723716639499

McArthur, B. A., Tough, S., & Madigan, S. (2022). Screen time and developmental and behavioral outcomes for preschool children. *Pediatric Research, 91*, 1616–1621. https://doi.org/10.1038/s41390-021-01572-w

Medawar, J., Tabullo, Á. J., & Gago-Galvagno, L. G. (2023). Early language outcomes in Argentinean toddlers: Associations with home literacy, screen exposure, and joint media engagement. *British Journal of Developmental Psychology, 41*, 13–30. https://doi.org/10.1111/bjdp.12429

Mendelsohn, A. L., Berkule, S. B., Tomopoulos, S., Tamis-LeMonda, C. S., Huberman, H. S., Alvir, J., & Dreyer, B. P. (2008). Infant television and video exposure associated with limited parent-child verbal interactions in low socioeconomic status households. *Archives of Pediatric & Adolescent Medicine, 162*(5), 411–417. https://doi.org/10.1001/archpedi.162.5.411

Mendelsohn, A. L., Brockmeyer, C. A., Dreyer, B. P., Fierman, A. H., Berkule-Silberman, S. B., & Tomopoulos, S. (2010). Do verbal interactions with infants during electronic media exposure mitigate adverse impacts on their language development as toddlers? *Infant & Child Development, 19*(6), 577–593. https://doi.org/10.1002/icd.711

Müller-Brauers, C., Miosga, C., Fischer, S., Maus, A., & Potthast, I. (2020). Narrative potential of picture-book apps: A media- and interaction-oriented study. *Frontiers in Psychology, 11*. https://doi.org/10.3389/fpsyg.2020.593482

Munzer, T. G., Miller, A. L., Weeks, H. M., Kaciroti, N., & Radesky, J. (2019). Differences in parent-toddler interactions with electronic versus print books. *Pediatrics, 143*(4), e20182012. https://doi.org/10.1542/peds.2018-2012

Mustonen, R., Torppa, R., & Stolt, S. (2022). Screen time of preschool-aged children and their mothers, and children's language development. *Children, 9*(10), 1–13. https://doi.org/10.3390/children9101577

Myers, L. J., Crawford, E., Murphy, C., Aka-Ezoua, E., & Felix, C. (2018). Eyes in the room trump eyes on the screen: Effects of a responsive co-viewer on toddlers' responses to and learning from video chat. *Journal of Children and Media, 12*(3), 275–294. https://doi.org/10.1080/17482798.2018.1425889

Myers, L. J., Keyser, H., & Cors, M. (2019). Co-viewers support participation in video chat interactions, but live experiences promote richer word learning for 24- to 36-month-olds in the USA. *Journal of Children and Media, 13*(4), 415–432. https://doi.org/10.1080/17482798.2019.1646294

Myers, L. J., LeWitt, R. B., Gallo, R. E., & Maselli, N. M. (2017). Baby FaceTime: Can toddlers learn from online video chat? *Developmental Science, 20*, e12430. https://doi.org/10.1111/desc.12430

Okumura, Y., & Kobayashi, T. (2021). Contingent experience with touchscreens promotes parent-child conversations. *Cognitive Development, 60*, 101100. https://doi.org/10.1016/j.cogdev.2021.101100

Ozturk, G., & Hill, S. (2020). Mother-child interactions during shared reading with digital and print books. *Early Child Development and Care, 190*(9), 1425–1440. https://doi.org/10.1080/03004430.2018.1538977

Parish-Morris, J., Mahajan, N., Hirsh-Pasek, K., Golinkoff, R. M., & Collins, M. F. (2013). Once upon a time: Parent–child dialogue and storybook reading in the electronic era. *Mind, Brain, and Education, 7*, 200–211. https://doi.org/10.1111/mbe.12028

Pempek, T. A., Demers, L. B., Hanson, K. G., Kirkorian, H. L., & Anderson, D. R. (2011). The impact of infant-directed videos on parent–child interaction. *Journal of Applied Developmental Psychology, 32*(1), 10–19. https://doi.org/10.1016/j.appdev.2010.10.001

Pempek, T. A., Kirkorian, H. L., & Anderson, D. R. (2014). The effects of background television on the quantity and quality of child-directed speech by parents. *Journal of Children and Media, 8*(3), 211–222. https://doi.org/10.1080/17482798.2014.920715

Radesky, J. S. (2021). Young children's online–offline balance. *Acta Paediatrica, 110*(3), 748–749. https://doi.org/10.1111/apa.15649

Ramírez, N. J., Hippe, D. S., & Shapiro, N. T. (2021). Exposure to electronic media between 6 and 24 months of age: An exploratory study. *Infant Behavior and Development, 63*, 101549. https://doi.org/10.1016/j.infbeh.2021.101549

Rocha, H. A. L., Correia, L. L., Leite, Á. J. M., Machado, M. M. T., Lindsay, A. C., Rocha, S. G. M. O., Campos, J. S., Cavalcante e Silva, A., & Sudfeld, C. R. (2021). Screen time and early childhood development in Ceará, Brazil: A population-based study. *Biomedical Central Public Health, 21*(2072), 4–11. https://doi.org/10.1186/s12889-021-12136-2

Romeo, R. R., Leonard, J. A., Robinson, S. T., West, M. R., Mackey, A. P., Rowe, M. L., & Gabrieli, J. D. E. (2018). Beyond the 30-million-word gap: Children's conversational exposure is associated with language-related brain function. *Psychological Science, 29*(5), 700–710. https://doi.org/10.1177/0956797617742725

Roseberry, S., Hirsh-Pasek, K., & Golinkoff, R. M. (2014). Skype me! Socially contingent interactions help toddlers learn language. *Child Development, 85*, 956–970. https://doi.org/10.1111/cdev.12166

Roseberry, S., Hirsh-Pasek, K., Parish-Morris, J., & Golinkoff, R. M. (2009). Live action: Can young children learn verbs from video? *Child Development, 80*, 1360–1375. https://doi.org/10.1111/j.1467-8624.2009.01338.x

Rothstein, J. D., Buckland, A. J., Gagnier, K., Ochoa, M., Allen-Valley, A., Jivapong, B., Cabrera, L. Z., Leontsini, E., & Fisher, K. R. (2021). Assessing the play and learning environments of children under two years in peri-urban Lima, Peru: A formative research study. *BMC Public Health, 21*(1), 1–15. https://doi.org/10.1186/s12889-020-10119-3

Rowe, M. L. (2012). A longitudinal investigation of the role of quantity and quality of child-directed speech vocabulary development. *Child Development, 83*(5), 1762–1774. https://doi.org/10.1111/j.1467-8624.2012.01805.x

Rowe, M. L., Leech, K. A., & Cabrera, N. (2016). Going beyond input quantity: Wh-questions matter for toddlers' language and cognitive development. *Cognitive Science, 41*(1), 162–179. https://doi.org/10.1111/cogs.12349

Rowe, M. L., Turco, R. G., & Blatt, J. H. (2021). Can interactive apps promote parent-child conversations? *Journal of Applied Developmental Psychology, 76*, 101326. https://doi.org/10.1016/j.appdev.2021.101326

Ruangdaraganon, N., Chuthapisith, J., Mo-suwan, L., Kriweradechachai, S., Udomsubpayakul, U., & Choprapawon, C. (2009). Television viewing in Thai infants and toddlers: Impacts to language development and parental perceptions. *BMC Pediatrics, 9*, 34. https://doi.org/10.1186/1471-2431-9-34

Rvachew, S. (2013). Language development and literacy—Synthesis. In R. E. Tremblay, M. Boivin, & R. D. V. Peters (Eds.), *Encyclopedia on early childhood development*. [Online] (2nd ed., pp. 1–94). Centre of Excellence for Early Childhood Development and Strategic Knowledge Cluster on Early Child Development. https://www.child-encyclopedia.com/language-development-and-literacy/synthesis

Schmidt, M. E., Rich, M., Rifas-Shiman, S. L., Oken, E., & Taveras, E. M. (2009). Television viewing in infancy and child cognition at 3 years of age in a US cohort. *Pediatrics, 123*(3), e370–e375. https://doi.org/10.1542/peds.2008-3221

Sosa, A. V. (2016). Association of the type of toy used during play with the quantity and quality of parent-infant communication. *JAMA Pediatrics, 170*(2), 132–137. https://doi.org/10.1001/jamapediatrics.2015.3753

Strouse, G. A., O'Doherty, K., & Troseth, G. L. (2013). Effective co-viewing: Preschoolers' learning from video after a dialogic questioning intervention. *Developmental Psychology, 49*(12), 2368–2382. https://doi.org/10.1037/a0032463

Strouse, G. A., Troseth, G. L., O'Doherty, K. D., & Saylor, M. M. (2018). Co-viewing supports toddlers' word learning from contingent and noncontingent video. *Journal of Experimental Child Psychology, 166*, 310–326. https://doi.org/10.1016/j.jecp.2017.09.005

Strouse, G. A., Troseth, G. L., & Stuckelman, Z. D. (2023). Page and screen: Storybook features that promote parent-child talk during shared reading. *Journal of Applied Developmental Psychology, 86*, 101522. https://doi.org/10.1016/j.appdev.2023.101522

Sundqvist, A., Koch, F.-S., Söderberg, M., Barr, R., & Heimann, M. (2022). Qualitative and quantitative aspects of child-directed parental talk and the relation to 2-year-old's developing vocabulary. *Infancy, 27*(4), 1–18. https://doi.org/10.1111/infa.12476

Tanimura, M., Okuma, K., & Kyoshima, K. (2007). Television viewing reduced parental utterance, and delayed speech development in infants and young children. *Archives of Pediatrics and Adolescent Medicine, 161*(6), 618–619. https://doi.org/10.1001/archpedi.161.6.618-b

Tatar, B. H., & Gerde, H. K. (2023). Partnering with families to use screen time for supporting early language and literacy. *The Reading Teacher, 76*(4), 439–450. https://doi.org/10.1002/trtr.2150

Tomasello, M. (2009). The usage-based theory of language acquisition. In E. L. Bavin (Ed.), *The Cambridge handbook of child language* (pp. 69–87). Cambridge University Press.

Troseth, G. L., Strouse, G. A., Flores, I., Stuckelman, Z. D., & Russo Johnson, C. (2020). An enhanced eBook facilitates parent–child talk during shared reading by families of low socioeconomic status. *Early Childhood Research Quarterly, 50*, 45–58. https://doi.org/10.1016/j.ecresq.2019.02.009

Turco, R. G., Lesaux, N. K., & Jones, S. M. (2023a). Home literacy in the digital era: The role of mobile screen media frequency in a U.S. state. *British Journal of Educational Technology, 54*(2), 513–533. https://doi.org/10.1111/bjet.13259

Turco, R. G., Rowe, M. L., & Blatt, J. H. (2023b). Exploring parent profiles in parent–child interactions with e-books. *First Language, 10*, 380. https://doi.org/10.1177/01427237231160242

van den Heuvel, M., Ma, J., Borkhoff, C. M., Koroshegyi, C., Dai, D. W. H., Parkin, P. C., Maguire, J. L., & Birken, C. S. (2019). TARGet kids! Collaboration: Mobile media device use is associated with expressive language delay in 18-month-old children. *Journal of Developmental & Behavioral Pediatrics, 40*(2), 99–104. https://doi.org/10.1097/DBP.0000000000000630

Vanderloo, L. M., Janus, M., Omand, J. A., Keown-Stoneman, C. D. G., Borkhoff, C. M., Duku, E., Mamdani, M., Lebovic, G., Parkin, P. C., Randall Simpson, J., Tremblay, M. S., Maguire, J. L., & Birken, C. S. (2022). Children's screen use and school readiness at 4–6 years: Prospective cohort study. *Biomedical Central Public Health, 22*, 1–11. https://doi.org/10.1186/s12889-022-12629-8

Varadarajan, S., Govindarajan Venguidesvarane, A., Ramaswamy, K. N., Rajamohan, M., Krupa, M., Bernard, S., & Christadoss, W. (2021). Prevalence of excessive screen time and its association with developmental delay in children aged <5 years: A population-based cross-sectional study in India. *PLoS One, 16*(7), 1–13. https://doi.org/10.1371/journal.pone.0254102

Vygotsky, L. S. (1984). *The social formation of the mind.* Martins Fontes.

Weizman, Z. O., & Snow, C. E. (2001). Lexical output as related to children's vocabulary acquisition: Effects of sophisticated exposure and support for meaning. *Developmental Psychology, 37*(2), 265–279. https://doi.org/10.1037/0012-1649.37.2.265

Yang, D., Xia, C., Collins, P., & Warschauer, M. (2022). The role of bilingual discussion prompts in shared E-book reading. *Computers & Education, 190*, 104622. https://doi.org/10.1016/j.compedu.2022.104622

Zack, E., & Barr, R. (2016). The role of interactional quality in learning from touch screens during infancy: Context matters. *Frontiers in Psychology, 7*, 1–12. https://doi.org/10.3389/fpsyg.2016.01264

Zimmerman, F. J., Gilkerson, J., Richards, J. A., Christakis, D. A., Xu, D., Gray, S., & Yapanel, U. (2009). Teaching by listening: The importance of adult-child conversations to language development. *Pediatrics, 124*(1), 342–349. https://doi.org/10.1542/peds.2008-2267

Zosh, J. M., Verdine, B. N., Filipowicz, A., Golinkoff, R. M., Hirsh-Pasek, K., & Newcombe, N. S. (2015). Talking shape: Parental language with electronic versus traditional shape sorters. *Mind, Brain, and Education, 9*(3), 136–144. https://doi.org/10.1111/mbe.12082

Chapter 9
Video Chat: A Tool for Young Children's Engagement and Early Social Learning

Georgene L. Troseth, Rachel F. Barr, Jennifer M. Zosh, Gabrielle A. Strouse, and Lauren J. Myers

The best is the enemy of the good

There is no doubt about it, human relationships are key to healthy child development. Responsive, high-quality caregiving helps infants and young children to thrive in the world (National Scientific Council on the Developing Child, 2004), and indeed, social relationships are central to human health and well-being (Umberson & Montez, 2010). Therefore, it is little wonder that every new technology that potentially disturbs those interactions tends to be met with alarm. In the 1500s, concerns arose about the printing press and easy access to books diverting time from person-to-person relationships (Bell, 2010). Today, widespread alarm about the use of handheld devices (tablets and smartphones) reflects the same central theme: that high-quality, responsive, emotionally warm human interaction is best and anything that stands in the way of that optimal interaction is bad.

G. L. Troseth (✉)
Vanderbilt University, Nashville, TN, USA
e-mail: georgene.troseth@vanderbilt.edu

R. F. Barr
Georgetown University, Washington, D.C, USA
e-mail: rfb5@georgetown.edu

J. M. Zosh
Pennsylvania State University, Brandywine, Media, PA, USA
e-mail: jzosh@psu.edu

G. A. Strouse
University of South Dakota, Vermillion, SD, USA
e-mail: gabrielle.strouse@usd.edu

L. J. Myers
Lafayette College, Easton, PA, USA
e-mail: myersl@lafayette.edu

G. B. Frizzo (ed.), *Digital Media and Early Child Development*,
https://doi.org/10.1007/978-3-031-69224-6_9

But is this the right approach? Big thinkers tend to highlight the error of this path. Voltaire suggested, "the best is the enemy of the good," and Confucius observed, "Better a diamond with a flaw than a pebble without" (Patel, 2017). By operating at extremes, we miss potential good. It may be preferable to have high-quality, human-to-human interaction, but constant interchange is frankly impossible and would prevent children from developing coping skills and the capacity to handle tolerable stress. The debate about children and screens may be falling victim to this same fallacy. By arguing that all screen time is bad because it is not as good as the most optimal in-person experience, we may miss out on beneficial experiences for children, such as the possibility that handheld screens may be a powerful tool to help support and strengthen today's families.

There are indicators that parents, pediatricians, and researchers are realizing that more nuance is needed when thinking about screen use, especially for young children (Kucirkova et al., 2023). Although children's media policy has held that babies and toddlers should have little exposure to screens, these guidelines now acknowledge that all screen use is not created equal. Current guidelines are based on the idea that social engagement is key and the affordances of some digital media, such as video chat, may allow for social connection (Reid Chassiakos et al., 2016). Here, we report what is known about the ability of infants, young children, and families to use video chat as a method to connect with the social world. Doing so requires us to reimagine what we know about infants' and young children's abilities to engage with and learn from screens. We must think more broadly about the types of beneficial experiences that make up the everyday lives of young children (age 3 and under)—with a nod to the list of unknowns that still exist.

In this chapter, we will explore the ability of infants, toddlers, and preschoolers to engage with video chat. Research to date suggests that video chat capitalizes on the social way that young children's brains engage in learning. As such, it appears to be a powerful source for social connection and for children to develop shared attention, play, learn words, and learn to take others' perspectives (Glick et al., 2022; McClure et al., 2015, 2018, 2020; McClure & Barr, 2017). During early childhood, learning initially is social, and video chat complements those early learning mechanisms.

Social Contingency Is Key

During video chat, a viewing child is exposed to social contingency from the person on the screen who can see, hear, and react to the child in real time. "Contingency" refers to the reliable relation between one event (such as a child's smile) and another (e.g., an adult's response). This kind of video is very different from watching television or pretaped home videos. The visual dimension of video chat allows the parties to respond to each other using nonverbal cues that are especially meaningful for very young children, including facial expressions, gaze direction, and gestures. Unlike a phone call, video chat provides the viewer with visual information (e.g., facial expressions and body language) that, beyond the voice, can convey additional information about warmth and emotion.

During video chat, both parties can also see the distant partner's surrounding physical context, which enables *virtual triadic interactions* (McClure et al., 2018; Myers et al., 2024). For example, video chat can show what an on-screen partner is looking at in their own environment (such as a grandmother holding up, looking at, and labeling a peach she is eating), and it presents audible and visual information such as the on-screen partner's social responses "in real time" (e.g., when the infant points at the piece of fruit on the screen and vocalizes, the grandmother can immediately and contingently respond with, "Yes, I'm eating a *peach*!").

Unlike video chat, pretaped video may violate infants' and toddlers' expectations of contingency from people who appear to be looking at and talking to them, leading them to discount this kind of media as a viable source of information with any relevance to them. In contrast, the social contingency of video chat may increase the meaningfulness of screen-based information for the child and increase both engagement and learning (Strouse et al., 2018; Troseth et al., 2006, 2018).

For Engagement

Infants notice and respond to face-to-face social contingency from a very young age. In a study with 3-month-olds, a researcher who was in the room with the infant either responded to the infant's vocalizations by smiling and saying "Hi, [infant's name]," or the same responses were timed to follow the recorded vocalizations of another infant (delivered to the researcher via earphones—a "yoked" condition). Infants responded to the contingent adult by producing a higher proportion of speech-like vocalizations than infants did in the noncontingent, yoked condition (Bloom et al., 1987). Bloom et al. (1987) reasoned that adult turn-taking may have incited infants to mimic the character of the adult's speech, or it may have increased the infants' arousal and attention to the adult's behavior. In another study, when an adult who was facing an infant suddenly adopted a "still face" (not responding at all to the infant), 5-month-olds attempted to regain the adult's attention by vocalizing when the adult was unresponsive to their social bids: they had "learned the social efficacy of their vocalizations on caregivers' behavior" (Goldstein et al., 2009, p. 636).

Video chat allows these same types of socially contingent interactions to take place at a distance, through screens. The groundwork for studying video chat and development began in the 1980s and 1990s as researchers examined infants' responses to live, contingent video and prerecorded, noncontingent video compared to their responses to real-world events. In one study, 2-month-olds responded the same to prerecorded and to live, closed-circuit video of their talking and smiling mothers, as if they noticed no lack of contingent responsiveness in the prerecorded video (Marian et al., 1996). However, in other research, infants of this age behaved in a way that suggested they did notice the lack of contingency: they displayed negative affect during noncontingent video playback of their mother's or a researcher's smiling and talking face (Nadel et al., 1999; Soussignan et al., 2006). By 3–8 months, infants clearly noticed when interpersonal contingency was disrupted; they paid attention to, responded more to, and/or better remembered and preferred the person on the screen when watching live events (Bigelow et al., 1996; Hains & Muir, 1996; McClure et al., 2020) or contingent, closed-circuit video (Bigelow, 1996; Bigelow et al., 1996; Gusella et al., 1988; Hains & Muir, 1996) compared to recorded video.

Contingency may play an important role in maintaining infants' attention. In general, experimental studies have shown that infants, toddlers, and preschoolers are more engaged and responsive during video chat than when watching video recordings (Gaudreau et al., 2020; Hains & Muir, 1996; Myers et al., 2017, 2019; Strouse et al., 2018). For example, 4- to 6-month-old infants displayed less attention to a prerecorded video of an adult smiling and talking than to the same person interacting with them via closed-circuit video (Hains & Muir, 1996).

Because video chat allows adults and children to communicate responsively with one another, it also may support developing closeness with the person on the screen. In several studies, infants (6–12 months) responded with positive affect to high-quality, warm, contingent interactions via video chat with their mothers (McClure et al., 2020) and their grandmothers (Roche et al., 2022). In another study, 8-month-old infants smiled more at their mothers in a contingent video chat condition than in a noncontingent condition, so long as their mothers established social contingency by saying hello (or similar) and pausing for a response (McClure et al., 2020). When interacting with a grandparent on video chat, 6- to 18-month-olds paid more attention when grandparents sensitively responded to them (McClure et al., 2018; Myers et al., 2024).

Young children also can use video chat to *establish* relationships (McClure et al., 2015; McClure & Barr, 2017; Myers et al., 2017). After six video chat interactions with a researcher whom they had never met in person, toddlers (17–24 months) recognized and preferred to play with this researcher when visiting their lab (Myers et al., 2017). In contrast, children who had viewed a noncontingent researcher during six prerecorded video sessions showed no such recognition or preference for the researcher.

Research with older infants, toddlers, and preschoolers indicates that the combination of contingent audio and video can provide a sense of social connectedness for children. Tarasuik et al. (2011) used an adaptation of the Strange Situation protocol (Ainsworth & Wittig, 1969) to investigate whether children from 17 months to 5 years of age who were left alone in a playroom had a sense of emotional security when they could see and hear their mothers on video chat, compared to when they did not have this access. With video chat, the children were content for longer and played for a greater percentage of the time. In a replication and extension, Tarasuik et al. (2013) found that the responsive audio and video streams of video chat gave 2- and 3-year old children a "sense of proximity" to their mothers that was not produced when the children merely could hear audio of their mothers while left alone in the playroom, in line with the finding that children up to age 7 tend to have difficulty using the telephone to communicate successfully (Ballagas et al., 2009). Ballagas et al. (2009) suggest that a visual medium such as video chat would be a developmentally appropriate alternative to traditional phone calls for family connection with young children.

For Learning

The lack of contingent audio and video also may impair infants' learning from pretaped video such as television. A 1-month-long study focused on the period of "perceptual narrowing" when infants lose the ability to perceive speech differences in any language. American 9-month-olds (whose parents spoke English) were exposed to 5 total hours of Mandarin as adult speakers in the room or on recorded video read books and showed them toys (Kuhl et al., 2003). At the study's end, the then 10-month-olds who had seen the speakers "in person" could distinguish Mandarin sound differences, but the infants who had watched the videos could no longer tell the sounds apart. Kuhl et al. (2003) concluded that gaze direction and other social cues available in the direct interaction but missing from the video were vital for infants' learning: they kept infants' attention and indicated what the people were talking about. Because Kuhl and colleagues did not have a condition with speakers on video chat, further research was needed to examine the specific social contingencies that did and did not support learning from video.

In the early 2000s, studies probed toddlers' learning from a responsive person on closed-circuit video that was similar to the video chat of today. In these studies, an on-screen adult highlighted the social contingencies of the closed-circuit setup, as most children did not have much experience with live video. To do so, she personalized the experience by referring to the child by name and commenting on their surroundings; she played interactive games (e.g., "Simon Says") that highlighted that she could see and hear the child; she also encouraged the child's parent to participate in these demonstrations (Nielsen et al., 2008; Troseth et al., 2006). Then, she gave the toddlers information to solve the study task (imitating a modeler's actions to open a box in one case; finding a hidden object in the other). The 24-month-olds were more likely to use the information from the contingent, responsive researcher than toddlers who watched a yoked, noncontingent video recording of the researcher's responses from a prior participant's closed-circuit session. In Troseth et al.'s (2006) study, children who were exposed to the contingency of closed-circuit video also were about three times more successful at using the information from the person on video to solve the finding game compared to children who heard the same information from a person on video who had not established contingency.

In other research, Roseberry et al. (2014) taught 24- to 30-month-old toddlers novel verbs in one of three conditions: face-to-face interaction, socially contingent video chat, or noncontingent video. Toddlers learned from the contingent video chat but showed significantly less learning in the noncontingent condition. The researchers concluded that learning in the closed-circuit conditions was similar to the way children learned when interacting face-to-face with the researcher. These initial studies showed that video interactions involving social contingency between the child and a person presenting information on video could support social learning.

More recent studies (Myers et al., 2017; Strouse et al., 2018; Troseth et al., 2018) have focused on particular aspects of closed-circuit video interactions that may be key for successful learning. One change has involved using an ask-and-wait style of prerecorded video for control conditions (e.g., similar to the way the TV character *Dora the Explorer* pauses and waits for a response when she asks a question) rather than comparing closed-circuit video to a recording of another child's session. This controls for irrelevant or inaccurate information in yoked recordings. Other changes have involved matching aspects of the training games across conditions by removing personalization that cannot be prerecorded, removing the training games entirely, and varying whether support from the co-viewing parent is requested or eliminated.

From these follow-up studies, we have learned that both the supportive parent who co-views and the training games that emphasize social contingency likely contributed to children's learning in the initial studies. Roseberry et al. (2014) found that 24- to 30-month-old children who participated over Skype and were introduced to the contingency of the video with training games learned more than those who watched a previous participant's recording in the absence of co-viewer support (parents wore dark glasses and did not participate). On the other hand, several studies have reduced the contingency training or made it less personal and found that 2-year-olds failed to learn new words unless they had a participatory co-viewing adult (Myers et al., 2018; Strouse et al., 2018; Troseth et al., 2018). A recent meta-analysis of studies that compared contingent video (i.e., closed circuit, live feed, and video chat) to unmediated face-to-face learning found no difference across several types of tasks (Strouse & Samson, 2021). Therefore, it seems that video chat can be a successful learning tool, especially if the on-screen partner *or* someone in the room provides support. For instance, in-person social partners who are with the child during video chat can model paying attention to the screen and can demonstrate responsiveness to the on-screen partner that the child can imitate.

Limitations of Video Chat

Although video chat offers opportunities for engagement and learning, it is also important to consider potential challenges of using this medium with young children. In other words, while the best might be the enemy of the good, good is not perfect. There may be lessons learned by examining those imperfections. Below, we explore some of these challenges and then discuss compensatory approaches that might help families overcome these challenges.

Perceptual Limitations and Conceptual Challenges

Despite the promises of video chat for interaction, it may be difficult for the youngest children to fully interact with loved ones via video chat due to inherent constraints of the medium. Perceptual and conceptual factors that make it difficult for very young children to connect between any video and reality are also present during video chat. When watching a video, there is a perceptual mismatch between encoding of the flat, two-dimensional scene (e.g., Grandma on the screen) compared to the three-dimensional world (e.g., Grandma that we visited in her house). Additionally, the size of objects on screen tends to be smaller or larger than the actual objects, depending how close to the camera they are. These perceptual limitations may make it challenging for children to align their memories of what happened on the screen with their experience of the real world and to transfer and use information from the screen (Barr, 2019). Furthermore, through exposure to television and online videos, children see many on-screen events that are noncontingent, distant in time or location, or fantastical and pretend. The many ways that video can relate to (or not relate to) reality creates a conceptual challenge for children, requiring them to identify when on-screen events and people are real and relevant to them (Strouse et al., 2018; Troseth et al., 2006). Additionally, people and items on video chat are physically inaccessible, and the actual location of the depicted people and objects is not always obvious. Because video images are representations (or symbols), children need adult support to learn how to interpret video images, including video chat (Strouse et al., 2018; Troseth et al., 2019).

Virtual Interactions Do Not Happen in the Same Physical Space

A number of features of face-to-face interaction are diminished in video chat. Besides any delays in social contingency, the loss of physical contact and the misalignment of gaze can contribute to poorer social interactions compared to interacting face-to-face in the same room (Parkinson & Lea, 2011). What the camera can see and convey to the partner on the other side of the screen limits the movement a video chat partner can make and still be visible, and users are restricted to a head-on orientation toward the camera (and one another). The frame of the screen also presents a limited range of sight, and video chat does not convey olfactory signals (e.g., the smell of a ripe peach) that are present when both parties are in the same space. Typical physical contact that would take place between adults and young children in a face-to-face interaction is most certainly compromised in video-mediated interactions (Stack, 2004).

Technology Disruptions

Outdated devices and Internet connectivity problems can also present challenges for family interaction using video chat. Technology disruptions due to poor bandwidth may result in reduced effectiveness of social contingency. A minimal and often undetectable timing delay of less than 150 milliseconds reduces optimal communication (Roberts et al., 2009). With good connectivity, frame rates are currently 30 frames per second, and such delays are now unlikely. However, more noticeable delays due to poor connectivity may disrupt infant–adult video chat interactions. For example, after being presented with offset audio and visual content compared to synchronous content, 5-month-old infants showed less recall of the asynchronous content (Bahrick & Lickliter, 2000). Because poor Internet stability and connectivity often results in a loss of audio or visual information, infants may find this aversive or may become inattentive (McClure & Barr, 2017).

Challenges of Eye Contact in Virtual Spaces

Direct eye contact and joint visual attention (JVA), including pointing as a communicative gesture, can also be affected in video chat. JVA is simply "looking where someone else is looking" or, more subtly, "following the direction of attention of another person to the object of their attention" (Bakeman & Adamson, 1984, p. 213). Before 9 months, parents support JVA by adjusting their own gaze to the infant's attention (Bakeman & Adamson, 1984). Starting around 9 months, face-to-face JVA becomes coordinated, and the infant begins to more frequently initiate the exchange of attention, refer to objects (e.g., by looking and pointing at them), and follow the adult's gaze (Bakeman & Adamson, 1984). Unfortunately, with currently available technology at the time of this writing in 2024, direct eye contact is compromised in video chat. Cameras tend to be located above computer monitors and at the top of smartphones, while faces of the on-screen partner are usually displayed in the center of the screen. During video chat, when a person attempts to make eye contact with the face as presented on the screen, that person is directing his or her gaze below the camera's aperture. Therefore, the image that is transmitted to the user's partner is that of the user gazing below the receiver's eye level (Grayson & Monk, 2003). It is also difficult for the video chat partner to interpret if a child points to an object on the screen (that is, to an object in the environment of the video chat partner) due both to the closeness of the child to the screen and the relative position of the camera.

McClure et al. (2018) documented two different primary types of JVA during video chat while observing mothers and their infants in their homes as they video chatted with the infant's remote grandmother. First, *within-screen JVA* was defined as when the JVA initiator directs a partner's attention to an object or person on the initiator's side of the screen (e.g., an infant brings a toy to the screen to show the grandparent; a grandmother shows the infant a peach growing on the grandmother's peach tree). Within-screen JVA is similar to traditional in-person JVA: detecting the initiator's referential visual cues (gaze direction, point, etc.) to something in their own environment is less affected by camera location and visual angles. This shared behavior contrasts with *across-screen JVA*, defined as when the initiator directs a partner's attention to an object or person on the other side of the screen (e.g., the infant points *on the screen* to her remote grandmother's dog). From the point of view of the remote partner, the infant is gazing and pointing from the screen, but the infant's gaze direction and point (actually directed toward the picture on the screen) may or may not align with its referent in the other space (e.g., Grandma's dog in her house), depending on factors such as the infant's and the dog's distance from the respective screens/cameras and the position of the device camera relative to the viewing screen. Across-screen JVA also is more complicated because the participants must coordinate attention, not just between a person and a shared object of interest, but between their separate environments mediated by the screen.

Solutions and Adaptations

Although each of the limitations presents significant challenges to the effectiveness of video chat for engagement and learning, a potential solution involves the value of social relationships for children's early development and how they can be leveraged to solve each problem. Socially contingent adults on both sides of the video chat (that is, the remote partner and the co-viewing parent) can dynamically adapt the typical social supports they use in face-to-face interaction to enable social connection with very young children across a screen. Thus, not only are family social interactions facilitated by video chat, but social supports act as a scaffold for virtual interactions.

Proxy for Navigating the Screen

Given that young infants are unable to control the video chat technology themselves and on-screen partners are limited in their ability to assist, one way to overcome the challenges associated with orienting to information across the screen is to have adults on both sides of the screen to help navigate the space. For instance, in Fig. 9.1, the parent in the room with the child may ask if the child wants to "wear a hat [a cup] like Grandpa on the screen." The adult who is present in the room can be available to interpret any referential markers, reduce perceptual confusion, and fill in details due to connectivity issues or missed social cues that arise during video chat. If the infant points and looks at something that is off screen from the remote partner's perspective or moves the object of reference so close to the screen (the apparent location of the partner) that the object cannot be seen by the on-screen partner, the adults can offer assistance so focus on the object can be shared (McClure &

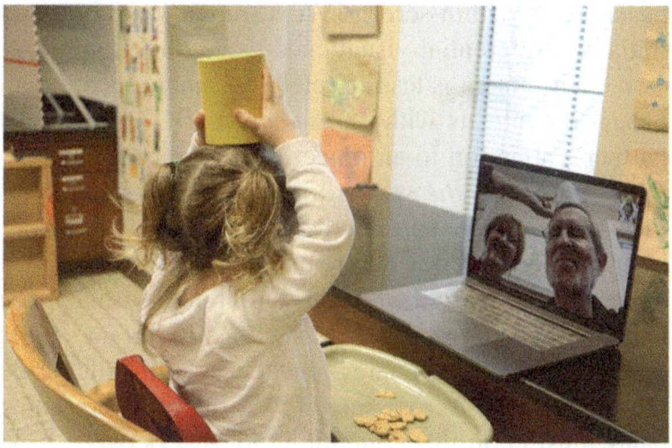

Fig. 9.1 Real-time social game via video chat: imitating on-screen grandparents

Barr, 2017). To make sense of potentially confusing media experiences, children depend on trusted adults who can scaffold the interaction through co-engagement with the medium, helping children understand what happens on the screen (Stevens & Takeuchi, 2011; Strouse et al., 2018). A sensitive adult co-viewer can support children's video chat interactions by making in-the-moment modifications to clarify referential and perceptual confusion. For example, parents may label the on-screen referent of the remote partner's attention or emphasize connections between the two-dimensional image on the screen and three-dimensional reality by reminding children about objects and people they have seen in the real world (e.g., "at Grandma's house") when they appear on the screen—adult support termed "instruction" in DeLoache's theoretical model of symbolic reasoning (DeLoache, 1995; Troseth et al., 2019). Parents may also help to illustrate the utility and relevance of interacting with people on screen by modeling contingent interactions with them (Strouse et al., 2018).

Proxy to Bridge Across Physical Spaces

Naturalistic research has shown that infants make up for the loss of physical contact with the partner on the screen by interacting physically with the person in the room with them (McClure & Barr, 2017). Remote adults and children can simply pretend to touch one another via a virtual high five or pretend to share physical items (including toys and food), and physically present adults can also offer themselves as proxies for physical contact between the remote partner and the child. Caregivers also have been observed acting as a proxy playmate for a remote partner, running after the child with the device in a game of tag, or enabling a game of "This Little Piggy" with the child by acting as the remote partner's hands (McClure & Barr, 2017).

During the COVID-19 pandemic, extended physical separations led families to engage in cultural exchange by means of video chat. They shared meals and family holidays together, passed wisdom about infant care across the generations to sleep-deprived new parents, and took part in a culture of care by using technology to adapt to social distancing (Piper et al., 2023). Access to stable high-speed Internet provided a benefit to family well-being, maintaining multigenerational links with frequent video chat contact during the pandemic (Roche et al., 2022; Strouse et al., 2021).

Social Bridges for Technology Disruption

Caregivers can help support children in situations when, due to technical limitations, a video chat partner appears less responsive than an in-person partner would be. For example, if a screen freezes, a parent might describe poor Wi-Fi as the reason; if the session gets disconnected, parents might reframe as, "Where did Grandma go?" and then, "She'll be right back!" and finally, "There she is!" so that children know what is happening. During family video chat sessions that were part of a longitudinal study, parents and grandparents often successfully navigated Internet disruptions by talking to the child about technology problems (Piper et al., 2023).

Another common challenge, even when families had few disruptions due to connectivity, were disruptions due to calls being ended by the infant pressing a button on the device. Families often quickly recovered from such disruptions by restarting the call or moving the device slightly out of the infant's reach before the call was disconnected. Having an adult co-viewer with the child during video chat served as a social bridge to minimize tech disruptions (Piper et al., 2023).

Adaptation: Virtual Joint Visual Attention (JVA) Is Possible Via Video Chat

A prime example of families' adaptation to the limitations of video chat, while benefiting from the social contingency of video chat, is how they engage in *virtual* JVA (see Fig. 9.2). Due to adults' and infants' adaptability, researchers have observed instances of within-screen JVA on video chat with infants beginning around 8 months of age (McClure et al., 2018; Myers et al., 2024) at the same time as infants' first initiations of traditional JVA at around 9 months (Butterworth, 2004). At 11–12 months of age, infants followed a researcher's head turn and gaze toward an object that was beside the researcher on video chat when the person's eyes were open but not when their eyes were closed (Capparini et al., 2023), showing that babies of this age rely on the appropriate social cue of gaze direction visible on a screen to participate in within-screen JVA.

Successfully establishing across-screen JVA can be more difficult, however, because it requires the responding individual to follow the gaze or other cues they see given by an initiator on screen to a referent in the responding individual's own

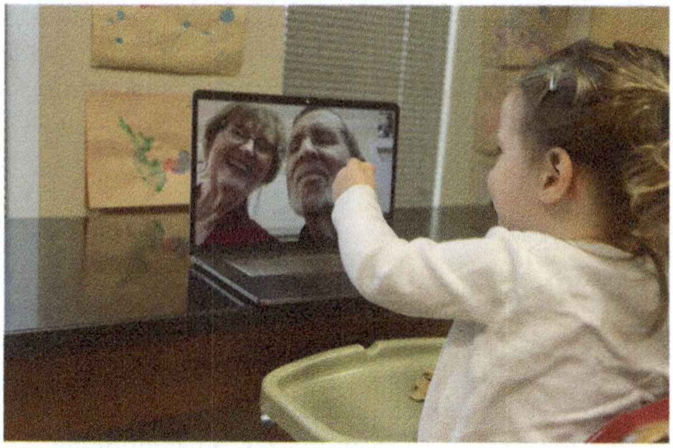

Fig. 9.2 Example of within-screen JVA: a 2-year-old child shows an object to her grandparents on FaceTime

environment. In Myers et al.'s (2024) observations of video chat sessions with infants between 4 and 20 months, the number of sessions that included infant initiations of within-screen JVA was more than three times the number that included any infant initiations of across-screen JVA. To support infant initiations of the more challenging across-screen JVA, a person in the room with the infant might describe to the person across the screen what the infant is pointing to or looking at. When the JVA initiator is an adult who is across the screen from the infant (such as a grandfather referring to the dinosaur on a child's shirt), the adult in the room with the infant may offer support by pointing at or touching the dinosaur to draw the infant's attention to the grandfather's object of reference, in addition to talking about it. They may also touch the infant to redirect their attention. Suarez-Rivera et al. (2019) showed that infants' looks during JVA were longer if the JVA episode included multiple components (e.g., mutual eye gaze, touch, and talk). To support across-screen JVA, these multimodal cues may be provided by adults on both sides of the screen.

Piper et al. (2023) found that families adapted a number of rituals to fit the visual and space parameters of video chat as well. For example, when acting out nursery rhymes, families ensured that dances or gestures remained within the constraints of the screen. One family changed the interactive song "Head, Shoulders, Knees, and Toes" by replacing "Toes" (which could not be seen on the screen) with "Belly button." In this way, families adapted to support interaction based on JVA so that both infants and remote grandparents could participate together.

Unknowns and Future Directions

With increased use of video chat by society, children are getting more exposure to contingent, responsive video of distant relatives and other familiar people, which differs from pretaped video and television in important ways (Troseth et al., 2019). In this new media context, children experience video images that represent real events in real time (e.g., Grandma really is waving at you right now), yet in a distant physical location (e.g., she is not here in the room; she is in her house across town, or across the state, or across the globe). Young children are challenged with learning what aspects of this new kind of social interaction are the same as when the person is present and which are changed by the screen-mediated context. They must learn new social conventions, adapt to the physical limitations for interacting with a person who is not physically present, and learn to engage in a new kind of pretend play involving virtual interaction.

A general category of behaviors that reflect these challenges has been termed "media errors" (Rosengren et al., 2021), instances where children attempt to perform a normally logical action that is impossible with screen media. A famous example of a media error was produced by an empathetic Japanese toddler in 2014: on seeing a disgraced, crying politician (who had been caught in a scandal) on television, the child attempted to wipe his tears with a tissue through the TV screen (Miller, 2015). Media errors were reported frequently by parents of children 1–4 years old, peaking around the beginning of the third year and then declining (Rosengren et al., 2021).

Rosengren and colleagues did not include as media errors behaviors that appeared to be pretend play or that were suggested by an adult. Yet, the physical constraints on interaction using video chat may provoke both spontaneous and adult-supported pretense as well as media errors and new conventional behaviors that are required by the limits of interacting through a screen. For instance, in the context of video chat, it is not possible to share a snack with Grandma or give her a goodbye hug, so what do you do? Parents may suggest and support doing impossible things as a form of engagement with the virtual partner, such as feeding a grandparent on the screen a snack or kissing her through the screen. But do children realize that the grandparent on the other side of the screen is real, or do they view the person as they do a character on TV and possibly develop a "parasocial" relationship (Richards & Calvert, 2017) with this screen-based grandparent? A few examples demonstrate that young children's understanding of these interactions is an area ripe for investigation.

One caregiver shared that their toddler dropped the phone while video chatting with a grandparent, picked up the phone, and asked their grandmother if she was ok. In this case, it appears that the child understood that they were talking to a real human being but did not understand the physical reality of where that grandmother was and how she could (or could not) be hurt by the phone being dropped while video chatting. Another family gave an example of a child video chatting with a grandparent and "sharing" a snack by placing a cracker behind their mother's phone on which the grandparent's face appeared. Did this child assume that the grandparent on the screen could physically access that snack? Similarly, a child who had never met their grandparent in real life due to the pandemic but had video chatted exclaimed, when meeting in person for the first time, "Grandma! You are out of the box!" It is not clear how young children conceptualize the physical reality of their video chat partners, but it is likely that their understanding changes over the course of development.

A colleague reported to us that her 18-month-old toddler, while video chatting with his aunt, took the phone from his mother and placed it on a toy train for a ride as the train went around the room. Our colleague cannot recall whether this was her son's spontaneous pretend play or pretense that she suggested. Whichever was the case, through feedback from his aunt on the phone screen, the child learned that his aunt could see the circuit of the room that the train was making from her (video-augmented) vantage point on the train!

Research on children's developing understanding of pretense and of perspective taking suggests that this kind of video-mediated situation is one that toddlers would not fully understand without adult support. According to Harris (2022), most children begin engaging in pretend play by 24 months, reenacting everyday scenes such as pouring imaginary tea from a teapot or putting a doll to bed. Pretense emerges across cultures at about the same time, whether or not adults actively support it (Callaghan et al., 2011; Harris & Jalloul, 2013), but adult suggestions and modeling, along with offering relevant props, increase the sophistication of children's pretense (Kalkusch et al., 2021). Research by Tomasello et al. (1999) suggests that toddlers under age 2 accurately interpret an adult's pretend gesture (flapping arms to indicate a bird) but have difficulty with a novel pretend identity that an adult might assign to an object (putting a cup on their head, pretending it is a hat). Between the ages 2 and 3, children begin to understand and collaborate with others' pretense (Harris et al., 1993), adopt pretend identities, and interact with imaginary characters who initially are treated as "a sentient but passive recipient of their ministrations" (Harris, 2022, p. 9) but whom older children endow with agency, personalities, and perspectives (Harris, 2000). Thus, with age, children will need less support to understand the kinds of pretense that their parent or grandparent might suggest as a work-around to interact through video chat.

Another aspect of children's development that is relevant to our examples is perspective taking. Preschool children (age 3–6 years) have trouble taking another person's visual perspective to infer what they can see and know (Kampis et al., 2023), but training can help them overcome an egocentric perspective. Researchers have begun to examine how a co-viewing parent supports 2-year-old children's perspective taking in the context of video chat, defined as moving the video chat device to a toy they are trying to show the remote partner or holding the toy up to the camera (Neer et al., 2022).

A different kind of behavior that families engage in and teach their children involves conventional gestures—culturally meaningful emotion-signaling behaviors that are distinct from pretend behaviors. Conventional gestures emerge in infancy, are learned from parents, and reflect exposure to the gestures that are meaningful in a child's culture (Kwon et al., 2018). Over the course of a brief longitudinal video chat study (Piper et al., 2023), parents and grandparents frequently engaged in conventional gestures. Within the new setting of video chat, families typically started and ended their video chat calls with a greeting, and grandparents waved at the child. In turn, parents encouraged their children to "wave to Grandma," in line with the finding that parents' encouragement and "coaching" of their toddlers' practicing of conventional actions supports the adoption of new conventional behaviors (Brezack et al., 2021).

Just as blowing a kiss is a conventional gesture used to express affection when the parties are no longer within arm's reach (e.g., family at the curb blowing kisses to departing loved ones pulling away in the car), families adapted and developed rituals to express emotional closeness within the physical constraints of video chat. Besides commonly blowing a kiss to family members on the other side of the screen, some participants kissed the image of the person on the screen. Family members on both sides of the screen sometimes raised their drinking glasses and said "cheers" in unison, and infants typically also engaged in these conventional gestures (Piper et al., 2023).

Researchers have asked preschoolers what they think about digital social interactions to clarify their understanding of some aspects of this new medium. Bennette et al. (2021) asked 4-year-olds whether they believed that people on video chat could see, hear, feel, or physically interact with someone through the screen. Most children believed the person could see (80%) and could not feel (77%) things on the other side of the screen. They were more split on whether the person could hear (50%) or physically interact (36%) across the screen. Children's responses in comparison conditions in which they were asked about in-person interactions and photographs indicated that children did differentiate video chat from other interactions and images. Thus, before they reach school age, children understand quite a bit about the perceptual affordances of video chat. Adult support in discussing what is possible in unusual situations (such as when a person, not physically present but visible on a screen, can respond contingently to a child) will support children's gradually emerging ability to distinguish what is and is not possible (Nolan-Reyes et al., 2016).

Conclusion

Although best may be the enemy of good when it comes to use of screens by young children, we suggest in this chapter that video chat represents a powerful tool for supporting today's families in building and sustaining relationships. Further, the use of this medium indicates that young children's abilities to engage and learn from others via screens exceed what one might have anticipated based on earlier understanding of young children's social and representational abilities. Research to date shows that families are learning how to support the use of video chat, despite challenges. But one could also argue that while best may be the enemy of the good, perhaps video chat allows young children to engage with *the best that families have to offer*—supportive and contingent interactions with loved ones, even those who are physically apart from us. In this way, video chat allows "the best" to enter the lives of young children in new and dynamic ways that represent a tremendous opportunity for supporting and sustaining social relationships. Both policy and clinical guidance need to reflect nuance not only in children's media guidelines but also in advice shared with families, such that we focus on both in-person *and* virtual ways to foster high-quality supportive relationships in the digital age.

References

Ainsworth, M. D., & Wittig, B. A. (1969). Attachment and exploratory behavior of one-year-olds in a strange situation. In B. M. Foss (Ed.), *Determinants of infant behavior* (Vol. 4, pp. 113–136). Methuen.

Bahrick, L. E., & Lickliter, R. (2000). Intersensory redundancy guides attentional selectivity and perceptual learning in infancy. *Developmental Psychology, 36*(2), 190–201. https://doi.org/10.1037/0012-1649.36.2.190

Bakeman, R., & Adamson, L. (1984). Coordinating attention to people and objects in mother-infant and peer-infant interaction. *Child Development, 55*(4), 1278–1289.

Ballagas, R., Kaye, J. J., Ames, M., Go, J., & Raffle, H. (2009). *Family communication: Phone conversations with children* (pp. 321–324). Proceedings of the 8th International Conference on Interaction Design and Children. https://doi.org/10.1145/1551788.1551874

Barr, R. (2019). Growing up in the digital age: Early learning and family media ecology. *Current Directions in Psychological Science, 28*(4), 341–346. https://doi.org/10.1177/0963721419838245

Bell, V. (2010, February 15). Don't touch that dial! A history of media technology scares, from the printing press to Facebook. *Slate Magazine*. https://slate.com/technology/2010/02/a-history-of-media-technology-scares-from-the-printing-press-to-facebook.html

Bennette, E., Metzinger, A., Lee, M., Ni, J., Nishith, S., Kim, M., & Schachner, A. (2021). Do you see what I see? Children's understanding of perception and physical interaction over video chat. *Human Behavior and Emerging Technologies, 3*(4), 484–494. https://doi.org/10.1002/hbe2.276

Bigelow, A. E. (1996). Infants' memory for contingently responding persons. *Infant Behavior and Development, 19*, 334. https://doi.org/10.1016/S0163-6383(96)90388-4

Bigelow, A. E., MacLean, B. K., & MacDonald, D. (1996). Infants' response to live and replay interactions with self and mother. *Merrill-Palmer Quarterly, 42*(4), 596–611.

Bloom, K., Russell, A., & Wassenberg, K. (1987). Turn taking affects the quality of infant vocalizations. *Journal of Child Language, 14*(2), 211–227. https://doi.org/10.1017/S0305000900012897

Brezack, N., Radovanovic, M., & Woodward, A. L. (2021). Everyday interactions support toddlers' learning of conventional actions on artifacts. *Journal of Experimental Child Psychology, 210*, 105201. https://doi.org/10.1016/j.jecp.2021.105201

Butterworth, G. (2004). Joint visual attention in infancy. In J. G. Bremner & A. Fogel (Eds.), *Blackwell handbook of infant development* (pp. 213–240). Blackwell.

Callaghan, T., Moll, H., Rakoczy, H., Warnek, F., Liszkowski, U., Behne, T., & Tomasello, M. (2011). Early social cognition in three cultural contexts. *Monographs of the Society for Research in Child Development, 76*(2), 1–142.

Capparini, C., To, M. P. S., & Reid, V. M. (2023). Should I follow your virtual gaze? Infants' gaze following over video call. *Journal of Experimental Child Psychology, 226*, 105554. https://doi.org/10.1016/j.jecp.2022.105554

DeLoache, J. S. (1995). Early understanding and use of symbols: The model model. *Current Directions in Psychological Science, 4*, 109–113.

Gaudreau, C., King, Y. A., Dore, R. A., Puttre, H., Nichols, D., Hirsh-Pasek, K., & Golinkoff, R. M. (2020). Preschoolers benefit equally from video chat, pseudo-contingent video, and live book reading: Implications for storytime during the coronavirus pandemic and beyond. *Frontiers in Psychology, 11*. https://doi.org/10.3389/fpsyg.2020.02158

Glick, A. R., Saiyed, F. S., Kutlesa, K., Onishi, K. H., & Nadig, A. S. (2022). Implications of video chat use for young children's learning and social–emotional development: Learning words, taking turns, and fostering familial relationships. *WIREs Cognitive Science, 13*(5), e1599. https://doi.org/10.1002/wcs.1599

Goldstein, M. H., Schwade, J. A., & Bornstein, M. H. (2009). The value of vocalizing: Five-month-old infants associate their own noncry vocalizations with responses from caregivers. *Child Development, 80*(3), 636–644. https://doi.org/10.1111/j.1467-8624.2009.01287.x

Grayson, D. M., & Monk, A. F. (2003). Are you looking at me? Eye contact and desktop video conferencing. *ACM Transactions on Computer-Human Interaction, 10*(3), 221–243. https://doi.org/10.1145/937549.937552

Gusella, J. L., Muir, D., & Tronick, E. Z. (1988). The effect of manipulating maternal behavior during an interaction on three- and six-month-olds' affect and attention. *Child Development, 59*(7), 1111–1124.

Hains, S. M. J., & Muir, D. W. (1996). Effects of stimulus contingency in infant-adult interactions. *Infant Behavior and Development, 19*(1), 49–61. https://doi.org/10.1016/S0163-6383(96)90043-0

Harris, P. L. (2000). *The work of the imagination*. Blackwell Publishing Ltd..

Harris, P. L. (2022). *Children's imagination*. Cambridge University Press.

Harris, P. L., & Jalloul, M. (2013). Running on empty? Observing causal relationships of play and development. *American Journal of Play, 6*(1), 29–38.

Harris, P. L., Kavanaugh, R. D., Wellman, H. M., & Hickling, A. K. (1993). Young children's understanding of pretense. *Monographs of the Society for Research in Child Development, 58*(1), i. https://doi.org/10.2307/1166074

Kampis, D., Lukowski Duplessy, H., Askitis, D., & Southgate, V. (2023). Training self-other distinction facilitates perspective taking in young children. *Child Development, 94*, 956–969. https://doi.org/10.1111/cdev.13912.

Kalkusch, I., Jaggy, A.-K., Burkhardt Bossi, C., Weiss, B., Sticca, F., & Perren, S. (2021). Promoting social pretend play in preschool age: Is providing roleplay material enough? *Early Education and Development, 32*(8), 1136–1152. https://doi.org/10.1080/10409289.2020.1830248

Kucirkova, N. I., Livingstone, S., & Radesky, J. S. (2023). Faulty screen time measures hamper national policies: Here is a way to address it. *Frontiers in Psychology, 14*, 1243396. https://doi.org/10.3389/fpsyg.2023.1243396

Kuhl, P. K., Tsao, F.-M., & Liu, H.-M. (2003). Foreign-language experience in infancy: Effects of short-term exposure and social interaction on phonetic learning. *Proceedings of the National Academy of Sciences, 100*(15), 9096–9101. https://doi.org/10.1073/pnas.1532872100

Kwon, A. Y., Vallotton, C. D., Kiegelmann, M., & Wilhelm, K. H. (2018). Cultural diversification of communicative gestures through early childhood: A comparison of children in English-, German-, and Chinese- speaking families. *Infant Behavior and Development, 50*, 328–339. https://doi.org/10.1016/j.infbeh.2017.10.003

Marian, V., Neisser, U., & Rochat, P. (1996). *Can 2-month-old infants distinguish live from videotaped interactions with their mothers?* (33; Emory Cognition Project). Emory University.

McClure, E., & Barr, R. (2017). Building family relationships from a distance: Supporting connections with babies and toddlers using video and video chat. In *Media exposure during infancy and early childhood: The effects of content and context on learning and development* (pp. 227–248). Springer International Publishing AG. https://doi.org/10.1007/978-3-319-45102-2_15

McClure, E., Chentsova-Dutton, Y. E., Barr, R., Holochwost, S. J., & Parrott, W. G. (2015). "Facetime doesn't count": Video chat as an exception to media restrictions for infants and toddlers. *International Journal of Child-Computer Interaction, 6*, 1–6. https://doi.org/10.1016/j.ijcci.2016.02.002

McClure, E., Chentsova-Dutton, Y. E., Holochwost, S. J., Parrott, W. G., & Barr, R. (2018). Look at that! Video chat and joint visual attention development among babies and toddlers. *Child Development, 89*(1), 27–36. https://doi.org/10.1111/cdev.12833

McClure, E., Chentsova-Dutton, Y., Holochwost, S., Parrott, W. G., & Barr, R. (2020). Infant emotional engagement in face-to-face and video chat interactions with their mothers. *Enfance, 3*, 353–374. https://doi.org/10.3917/enf2.203.0353

Miller, K. K. (2015, November 29). Innocent child's reaction to seeing the bawling politician fills us with "d'awws." *Sora News 24*. https://soranews24.com/2015/11/29/innocent-childs-reaction-to-seeing-the-bawling-politician-fills-us-with-dawws/

Myers, L. J., LeWitt, R. B., Gallo, R. E., & Maselli, N. M. (2017). Baby FaceTime: Can toddlers learn from online video chat? *Developmental Science, 20*(4), e12430. https://doi.org/10.1111/desc.12430

Myers, L. J., Crawford, E., Murphy, C., Aka-Ezoua, E., & Felix, C. (2018). Eyes in the room trump eyes on the screen: Effects of a responsive co-viewer on toddlers' responses to and learning from video chat. *Journal of Children and Media, 12*(3), 275–294. https://doi.org/10.1080/17482798.2018.1425889

Myers, L. J., Keyser, H., & Cors, M. (2019). Co-viewers support participation in video chat interactions, but live experiences promote richer word learning for 24- to 36-month-olds in the USA. *Journal of Children and Media, 13*(4), 415–432. https://doi.org/10.1080/17482798.2019.1646294

Myers, L. J., Strouse, G. A., McClure, E., Keller, K., Neely, L. I., Stoto, I., Vadakattu, N., Kim, E., Troseth, G. L., Barr, R. F., & Zosh, J. M. (2024). Look at grandma! Triadic joint visual attention over video chat during the COVID-19 pandemic. *Infant Behavior and Development., 75*, 101934.

Nadel, J., Carchon, I., Kervella, C., Marcelli, D., & Reserbat-Plantey, D. (1999). Expectancies for social contingency in 2-month-olds. *Developmental Science, 2*(2), 164–173. https://doi.org/10.1111/1467-7687.00065

National Scientific Council on the Developing Child. (2004). *Young children develop in an environment of relationships*. Working Paper No. 1. http://www.developingchild.net

Neer, E. M., Glynn, S. S., & Sandhofer, C. M. (2022, July 7). *Toddler perspective taking during video chat interactions* [Poster]. XXIII International Congress of Infant Studies 2022 Developmental Cascades

Nielsen, M., Simcock, G., & Jenkins, L. (2008). The effect of social engagement on 24-month-olds' imitation from live and televised models. *Developmental Science, 11*(5), 722–731. https://doi.org/10.1111/j.1467-7687.2008.00722.x

Nolan-Reyes, C., Callanan, M. A., & Haigh, K. A. (2016). Practicing possibilities: Parents' explanations of unusual events and Children's possibility thinking. *Journal of Cognition and Development, 17*(3), 378–395. https://doi.org/10.1080/15248372.2014.963224

Parkinson, B., & Lea, M. (2011). Video-linking emotions. In A. Kappas & N. C. Krämer (Eds.), *Face-to-face communication over the internet: Emotions in a web of culture, language and technology* (pp. 100–126). Cambridge University Press. https://doi.org/10.1017/CBO9780511977589.007

Patel, D. (2017). *Why perfection is the enemy of done*. https://www.forbes.com/sites/deeppatel/2017/06/16/why-perfection-is-the-enemy-of-done/?sh=30fb94a94395

Piper, D., Malik, S., Badger, A.-N., Washington, C., Valle, B., Strouse, G. A., Myers, L. J., McClure, E., Troseth, G. L., Zosh, J. M., & Barr, R. (2023). Sharing culture in a tech world: Grandparent–grandchild cultural exchanges over video chat. *Translational Issues in Psychological Science, 9*, 289. https://doi.org/10.1037/tps0000358

Reid Chassiakos, Y. (Linda), Radesky, J., Christakis, D., Moreno, M. A., Cross, C., Council on Communications and Media, Hill, D., Ameenuddin, N., Hutchinson, J., Levine, A., Boyd, R., Mendelson, R., & Swanson, W. S. (2016). Children and adolescents and digital media. *Pediatrics, 138*(5), e20162593. https://doi.org/10.1542/peds.2016-2593

Richards, M. N., & Calvert, S. L. (2017). Measuring young U.S. children's parasocial relationships: Toward the creation of a child self-report survey. *Journal of Children and Media, 11*(2), 229–240. https://doi.org/10.1080/17482798.2017.1304969

Roberts, D., Duckworth, T., Moore, C., Wolff, R., & O'Hare, J. (2009). *Comparing the end to end latency of an immersive collaborative environment and a video conference* (pp. 89–94). 2009 13th IEEE/ACM International Symposium on Distributed Simulation and Real Time Applications. https://doi.org/10.1109/DS-RT.2009.43

Roche, E., Rocha-Hidalgo, J., Piper, D., Strouse, G. A., Neely, L. I., Ryu, J., Myers, L. J., McClure, E., Troseth, G. L., Zosh, J. M., & Barr, R. (2022). Presence at a distance: Video chat supports intergenerational sensitivity and positive infant affect during COVID-19. *Infancy, 27*(6), 1008–1031. https://doi.org/10.1111/infa.12491

Roseberry, S., Hirsh-Pasek, K., & Golinkoff, R. M. (2014). Skype me! Socially contingent interactions help toddlers learn language. *Child Development, 85*(3), 956–970. https://doi.org/10.1111/cdev.12166

Rosengren, K. S., Kirkorian, H., Choi, K., Jiang, M. J., Raimer, C., Tolkin, E., & Sartin-Tarm, A. (2021). Attempting to break the fourth wall: Young children's action errors with screen media. *Human Behavior and Emerging Technologies, 3*(4), 468–483. https://doi.org/10.1002/hbe2.273

Soussignan, R., Nadel, J., Canet, P., & Gerardin, P. (2006). Sensitivity to social contingency and positive emotion in 2-month-olds. *Infancy, 10*(2), 123–144. https://doi.org/10.1207/s15327078in1002_2

Stack, D. M. (2004). The salience of touch and physical contact during infancy: Unraveling some of the mysteries of the somesthetic sense. In G. Bremner & A. Fogel (Eds.), *Blackwell handbook of infant development* (pp. 351–378). Blackwell Publishing Ltd.. https://doi.org/10.1002/9780470996348.ch13

Stevens, R., & Takeuchi, L. M. (2011). *The new coviewing: Designing for learning through joint media engagement*. The Joan Ganz Cooney Center. https://www.scholars.northwestern.edu/en/publications/the-new-coviewing-designing-for-learning-through-joint-media-enga.

Strouse, G. A., & Samson, J. E. (2021). Learning from video: A meta-analysis of the video deficit in children ages 0 to 6 years. *Child Development, 92*(1), e20. https://doi.org/10.1111/cdev.13429

Strouse, G. A., Troseth, G. L., O'Doherty, K. D., & Saylor, M. M. (2018). Co-viewing supports toddlers' word learning from contingent and noncontingent video. *Journal of Experimental Child Psychology, 166*, 310–326. https://doi.org/10.1016/j.jecp.2017.09.005

Strouse, G. A., McClure, E., Myers, L. J., Zosh, J. M., Troseth, G. L., Blanchfield, O., Roche, E., Malik, S., & Barr, R. (2021). Zooming through development: Using video chat to support family connections. *Human Behavior and Emerging Technologies, 3*, 552. https://doi.org/10.1002/hbe2.268

Suarez-Rivera, C., Smith, L. B., & Yu, C. (2019). Multimodal parent behaviors within joint attention support sustained attention in infants. *Developmental Psychology, 55*(1), 96–109. https://doi.org/10.1037/dev0000628

Tarasuik, Galligan, R., & Kaufman, J. (2011). Almost being there: Video communication with young children. *PLoS One, 6*(2), 1–8.

Tarasuik, J., Galligan, R., & Kaufman, J. (2013). Seeing is believing but is hearing? Comparing audio and video communication for young children. *Frontiers in Psychology, 4*. https://doi.org/10.3389/fpsyg.2013.00064

Tomasello, M., Striano, T., & Rochat, P. (1999). Do young children use objects as symbols? *British Journal of Developmental Psychology, 17*(4), 563–584. https://doi.org/10.1348/026151099165483

Troseth, G. L., Saylor, M. M., & Archer, A. H. (2006). Young children's use of video as a source of socially relevant information. *Child Development, 77*(3), 786–799. https://doi.org/10.1111/j.1467-8624.2006.00903.x

Troseth, G. L., Strouse, G. A., Verdine, B. N., & Saylor, M. M. (2018). Let's chat: On-screen social responsiveness is not sufficient to support toddlers' word learning from video. *Frontiers in Psychology, 9*, 2195. https://doi.org/10.3389/fpsyg.2018.02195

Troseth, G. L., Flores, I., & Stuckelman, Z. (2019). When representation becomes reality: Interactive digital media and symbolic development. In J. Benson (Ed.), *Advances in child development and behavior* (Vol. 56, pp. 65–108). Elsevier.

Umberson, D., & Montez, J. (2010). Social relationships and health: A flashpoint for health policy. *Journal of Health and Social Behavior, 51*(1_suppl), S54–S66. https://doi.org/10.1177/0022146510383501

Chapter 10
Parental Overload and the Offer of Digital Media to Children During the COVID-19 Pandemic: A Study of Children's Increase in Usage Time and Introduction of a New Device

Helena Silveira Riter, Gabriela Vescovi, and Giana Bitencourt Frizzo

The use of digital media in childhood has been perceived as a frequent and intense phenomenon (Azevedo et al., 2022). The literature has reported the presence of digital media in more than 90% of families (Rideout & Robb, 2020), including in low- and middle-income countries like Brazil (Azevedo et al., 2022; Nobre et al., 2019). However, there are still significant gaps regarding the factors that promote the use of digital media during childhood. When it comes to infants and preschoolers up to 36 months, this gap is more intense (Azevedo et al., 2022; Nevski & Siibak, 2016). Early childhood is a fundamental period for the development of various capacities such as language, cognitive, and socioemotional abilities (Grantham-McGregor et al., 2007). The intensive use of digital media in early childhood, contrary to the recommendations of various pediatric societies and the World Health Organization (WHO, 2019), seems to have worsened with the COVID-19 pandemic (Carroll et al., 2020; Nyström et al., 2020; Sá et al., 2021). Linhares and Enumo (2020), considering the bioecological model (Bronfenbrenner, 2002) in the context of adversities, suggest that the pandemic and social isolation have modified the family system and the development of children in a disruptive way. Thus, it is possible that the pandemic brings changes in the pattern of digital media use, as well as in parental variables, such as mental health and the social support network (Carroll et al., 2020; Riter et al., 2021; Vescovi et al., 2021), which may represent a risk for child development (Cuartas, 2020; Linhares & Enumo, 2020).

The change in the child's pattern of digital media use is understood here as being composed of two aspects: an increase in usage time and the introduction of a new electronic device. The perception of the time spent in front of screens is the most frequently used way to assess the pattern of media use (Barr et al., 2020; Radesky

H. S. Riter · G. Vescovi · G. B. Frizzo (✉)
Universidade Federal do Rio Grande do Sul, Porto Alegre, RS, Brazil
e-mail: gabriela-vescovi@saude.rs.gov.br; giana.frizzo@ufrgs.br

G. B. Frizzo (ed.), *Digital Media and Early Child Development*,
https://doi.org/10.1007/978-3-031-69224-6_10

et al., 2020), and many studies demonstrate a larger usage time in the context of pandemic (Aguilar-Farias et al., 2020; Carroll et al., 2020; Cartanyà-Hueso et al., 2020; Horiuchi et al., 2020; Nyström et al., 2020; Orgilés et al., 2020; Sá et al., 2021), which can represent an excess in the media usage by children according to WHO recommendations. The introduction of a new device is not a variable commonly addressed in the literature. However, some studies indicate a relationship between a greater number of devices available to children and increased usage time (Dumuid et al., 2016). When it comes to early childhood, one might think that the introduction of a new device by the child could be linked not only to the development of new capabilities but also to a change in family routine, possibly leading to an increase in screen time and moments of use during the day.

Since caregivers mediate children's digital media use (Brito et al., 2017), this phenomenon had already been studied before the pandemic in relation to parents' mental health and loss of support. Regarding mental health, associations have been reported between maternal depressive symptoms and longer children's media usage time (Anand et al., 2014; Conners et al., 2007; Park et al., 2018). During the pandemic, the literature indicates moderate to severe levels of psychological stress among parents (Wang et al., 2020), as well as associations between the context of the pandemic and the risk of common mental disorders (CMD; Duarte et al., 2020), such as anxiety and depression (Martins et al., 2021; Vescovi et al., 2021). Positive associations were also found between symptoms of CMD in parents and intention to offer media to children during COVID-19 health emergency (Pedrotti et al., 2021) and greater use of screens by children of parents with higher levels of mental health issues (Orgilés et al., 2020).

In contrast, social support is a protective factor in stressful situations, promoting the quality of the parent–child relationship (Rapoport & Piccinini, 2006). Social support has been associated with opportunities for families to avoid excessive use of digital media by children (Conners et al., 2007; Lampard et al., 2013). Pre-pandemic research already reported that digital media can represent a resource that parents and mothers turn to in times of lack of support for childcare (Mallmann & Frizzo, 2019; Rosa et al., 2020). The closing of preschools and the loss of support networks for childcare were significant repercussions of the pandemic on family life (Cluver et al., 2020), representing an accumulation of care and work functions within the home. Thus, certain groups experienced the pandemic in particular ways, and among these are families with children (Holmes et al., 2020).

We conducted the present study considering that the use of digital media in early childhood is a relevant phenomenon that was increased by the COVID-19 pandemic and that parental mental health and the loss of social support have been a concern during the pandemic. The aim of this study was (a) to describe the parental perception of changes in the pattern of digital media use by infants and toddlers during the pandemic (i.e., increase in usage time and introduction of a new type of electronic device in the routine), as well as the following parental variables: loss of support due to the pandemic and symptoms of CMD, and (b) to verify differences between groups of children according to (1) the increase in usage time during the pandemic and (2) the introduction of a new device during the pandemic, regarding parental mental health, loss of support, and the child's age.

Method

This is a cross-sectional correlational study (Johnson, 2001). An online questionnaire was disseminated via social networks and the researchers' contact lists. Data collection was conducted in Brazil from May 27 to June 15, 2020. All ethical precautions for conducting research with human beings were met.

The participants of this study were 231 mothers (91.8%) and fathers aged 20–48 years (M = 33.84 years; SD = 4.84). Their children (55.4% female) were up to 36 months old (M = 17.02 months; SD = 9.88) and presented typical development as reported by their caregivers. Most of the participants lived with a partner (92.6%) and reported having only one child (74.5%). Regarding the time spent with the child during social isolation, 47.6% declared spending most of the day with the child but sharing the care with another adult, and 45.5% claimed to spend the whole day with the child without sharing.

Parents answered a sociodemographic questionnaire that included a question about their loss of support: *Due to the pandemic, did you lose any of these childcare supports? Check all that apply*. The options were *(a) Help from other family members and/or friends (grandparents, uncles, godmother, godfather, neighbors), (b) Daycare*, *(c) Nanny*, and *(d) I did not have any of these support before COVID-19.* Subsequently, the first three items were added together, indicating the loss of a support network due to the pandemic. Therefore, the score could vary between 0 and 3, and the higher the score, the more sources of support the family lost. Parents also answered the following questions about media use: *(a) During the quarantine, do you consider that your child's media use was greater, less, or the same as before the quarantine?* and *(b) During the quarantine, did your child start using any of these devices that they did not use before the quarantine? Check all that apply*. The options were *(a) Television*, *(b) Smartphone*, *(c) Tablet*, *(d) Computer*, and *(e) None*. Subsequently, the answers to the second question were dichotomized into yes (if the participant marked at least one of the four devices mentioned) and no (if the participant marked the "None" option). The instrument *Self-Reporting Questionnaire (SRQ-20)*, which assesses the presence of symptoms of common mental disorders, was also used.

The data were submitted to descriptive analyses (frequency, mean, and standard deviation) for sample characterization. With the aim of investigating to what extent the child's age (months), the loss of support during the pandemic, and the score of CMD symptoms were different in children who (1) increased their media use time during the pandemic compared to those who did not increase and (2) started using a new electronic device during the pandemic compared to those who did not start, we used Mann–Whitney *U*-test for independent samples.

Results

At the time of data collection, 88.7% of the sample considered themselves to be in social isolation due to the COVID-19 pandemic, with 61.9% reporting being engaged in work and/or study activities at home. The majority were middle-class and highly educated. Even so, 56.3% reported having decreased income due to the pandemic.

Regarding the change in the pattern of digital media use by children during the pandemic, 66.7% of participants stated that their child's usage time increased. In comparison, 33.3% stated that the time remained the same. Also, 42.9% reported having included at least one new type of digital media in the child's routine during the first months of social isolation. The loss of support sources was significant, and all families that had any of the evaluated support sources (80.1% of the total sample) faced losing at least one of these resources due to the pandemic (Table 10.1).

Regarding the SRQ-20 score, 46.3% of the participants were above the cut-off point for the presence of common mental disorder symptoms. The results of the group comparison (Table 10.2) showed that the children who increased their digital media usage time during the pandemic had a higher average age (M = 20.35 months; SD = 8.78); that is, they were older than the children who did not increase their usage time (M = 10.35 months; SD = 8.54).

The Mann–Whitney analysis indicated that there were differences only in the increase of usage time ($p < 0.001$) but not in the introduction of a new device ($p = 0.191$). Children who increased their usage time during the pandemic were older ($p < 0.001$) and had parents with higher averages of CMD symptoms ($p = 0.025$) and loss of support ($p < 0.001$). There was no interaction between the variables of increased time and device introduction.

Table 10.1 Reported loss of support ($N = 231$)

	N	%
Lost support source		
Daycare	114	49.4%
Help from relatives and/or friends	109	47.2%
Nanny	30	13.0%
None	46	19.9%
Number of lost support sources		
One	122	52.8%
Two	58	25.1%
Three	5	2.2%

Table 10.2 Mean and standard deviation of parental variables and child's age in relation to changes in usage pattern

	Changes in usage pattern	Group	*N*	Mean	SD	SE
SRQ score	Increase in time	Yes	154	7.65	4.21	0.34
		No	77	6.31	4.32	0.49
	Device insertion	Yes	99	7.85	4.11	0.41
		No	132	6.72	4.36	0.38
Loss of support	Increase in time	Yes	154	1.30	0.69	0.05
		No	77	0.67	0.59	0.06
	Device insertion	Yes	99	1.22	0.66	0.06
		No	132	1.00	0.76	0.06
Child's age	Increase in time	Yes	154	20.35	8.78	0.70
		No	77	10.35	8.54	0.97
	Device insertion	Yes	99	18.71	9.08	0.91
		No	132	15.74	10.29	0.89

Note. SD standard deviation, *SE* standard error

Discussion

The results of this study indicate a scenario of parental overload, with significant loss of support for childcare, as well as high rates of CMD symptoms, despite the medium-to-high socioeconomic level of the sample in the context of a middle-income country. Also, the increase in digital media usage time was present for most children, while the insertion of a new device during the pandemic was less frequent.

Regarding the increase in usage time during the pandemic, the results corroborate other studies that have verified the same phenomenon (Aguilar-Farias et al., 2020; Carroll et al., 2020; Nyström et al., 2020; Sá et al., 2021). The increase ranged from 74.9% (Sá et al., 2021) to 87% (Carroll et al., 2020) or reported an increase of 30 minutes (Nyström et al., 2020) to 1.4 h (Aguilar-Farias et al., 2020).

Considering the age of the children, the results pointed out that those who increased their usage time during the pandemic were older than those who did not have this increase. This result has been corroborated by different studies, which also suggest that children in the second year of life would be more prone to an increase in media exposure (Aguilar-Farias, 2021; Ribner & McHarg, 2021; Pedrotti et al., 2021), possibly due to developmental aspects. These data draw attention to the need for early interventions since the pattern of media use throughout life is established in early childhood (McArthur et al., 2020).

Regarding the introduction of a new device into the routine, no research was found that evaluated this variable during the pandemic. Most of the research conducted during this period only evaluated the usage time (Aguilar-Farias et al., 2020; Carroll et al., 2020; Nyström et al., 2020; Sá et al., 2021). The literature in the field has reflected on measures related to the use of digital media since considering only the usage time does not seem to contemplate the phenomenon's complexity (Barr et al., 2020; Radesky et al., 2020). Thus, this study sought to contribute to the field, including another variable to evaluate the pattern of media use by young children.

Both variables of change in the pattern of use (increase in time and introduction of device) are related to the demands that arise from social distancing, such as educational purposes, maintaining bonds with family and friends, and carrying out extracurricular activities, besides the use for distracting the children so that parents can perform other tasks (Dore et al., 2021; Carroll et al., 2020). According to these authors, the use of digital media for the abovementioned purposes occurred because of social isolation, not being common activities before the pandemic. Despite this, the insertion of a new device did not show significant results in this sample.

This discussion is related to the significant loss of support found in this study, demonstrating the need to reorganize the care for children, as pointed out in the literature (Cluver et al., 2020; Vescovi et al., 2021). Most caregivers reported carrying out work and/or study activities at home (61.9%), suggesting an accumulation of demands for parents. Previous studies have demonstrated the relevance of social support in terms of parents' ability to implement parenting practices that promote children's development (Rapoport & Piccinini, 2006; Serrano-Villar et al., 2017). Thus, these results seem to meet the concerns of specialists about the effects of the pandemic and the need to consider families with children as a priority group for the development of intervention policies (Holmes et al., 2020).

The high prevalence (46.3%) of CMD symptoms found in the present study represents a worrying result. Studies prior to the pandemic that also used the SRQ-20 in samples of Brazilian mothers found lower prevalences: 23.1% (Bandeira et al., 2020) and 37.6% (Carmo et al., 2018). However, research conducted during the pandemic has also reported high prevalences of symptoms of depression and anxiety (Giordani et al., 2021; Martins et al., 2021). Also, according to the rapid systematic review by Vescovi et al. (2021), different studies found more symptoms of depression, anxiety, and stress in samples of parents, mothers, and pregnant women during the pandemic. The same result was found by Pedrotti et al. (2021), when comparing the mental health of mothers before and during the pandemic.

In general, the literature has reported stressors associated with parenting during the pandemic, such as the distancing from family and friends, closure of schools and online school activities, loss of support, accumulation of demands, and financial insecurity (Calvano et al., 2020; Carroll et al., 2020; Chung et al., 2020). From our results, it can be inferred that the participants of this study were exposed to similar distal stressors, as they had to meet work and care demands, having suffered financial losses and loss of support sources. Thus, according to the literature, the high prevalence of CMD symptoms found in this sample may be related to the context of parenthood in the pandemic, highlighting the need for support and public policies in order to protect the well-being of parents and children (Calvano et al., 2020; Carroll et al., 2020; Chung et al., 2020).

The group comparison results make it possible to perceive relations between parental overload and the expansion of children's media use in the pandemic. Children who increased their screen time during the pandemic had mothers and fathers with greater loss of support and worse mental health (more CMD symptoms). This change in children's media use pattern was more reported among parents with greater loss of support. It may demonstrate the need to use electronic resources at more moments of the day due to the accumulation of demands and loss of support. It is known that digital media represent a source of support in childcare (Rosa et al., 2020) and that excessive use of media by children may be associated with a lack of social support for parents (Conners et al., 2007; Lampard et al., 2013). Other studies with parents of infants and toddlers reported an association between the adult's need to entertain the child and the use of digital media (Azevedo et al., 2022; Kabali et al.,2015; Mallmann & Frizzo, 2019; Pedrotti et al., 2021).

Also, the literature already points to the relationship between parental mental disorders and the greater use of digital media by children. For example, children of fathers and mothers who report depressive symptoms are at risk for early exposure (Anand et al., 2014), use above the recommended guidelines (Conners et al., 2007; Park et al., 2018), and exposure to content inappropriate for their age (Conners et al., 2007). A systematic review of factors associated with screen use in children under 3 years found a positive correlation with parental depression (Duch et al., 2013). Thus, it is possible to note that factors more distal to the child, like the COVID-19 pandemic and parental overload (understood as a loss of support and presence of CMD symptoms), seem to be related to more proximal factors (Bronfenbrenner, 2002), like the offering of digital media.

Therefore, it is crucial to consider intervention programs that focus on parental overload since this may remain even after the pandemic has subsided. More overloaded parents and those with fragile support systems may resort to less adaptive parenting practices, such as offering more digital media to young children.

Final Considerations

The present study accessed the changes in the digital media use pattern by young children and its relations with parental overload in a stressful context like the pandemic. The results indicated changes in the usage pattern (increase in time and introduction of a new device) due to the pandemic. The increase in usage time was more common among older children and with more overloaded mothers and fathers (greater loss of support and worse mental health). Despite these relevant results, this study has as limitations the participants' high levels of education and income. The way of access via online data collection is probably related to this bias, not reaching families in a situation of greater social vulnerability. Even so, online collections were a safe option for conducting research during the COVID-19 pandemic. It is also necessary to consider that the study was conducted in the initial period of the pandemic in Brazil (June 2020), when the first peak in the number of deaths was happening, creating a scenario of anxieties and uncertainties.

The cross-sectional and retrospective design prevented the follow-up of changes in media usage patterns over time, which would provide relevant data. Thus, future studies may focus on longitudinal follow-ups, seeking to understand not only the changes in media use precipitated by the pandemic but also by the child's own developmental cycle. New studies, including participants with greater socioeconomic variability, should be conducted to assess how and what changes occurred and their impact on family life.

Focusing on parental mental health and loss of support, this study provides important information for interventions to support parenting and child development in the post-pandemic period. Furthermore, it advances the discussion around ways of accessing digital media usage patterns, including the variable of introducing a new device, which is not commonly evaluated in the literature.

References

Aguilar-Farias, N., Toledo-Vargas, M., Miranda-Marquez, S., Cortinez-O'Ryan, A., Cristi-Montero, C., Rodriguez-Rodriguez, F., Martino-Fuentealba, P., Okely, A. D., & Del Pozo Cruz, B. (2020). Sociodemographic predictors of changes in physical activity, screen time, and sleep among toddlers and preschoolers in Chile during the COVID-19 pandemic. *International Journal of Environmental Research and Public Health, 18*(1), 176. https://doi.org/10.3390/ijerph18010176

Anand, V., Downs, S. M., Bauer, N. S., & Carroll, A. E. (2014). Prevalence of infant television viewing and maternal depression symptoms. *Journal of Development and Behavior Pediatrics, 35*(3), 216–224. https://doi.org/10.1097/DBP.0000000000000035

Azevedo, E. C., da Riter, H. S., Pieta, M. A. M., & Frizzo, G. B. (2022). Digital media use on interactions between mother and child: Differences in infants' early years. *Paidéia (Ribeirão Preto), 32*, e3210. https://doi.org/10.1590/1982-4327e3210

Bandeira, D. R., Azevedo, E. C., Cattani, B. C., da Silva, M. A., Mendonça Filho, E., & Frizzo, G. B. (2020). Factors associated with mental health in mothers with children under seven. *Psicothema, 32*(3), 346–351. https://doi.org/10.7334/psicothema2019.71

Barr, R., Kirkorian, H., Radesky, J., Coyne, S., Nichols, D., Blanchfield, O., Rusnak, S., Stockdale, L., Ribner, A., Durnez, J., Epstein, M., Heimann, M., Koch, F. S., Sundqvist, A., Birberg-Thornberg, U., Konrad, C., Slussareff, M., Bus, A., Bellagamba, F., & Fitzpatrick, C. (2020). Beyond screen time: A synergistic approach to a more comprehensive assessment of family media exposure during early childhood. *Frontiers in Psychology, 11*(1283). https://doi.org/10.3389/fpsyg.2020.01283

Barreto do Carmo, M. B., Santos, L. M., Feitosa, C. A., Fiaccone, R. L., Silva, N. B., Santos, D. N., et al. (2018). Screening for common mental disorders using the SRQ-20 in Brazil: What are the alternative strategies for analysis? *Brazilian Journal of Psychiatry, 40*(2), 115–122. https://doi.org/10.1590/1516-4446-2016-2139

Brito, R., Francisco, R., Dias, P., & Chaudron, S. (2017). Family dynamics in digital homes: The role played by parental mediation in young children's digital practices around 14 European countries. *Contemporary Family Therapy, 39*(4), 271–280. https://doi.org/10.1007/s10591-017-9431-0

Bronfenbrenner, U. (2002). *A Ecologia do Desenvolvimento Humano: Experimentos naturais e planejados*. Artes Médicas (Original publicado em 1996).

Carroll, N., Sadowski, A., Laila, A., Hruska, V., Nixon, M., Ma, D. W. L., & Haines, J. (2020). The impact of COVID-19 on health behavior, stress, financial and food security among middle to high income Canadian families with young children. *Nutrients, 12*(8), 2352. https://doi.org/10.3390/nu12082352

Chung, G., Lanier, P., & Wong, P. Y. J. (2020). Mediating effects of parental stress on harsh parenting and parent-child relationship during coronavirus (COVID-19) pandemic in Singapore. *Journal of Family Violence*. https://doi.org/10.1007/s10896-020-00200-1

Cluver, L., Lachman, J. M., Sherr, L., Wessels, I., Krug, E., Rakotomalala, S., et al. (2020). Parenting in a time of COVID-19. *The Lancet, 395*(10231), e64. https://doi.org/10.1016/S0140-6736(20)30736-4

Conners, N. A., Tripathi, S. P., Clubb, R., & Bradley, R. H. (2007). Maternal characteristics associated with television viewing habits of low-income preschool children. *Journal of Child and Family Studies, 16*(3), 415–425. https://doi.org/10.1007/s10826-006-9095-0

Cuartas, J. (2020). Heightened risk of child maltreatment amid the COVID-19 pandemic can exacerbate mental health problems for the next generation. *Psychological Trauma: Theory, Research, Practice, Policy, 12*(S1), S195–S196. https://doi.org/10.1037/tra0000597

Dore, R. A., Purtell, K. M., & Justice, L. M. (2021). Media use among kindergarteners from low-income households during the COVID-19 shutdown. *Journal of Developmental & Behavioral Pediatrics, Publish Ahead of Print., 42*, 672. https://doi.org/10.1097/DBP.0000000000000955

Duarte, M. Q., Santo, M. A. S., Lima, C. P., Giordani, J. P., & Trentini, C. M. (2020). COVID-19 e os impactos na saúde mental: Uma amostra do Rio Grande do Sul, Brasil. *Ciência & Saúde Coletiva, 25*(9), 3401–3412. https://doi.org/10.1590/1413-81232020259.16472020

Duch, H., Fisher, E. M., Ensari, I., & Harrington, A. (2013). Screen time use in children under 3 years old: A systematic review of correlates. *International Journal of Behavioral Nutrition and Physical Activity, 10*, 1–10. https://doi.org/10.1186/1479-5868-10-102

Dumuid, D., Olds, T. S., Lewis, L. K., & Maher, C. (2016). Does home equipment contribute to socioeconomic gradients in Australian children's physical activity, sedentary time and screen time? *BMC Public Health, 16*, 736. https://doi.org/10.1186/s12889-016-3419-9

Giordani, J. P., Lima, C. P., Duarte, M. Q., Santo, M. A. S., Czepielewski, L. S., & Trentini, C. (2021). COVID-19 and Brazilian's mental health: Risk factors and related symptoms. *Psicologia: Teoria e Prática, 23*(1), 1–19. https://doi.org/10.5935/1980-6906/ePTPC1913993

Gonçalves, D. M., Stein, A. T., & Kapczinski, F. (2008). Avaliação de desempenho do self-reporting questionnaire Como instrumento de rastreamento psiquiátrico: Um estudo comparativo com o structured clinical interview for DSM-IV-TR. *Cadernos de Saúde Pública, 24*(2), 380–390. https://doi.org/10.1590/S0102-311X2008000200017

Grantham-McGregor, S., Cheung, Y. B., Cueto, S., Glewwe, P., Richter, L., Strupp, B., & International Child Development Steering Group. (2007). Developmental potential in the first 5 years for children in developing countries. *The Lancet, 369*(9555), 60–70. https://doi.org/10.1016/s0140-6736(07)60032-4

Holmes, E. A., O'Connor, R. C., Perry, V. H., Tracey, I., Wessely, S., Arseneault, L., et al. (2020). Multidisciplinary research priorities for the COVID-19 pandemic: A call for action for mental health science. *Lancet Psychiatry, 7*, 547–560. https://doi.org/10.1016/S2215-0366(20)30168-1

Johnson, B. (2001). Toward a new classification of nonexperimental quantitative research. *Educational Researcher, 30*(2), 3–13. https://doi.org/10.3102/0013189x030002003

Lampard, A. M., Jurkowski, J. M., & Davison, K. K. (2013). The family context of low-income parents who restrict child screen time. *Childhood Obesity, 9*(5), 386–392. https://doi.org/10.1089/chi.2013.0043

Linhares, M. B. M., & Enumo, S. R. F. (2020). Reflexões baseadas na Psicologia sobre efeitos da pandemia COVID-19 no desenvolvimento infantil. *Estudos de Psicologia (Campinas), 37*, e200089. https://doi.org/10.1590/1982-0275202037e200089

Mallmann, M. Y., & Frizzo, G. B. (2019). O uso das novas tecnologias em famílias com bebês: Um mal necessário? *Revista Cocar. Edição Especial. Dossiê: Crianças, mídias e mediações, 7*, 26–46.

Martins, C. R., Neiva, A. C. L., Bahia, A. F., Oliveira, C. X., Cardoso, M. I. S., & Abreu, J. N. S. (2021). Parents' mental health and children's emotional regulation during the COVID-19 pandemic. *Psicologia: Teoria e Prática, 23*(1), 1–19. https://doi.org/10.5935/1980-6906/ePTPC1913554

McArthur, B. A., Browne, D., Tough, S., & Madigan, S. (2020). Trajectories of screen use during early childhood: Predictors and associated behavior and learning outcomes. *Computers in Human Behavior, 113*, 106501. https://doi.org/10.1016/j.chb.2020.106501

Nevski, E., & Siibak, A. (2016). The role of parents and parental mediation on 0–3-year olds' digital play with smart devices: Estonian parents' attitudes and practices. *Early Years, 36*(3), 1–15. https://doi.org/10.1080/09575146.2016.1161601

Nobre, J. N. P., Santos, J. N., Santos, L. R., Guedes, S. C., Pereira, L., Costa, J. M., & Morais, R. L. S. (2019). Fatores determinantes no tempo de Tela de crianças na primeira infância. *Ciência & Saúde Coletiva [Periódico Na Internet]*. Retrieved from http://www.cienciaesaudecoletiva.com.br/artigos/fatores-determinantes-no-tempo-de-tela-de-criancas-na-primeira-infancia/17321

Nyström, D., Alexandrou, C., Henström, C., Nilsson, M. E., Okely, A. D., Wehbe El Masri, S., & Löf, M. (2020). International Study of Movement Behaviors in the Early Years (SUNRISE): Results from SUNRISE Sweden's Pilot and COVID-19 Study. *International Journal of Environmental Research and Public Health, 17*(22), 8491. https://doi.org/10.3390/ijerph17228491

Orgilés, M., Morales, A., Delvecchio, E., Mazzeschi, C., & Espada, J. P. (2020). Immediate psychological effects of the COVID-19 quarantine in youth from Italy and Spain. *Frontiers in Psychology, 11*(579038). https://doi.org/10.3389/fpsyg.2020.579038

Park, S., Chang, H. Y., Park, E., Yoo, H., Jo, W., Kim, S., & Shin, Y. (2018). Maternal depression and children's screen overuse. *Journal of Korean Medical Science, 33*(34), 1–10. https://doi.org/10.3346/jkms.2018.33.e219

Pedrotti, B. G., Mallmann, M. Y., Almeida, C. R. S., Marques, F. M., Vescovi, G., Riter, H. S., Almeida, M. L., Pieta, M. A. M., & Frizzo, G. B. (2021). Infants' and toddlers' digital media use and mothers' mental health: A comparative study before and during the COVID-19 pandemic. *Infant Mental Health Journal, 43*(1), 24–35. https://doi.org/10.1002/imhj.21952

Radesky, J. S., Weeks, H. M., Ball, R., Schaller, A., Yeo, S., Durnez, J., et al. (2020). Young children's use of smartphones and tablets. *Pediatrics, 146*(1), 1–10. https://doi.org/10.1542/peds.2019-3518

Rapoport, A., & Piccinini, C. A. (2006). Apoio social e experiência da maternidade. *Revista Brasileira de Crescimento e Desenvolvimento Humano, 16*(1), 85–96. https://doi.org/10.7322/jhgd.19783

Ribner, A. D., & McHarg, G. (2021). Screens across the pond: Findings from longitudinal screen time research in the US and UK. *Infant Behavior and Development, 63*, 101551. https://doi.org/10.1016/j.infbeh.2021.101551

Rideout, V., & Robb, M. B. (2020). *The common sense census: Media use by kids age zero to eight, 2020*. Common Sense Media.

Riter, H. S., Almeida, M. L., Vescovi, G., Marques, F. M., Pedrotti, B. G., Mallmann, M. Y., Pieta, M. A. M., & Frizzo, G. B. (2021). Symptoms of common mental disorders in Brazilian parents during the COVID-19 pandemic: Associated factors. *Psychological Studies Journal, 66*, 270. https://doi.org/10.1007/s12646-021-00609-8

Rosa, L. C., Pedrotti, B. G., Mallmann, M. Y., & Frizzo, G. B. (2020). O Papel da Coparentalidade e da Rede de Apoio Materna no Uso de Mídias Digitais por Bebês. *Contextos Clínicos, 13*(3), 786–806. https://doi.org/10.4013/ctc.2020.133.04

Sá, C. S. C., Pombo, A., Luz, C., Rodrigues, L. P., & Cordovil, R. (2021). COVID-19 social isolation in Brazil: Effects on the physical activity routine of families with children. *Revista Paulista de Pediatria, 39*(e2020159), e2020159. https://doi.org/10.1590/1984-0462/2021/39/2020159

Serrano-Villar, M., Huang, K. Y., & Calzada, E. J. (2017). Social support, parenting, and social emotional development in young Mexican and Dominican American children. *Child Psychiatry & Human Development, 48*, 597–609. https://doi.org/10.1007/s10578-016-0685-9

Vescovi, G., Riter, H. S., Azevedo, E. C., Pedrotti, B. G., & Frizzo, G. B. (2021). Parenting, mental health, and COVID-19: A rapid systematic review. *Psicologia: Teoria e Prática, 23*(1), 1–28. https://doi.org/10.5935/1980-6906/ePTPC1913554

Wang, C., Pan, R., Wan, X., Tan, Y., Xu, L., Ho, C. S., & Ho, R. C. (2020). Immediate psychological responses and associated factors during the initial stage of the 2019 coronavirus disease (COVID-19) epidemic among the general population in China. *International Journal of Environmental Research and Public Health, 17*(1729), 1–25. https://doi.org/10.3390/ijerph17051729

Chapter 11
Relationship Between Early Childhood Development and Digital Media Use During the COVID-19 Pandemic in Brazil

Mônia Aparecida da Silva, Clarice Oliveira Campos, Letícia Carvalho Leão, and Bruno Carlos Ferreira

Introduction

The worldwide COVID-19 pandemic has played a significant role in the adoption of technological resources and the proliferation of screens in households (Hatschbach Ourique et al., 2020). Screens have skyrocketed across the global population at an unprecedented pace and scale during social distancing and lockdowns (Santos et al., 2022). As people have spent extended periods at home, screen usage has surged to meet work-related and leisure/entertainment needs.

Simultaneously, screen usage among children has experienced a remarkable increase. Furthermore, the age at which children first engage with screens has decreased, contributing to early exposure (Choi et al., 2021; Yoo, 2021). Early exposure to screens and its consequences raise concerns among researchers, professionals, and policymakers across various fields (Ribner & McHarg, 2021), transforming into a pressing issue for global public policies (Hua et al., 2022). During the pandemic, children have become significantly more involved with screens (Ribner et al., 2021). Consequently, excessive screen time has raised substantial concerns,

The research in this chapter was conducted as part of the Clarice Oliveira Campos undergraduate research under the guidance of Mônia Aparecida da Silva, funded by The National Council for Scientific and Technological Development (CNPq).

M. A. da Silva (✉) · L. C. Leão · B. C. Ferreira
Universidade Federal de São João del Rei, São João del Rei, Brazil
e-mail: monia@ufsj.edu.br; brunobps58@aluno.ufsj.edu.br

C. O. Campos
Universidade Federal de São João del Rei, São João del Rei, Brazil

Universidade do Algarve, Faro, Portugal
e-mail: cocampos@ualg.pt

G. B. Frizzo (ed.), *Digital Media and Early Child Development*,
https://doi.org/10.1007/978-3-031-69224-6_11

particularly in early childhood (Rocha & Nunes, 2020; Portugal et al., 2023; Varadarajan et al., 2021), a critical phase characterized by intensified brain development and the formation of complex neural connections. This period is susceptible to beneficial and detrimental environmental influences, making variables such as screen usage particularly impactful on development (Crespi et al., 2023).

Current studies indicate that families and children are not adhering to the screen usage recommendations and guidelines provided by institutions such as the American Academy of Pediatrics (AAP, 2016) and the World Health Organization (WHO, 2019). For instance, a study by Durham et al. (2021) involving 630 German children aged 12 months found that 45% of the participants had already been exposed to screens before their first birthday. Similarly, a study by Varadarajan et al. (2021) revealed that 89% of 718 Indian children had been exposed to at least one type of screen before 24 months. In Brazil, research conducted by Nobre et al. (2021) with children aged 24–42 months found that the average daily screen time exceeded 2 h. Another Brazilian study by Arantes and Morais (2022) emphasized that out of 102 participating children in early childhood, all had been exposed to screen devices before age 2, with 83% initiating screen usage before their first year.

Beyond the prevalence of screen usage in childhood, attention has been given to the consequences of screen time on development. Development is how each child evolves from helpless infancy to independent adulthood. It involves growth and development usually divided into five main domains: performance and cognition, gross and fine motor skills, speech and language, socio-emotional development, and adaptive behavior (Bellman et al., 2013). Some research findings have already indicated associations between screen use in childhood and various developmental domains. Kim et al. (2021) identified that excessive screen usage was negatively associated with the social, emotional, and cognitive development of 2- to 5-year-old children in South Korea. Similarly, a study in South Korea concluded that excessive screen exposure was linked to behavioral, emotional, and social problems (Choi et al., 2021). Owenz and Fowers (2020) found that continuous daily screen time of more than 2 h was associated with poor sleep quality, language acquisition difficulties, and attention problems in young children. Moreover, screen time exceeding 2 h was negatively correlated with children's mental and physical health (Owenz & Fowers, 2020). In a study by Hosokawa and Katsura (2018) conducted in Japan with 5- and 6-year-old children, excessive smartphone and tablet use was associated with a higher likelihood of behavior problems, increased social isolation, and negative impacts on social skills.

Within the Brazilian context, a study conducted by Rocha et al. (2021) with a sample of 3155 children aged 0–60 months (0–5 years) concluded that 7 out of 10 children were excessively exposed to screen time when considering the recommendations of the WHO (2019) and the Brazilian Society of Pediatrics (BSP; Sociedade Brasileira de Pediatria, 2019). Furthermore, increased screen time was associated with poorer outcomes in communication, problem-solving, and personal-social development domains, as assessed by the Brazilian version of the Ages and Stages Questionnaire (ASQ-3) (Rocha et al., 2021). It is important to note that most studies have solely focused on screen time, potentially overlooking important information when evaluating screen usage. The effects of screen time also depend on its context of use (Viner et al., 2019), which means that in addition to time, the content and types of devices can impact child development differently (Rocha & Nunes, 2020). The co-engagement and mediated use of screens by adults can influence the outcomes of screen usage, leading to either negative or positive consequences for development (Gaudreau et al., 2020; Rocha & Nunes, 2020).

To further expand studies on this topic in Brazil, this chapter presents a mixed methodology design that explores how digital media was used in families with infants and children up to 42 months old and its relationship with infant development during the COVID-19 pandemic. The quantitative approach aimed to establish associations between variables, while the qualitative design aimed to understand the experiences and perceptions of families regarding technology use. The study has investigated different aspects of digital media use, including screen media type, its relation to children's development, and the connection between parental use and children's use. As part of the qualitative design, focus groups were conducted with mothers of children aged 12–36 months. The objective was to shed light on the impact of digital media use on child development and understand the dynamics and experiences within these families.

Carrying Out this Study

The quantitative sample comprised 53 mothers and 1 father of infants and children up to 42 months old. The average age of the caregivers was 31.12 years (SD = 5.69). The sample was convenience-based; all participants resided in the countryside of Minas Gerais, a state in Southeastern Brazil. The average age of the children was 21.8 months (SD = 9.45), with 53.7% of them being female. None had been diagnosed with developmental disorders, and only 14.8% attended early childhood education or daycare.

Regarding the caregivers' education level, 33.3% had completed high school, and 31.5% had completed college. Of them, 24.1% reported having postgraduate education. Most participants had a monthly family income between one and two minimum wages on data collection time (between 1045.00 and 2092.00 Brazilian Reais). In 88.9% of the families, three (57.4%) or four (31.5%) people depended on this income, and 94.5% of the participants had one (63%) or two children (31.5%). The study used a version of the *Zero to Eight: Children's Media Use in America 2013* (Common Sense Media, 2013)—translated to the Brazilian context for *Núcleo de Pesquisa e Intervenção em Famílias com Bebês e Crianças* (Research and Intervention Center for Families with Infants and Children) from Federal University of Rio Grande do Sul in 2018. To understand the child and family's media use, the Common Sense Media questionnaire was administered, which covers the following: (1) access to household media platforms, such as television, computers, smartphones, tablets, gaming consoles, and e-readers; (2) usage patterns, average time spent watching television, using electronic devices, playing video games, and interacting with other forms of media; (3) content preferences, preferred genres, including television programs, movies, video games, apps, websites, and books; (4) parental involvement, co-viewing practices, parental media use restrictions, and parental attitudes regarding media content appropriateness for children; and (5) educational content, educational television programs, apps, websites, and interactive games, aiming to assess perceived educational value and parental attitudes toward such content.

Child development was evaluated through the *Inventário Dimensional de Avaliação do Desenvolvimento Infantil* (Dimensional Inventory for Child Development Assessment) *called* IDADI. IDADI is a multidimensional instrument for child development assessment, constructed and validated and standardized in Brazil by Silva et al. (2020) to evaluate children from 4 to 72 months of age. It consists of 435 items that assess aspects of development in the cognitive, communication and language (expressive and receptive), motor (gross and fine), socio-emotional, and adaptive behavior domains, based on parental reports. The items are divided into age groups according to the babies' and children's skill levels and are administered according to age, as developmental milestones vary across age ranges. Norms of interpretation were established for 17 age groups. A sociodemographic questionnaire was utilized to gather information about participants and their families, including the ages of both children and parents, education levels, housing conditions, and income. Moreover, questions pertaining to COVID-19 were incorporated to capture data regarding the pandemic's influence on family routines.

Quantitative data were analyzed using the Statistical Package for the Social Sciences (SPSS) software version 22.0. Descriptive statistical analyses were performed to describe the families' characteristics and technology use and classify the participating children's development in the different IDADI domains. To compare the developmental domains among children who used digital media and those who did not, we employed the Student's t-test, followed by Cohen's d effect size statistic (Cohen, 2016). Pearson correlational analyses were conducted to explore the relationship between screen use by parents and children.

For the qualitative segment of the study, two mothers aged 22 and 29, with children aged 12–36 months, who had previously completed the quantitative survey, took part in the focus group. Participant selection was based on convenience criteria, inviting mothers who were interested in the research topic, had access to the Internet and videoconferencing, and were available to participate following initial contact. The focus group technique was chosen for this stage. Due to the period of social isolation, we opted for a small sample, since too many people in one call would make the discussion unfeasible. The two mothers participated in a semi-structured video call lasting 1 h and 7 min. Two authors conducted this interview in a single meeting on August 10, 2021, exploring how the children and their parents used digital media and their perspectives on this usage. Some trigger questions were formulated beforehand, based on literature, to initiate and guide the dialogue among the participants. The questions were asked to guide situations where the topic was not addressed. If the topic arose spontaneously, it could be skipped. The questions were:

1. What are your thoughts on technology use by infants and children? In a more general sense, what is your opinion on this matter?
2. What does your child watch? For what purposes do they use screens? In what situations does this usage occur?
3. Who provides the screen-based media for the child? (Only the parents, external individuals, caregivers, etc.). If others besides the parents provide media, are there any agreements or restrictions?
4. How is screen-based media used by your family? (Frequency, number of hours, purposes, etc.)
5. Do you believe the pandemic has impacted media usage for you and your child? If so, how?
6. What advantages and disadvantages do you see in children's use of technology?
7. Have you noticed any changes in your child's behavior due to technology usage?
8. What are your thoughts on newspaper articles, magazine pieces, and internet articles criticizing parents who offer technology to their children?
9. Do you believe that the use of technology impacts your child's development?
10. Do you believe that screen usage affects your relationship with your child, and if so, how?
11. Have you received any information from a health professional regarding your children's technology usage?

The *Interface for Multidimensional Analysis of Texts and Questionnaires* (IRaMuTeQ) software was employed for data analysis. The main objective of the software is to analyze the structure and organization of discourse, allowing for the identification of relationships between the lexical words most frequently enunciated by the participants (Camargo & Justo, 2013). The hierarchical descending classification (CHD) was performed to recognize the dendrogram with emerging classes, where higher χ^2 values indicate stronger word associations with the class, while words with $\chi^2 < 3.80$ ($p < 0.05$) were disregarded.

Exploring Digital Media Usage Patterns in Families During the COVID-19 Pandemic: Unveiling Relationships with Infant Development

During the COVID-19 pandemic, 35.5% of Brazilian participants reported experiencing social isolation previously, but they were no longer going through it at the time of data collection. Among all participants, 27.8% reported being in isolation and performing work or study activities remotely at the study time. Additionally, 13% of participants reported having suspected COVID-19 at some point since the beginning of the pandemic, while 9.3% reported that someone close, residing in their household, also had the COVID-19 suspicion. Of the participants, 14.8% said being part of the highest-risk group of getting very sick from COVID-19, and 18.5% were living with someone from this highest-risk group. Furthermore, due to the pandemic, 38.9% of mothers lost the support of family and friends in caring for the baby, 16.7% lost the support of daycare, and 3.7% lost the support of babysitters. Nevertheless, 9.3% of mothers reported that their children were engaged in remote school-related activities, receiving school tasks at home.

Regarding media usage profile, participants said that during the isolation time, their child's use was either higher (44.4%) or the same (46.3%) as before the pandemic. The most used devices by the children in the present sample were television (TV) (83.3%) and smartphones (59.3%). Only 11.1% of participants reported their children using tablets, and only 9.3% used computers. Many children use multiple types of devices simultaneously, and this factor could influence the accuracy of the mothers' reported estimates of screen use.

Regarding the moments when caregivers needed to offer technology to their children, the following were highlighted: during household activities (68.5% offered TV and 37% offered smartphones) or while in the home office (48.1% offered TV and 22% offered smartphones). Additionally, it was identified that caregivers most often offered technology during the child's routine activities, such as during mealtime (24.1% offered TV and 29.6% offered smartphones) and bedtime (20.4% offered TV and 14.8% offered smartphones). Regarding offering TV, caregivers justified its use to keep their children entertained while they performed household tasks (72.2%) or for educational purposes (38.9%). Concerning the purpose of offering smartphones, in addition to the reasons mentioned above, caregivers also provided them to soothe their babies (20.4%), especially when they were in public.

Regarding child development profiles evaluated by the Dimensional Inventory for Child Development Assessment (IDADI), most of the children assessed demonstrated typical or above-average development according to the standard classification criteria (standardized score of 85 or higher). However, a percentage of children still exhibited developmental delays. For the cognitive domain, 88.8% of the children showed developmental classification within the average range or higher, while 11.2% experienced identifiable developmental delays. For the remaining domains, the breakdown of development within the average range and higher, as well as delays, is as follows: socio-emotional domain, 90.2% within average range and higher and 9.8% below average with delays; expressive communication and language, 88.5% within average range and higher and 11.5% below average with delays; receptive communication and language, 94.3% within average range and higher and 5.7% below average with delays; gross motor skills, 91.9% average and higher and 8.1% below average with delays; fine motor skills, 96.2% average and higher and 38% with delays; adaptive behavior, 76.9% average and higher and 23.1% below average with delays. The adaptive behavior domain is highly dependent on the context and caregivers' encouragement of the child's autonomy. This may explain a more significant percentage of delays in this domain.

To analyze the associations between digital media usage and child development, the groups were compared based solely on the usage and non-usage of TV and smartphones, as the frequency of children using tablets and computers was low. The results indicated that, except for gross motor skills and adaptive behavior, there was a developmental difference in all domains of IDADI between infants who watched

TV and those who did not, favoring the latter group. The domains most impacted by TV usage were socio-emotional ($p = .002$; effect size [*Cohen's d*] = 1.39), receptive language and communication ($p = .010$; *Cohen's d* = 1,08), fine motor skills ($p = .018$; *Cohen's d* = 1.06), and cognitive ($p = .017$; *Cohen's d* = 1.01). As confirmed by Cohen's d (Cohen, 2016), the effect size of the comparison of the mean difference was large.

Regarding smartphones, a statistically significant difference was also found between infants using and those not using this media for the cognitive ($p = .019$; *Cohen's d* = .68) and fine motor skills domains ($p = .020$; *Cohen's d* = .72), favoring the non-users. The effect size for the difference between the means was moderate. For the other domains of IDADI, no significant differences were found between children concerning the use or non-use of this digital media. These results suggest that watching TV could more harm child development across different domains than using smartphones. However, using both devices can be related to some developmental impairments.

The relationship between screen use by parents and children was assessed through correlation analyses, which demonstrated significant results. It was observed that the more parents watched videos, movies, or programs, the more time children spent watching videos, movies, or programs ($r = 0.37$; $p = .02$). Additionally, the more time parents used devices to search for information about COVID-19, the more time children spent on digital media listening to stories ($r = .43$, $p = .03$), listening to music ($r = .34$, $p = .04$), watching videos ($r = .37$, $p = .01$), and drawing or coloring on screens ($r = .93$; $p = .007$).

Qualitative data were analyzed using Textual Statistics and Descending Hierarchical Classification (DHC). Through DHC, the study explored the most pertinent words in the mothers' statements and their correlation with the research topic to establish distinct classes. The analysis of the subject discourse was then employed to identify key words and expressions and quantify them, facilitating the identification of central ideas. This process enabled the formation of distinct classes, as illustrated in the dendrogram (see Fig. 11.1).

The analysis corpus comprised two texts, each containing the speech of one participant, divided into 191 text segments (TS), with 162 TS utilized of the initial corpus (84.82%). A total of 6830 occurrences (words, forms, or terms) emerged, encompassing 1155 distinct words and 591 occurring only once. The analyzed content was categorized into five classes: Class 1 "Parents and screen media use: role-modelling"; Class 2 "Impacts on child development"; Class 3 "Type of device and content assessed by the child"; Class 4 "Home office: reflections of social distancing on family dynamics"; and Class 5 "Professional Information Seeking."

Class 1, *Parents and screen media use: role-modelling*, comprises 15.04% and 25 text segments of the total analyzed corpus. It consists of words and stems ranging between $\chi^2 = 4.30$ (give) and $\chi^2 = 27.69$ (Doctorate). The frequent words in this class include "computer," "work," "ask," "mother," "need," "class," "game," and "pandemic." This class discusses the use of digital media by parents, the parental model, and their perception of its implications on their children's media use. Overall, it is evident that mothers believe their children imitate their behavior in work-related

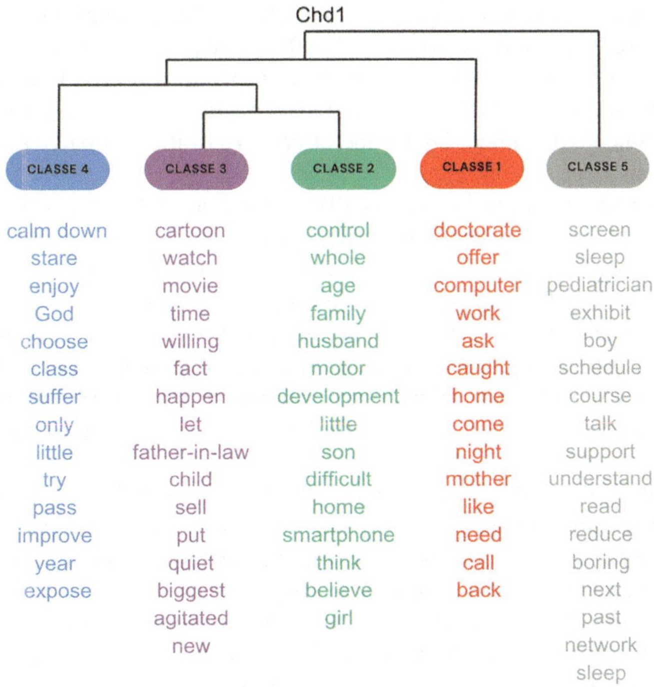

Fig. 11.1 Dendrogram of DHC classes

and leisure activities, such as when the children "play" that they are typing, playing games, and working. Some vignettes from this class include:

> I think we are examples all the time, right? So, they look up to us all the time, so when they see us using it, they want to use it too. Luca occasionally sits down and comes over to give my computer a few squeezes. We've caught him playing with it several times and he says "I'm working, I'm working. (Participant 01)

> I stay at home on the computer, and when I need (to work) at night, dealing with my doctoral things, he watches me using the computer. (Participant 01)

> ...she even turns on the computer by herself, opens it, and starts tapping with her little hand, pretending she's typing like this... They observe and do the same, I guess. (Participant 02)

Class 2, *Impact on Child Development*, comprises 20.99% of the analysis corpus and 34 text segments of the total analyzed. It consists of words and stems ranging between $\chi^2 = 19.42$ (control)—"dosar" in Portuguese—and $\chi^2 = 3.85$ (crazy). The class includes frequent words such as "motor," "development," "little," "smartphone," "Netflix," and "content."

The class content is related to mothers' perceptions of the impacts of media use on child development, with a particular focus on motor and psychological development. Mothers mentioned that media helps to "calm" their children, but they also express concerns about potential long-term consequences. To address this, they try to "control" media usage by setting limits believing that doing so will reduce some adverse effects. Examples of statements from this class include:

> ...I think it hinders motor development, mainly, you know? (Participant 01)

> I believe it has an impact on motor development, cognitive development, and psychological development. I think it affects various aspects negatively. (Participant 01)

> ...and then, we found ourselves in this conflict with Esther. I was thinking: will she also become obsessed with smartphones as she grows up, or can we find a way to regulate it somehow, you know? (Participant 02)

Class 3, *Media type and content accessed by children*, comprises 24.07% of the analyzed corpus, with 39 text segments. It includes words and word frequency ranging from $\chi^2 = 39.97$ (cartoon) to $\chi^2 = 5.17$ (new). Words frequently found in this class include "watch," "movie," "hour," "happen," "allow," "childish," and "restless."

This class focuses on the type of media and content children access. Parents' use of smartphones and television stands out, with a preference for cartoons, movies, and children's music. Narratives suggest simultaneous screen-based media use by children and their family during specific daily moments. Representative speech vignettes of this class include:

> When I was a child, if I wanted to watch a cartoon, it had a specific time on TV and a particular channel. I had to wait for it to happen; I didn't have control over it. I would watch it if available then. (Participant 2)

> Esther watches more... She watches on the smartphone... When she was younger, I used to put it on TV through Chromecast for her to watch, and I selected what she watched, usually cartoons with those children's songs. (Participant 02)

> We have a way of connecting even while doing different things, even watching other videos, like me studying and her watching cartoons. We often do this together, and it's good. (Participant 02)

Class 4, *Home office: reflections of social distancing on family dynamics*, comprises 24.07% (f = 39 ST) of the total analyzed corpus. It consists of words and roots within the range of $\chi^2 = 23.58$ (calm down) and $\chi^2 = 4.02$ (improve). This class includes words such as "to calm down," "enjoy," "to choose," "class/lesson," "to suffer," "a little," and "TV."

The class content highlights the sense of restlessness experienced by children in response to the new context brought about by the pandemic. Mothers shared their experiences concerning work and study routines during this period and the challenges of having limited access to support networks. When both parents worked from home, the children had to use screens on certain days. Relevant speech vignettes of this class include:

> "...mom, mom, mom" and I respond, "please, wait for just a little, I'm busy"...and it's like, I have to take deep breaths, calm myself, and this whole profound breathing thing is getting heavier every day. (Participant 02)

> Previously, Luca didn't have much exposure to it, but now I find myself more flexible with Tom around. Luca watches a little, although he is not particularly fond of it. But since Tom is one year old, he ends up watching by default, doesn't he? (Participant 01)

> Look, Tom was born on Wednesday, and I had a class… I presented a work, which I can say was the most difficult work I have ever presented in my Ph.D., on Friday. (Participant 01)

Class 5, *Professional information seeking*, encompasses 24.69% ($f = 40$ ST) of the total corpus analyzed. It consists of words and roots ranging between $\chi^2 = 11.45$ (screen) and $\chi^2 = 4.14$ (week). This class comprises words such as "understand," "reduce," "past," "sleep," "expose," "child," and "begin."

The principal subject matter of this class pertains to the search for information regarding access to digital media and its impacts, mainly concerning sleep. Both mothers mentioned being aware of the recommendations (from the World Health Organization) regarding restricting media usage for children under age 2. The most consulted sources involved healthcare professionals through face-to-face consultations, social media profiles, the Internet, or books. One of the mothers also noted a regression in her child's sleep quality after introducing digital media. Representative speech vignettes include:

> I remember reading a lot about this issue on social media as well, some pediatricians I follow discuss the topic of screen exposure for children under two years old. (Participant 01)

> …Esther's pediatrician, I always had a lot of confidence in her, and whenever she noticed something different, and we talked about it, she would say, "Could it be the screen? Let's reduce screen time?" (Participant 02)

> I had a thorough conversation with her [the doctor] about the importance of children's sleep periods, you know, having them sleep earlier and limiting screen exposure close to bedtime. (Participant 01)

Summary of the Chapter's Findings Considering Previous Research

This chapter presented data on the usage of digital media in families with babies and children up to 42 months old during the COVID-19 pandemic in cities in the interior of Minas Gerais. Additionally, a quantitative design was used to demonstrate associations between the usage of TVs and smartphones with domains of child development and the relationship between parents' and children's digital media usage. The qualitative design helped delve deeper into the quantitative results, uncovering relevant content categories regarding the perceptions of two mothers of children aged 1–3 years regarding screen usage and its correlates.

The quantitative study results indicated that watching TV and using smartphones were associated with lower average levels of child development in various domains. Specifically, TV usage was linked to greater developmental impairments. TVs are considered passive digital media, involving information consumption without direct social interactions. Sweetser et al. (2012) hypothesize that, on average, watching television generates lower levels of physical and cognitive activity compared to more active media like computers or video games. The drawbacks of excessive passive use of digital media are also discussed due to the lack of interaction and activity. Sweetser et al. (2012) state that children who only receive information without actively participating tend to become passive viewers, merely absorbing information. The reports from the participants in the focal group reinforced this understanding, as they revealed a high pattern of passive digital media consumption by children during the pandemic. One of the participants mentioned that her daughter predominantly watched content on mobile devices, such as a smartphone, chosen by the child herself. This passive use of screens was a distraction for the child so that the mother could engage in other activities. Differential effects between the type and amount of screen time and child development are likely to occur, as observed in this study. However, additional studies are necessary on this topic, given the divergent results in previous research.

The data from this chapter revealed associations between greater impairments in socio-emotional development, receptive communication and language, fine motor skills, and cognitive development among children who watched TV compared to those who did not. Impairments in communication and language were also associated with higher TV usage in Rocha et al.'s (2021) study with children aged 0–60 months. Increased screen time was also linked to lower language scores in studies conducted by Operto et al. (2020) and Sundqvist et al. (2021). These authors considered the combined screen time from different devices and found an association between higher exposure time and language deficits.

In contrast to this study, which did not find a significant relationship between smartphone usage and socio-emotional development, the findings of Hosokawa and Katsura (2018) and Lin et al. (2020) showed negative effects in this domain among children with higher smartphone and tablet usage. Specifically, in children under 2 years old, when daily screen time exceeded 1 h, it was found that greater screen exposure was significantly associated with developmental delays in all domains, especially language (Varadarajan et al., 2021). Kim et al.'s (2021) study revealed a negative association between smartphone usage and children's cognitive development. Since the sample size of the quantitative study is small, no age comparisons were made, which could provide new insights into the obtained results. However, concerns were raised by a participant in our study due to the on-demand nature of screen usage, meaning children have unrestricted access to various cartoons, movies, and shows and can choose what and when to watch. According to the participant, this could lead to difficulties in the child's behavior regulation and emotional control when facing frustrations. This concern is legitimate and supports findings in the literature that highlight behavioral and emotional control impairments associated with increased screen time (Hosokawa & Katsura, 2018; Kim et al., 2021; Radesky et al., 2014). In light of these results, this chapter raises the following question: is it possible that the immediacy of screen usage and even the provision of screens as a mechanism for emotional control may longitudinally impair a child's self-regulation? This is a question that deserves further investigation in future research.

The parental model emerged as an important variable associated with children's media usage in the current chapter, both quantitative and qualitative. The correlation between maternal screen time and that of infants and toddlers has been extensively explored in scholarly literature, as evidenced by the studies conducted by Nobre et al. (2019), Poulain et al. (2019), and Pedrotti et al. (2021). A consistent finding in these studies indicates that a mother's engagement with digital media is associated with a corresponding increase in screen time among her young children. Domoff et al. (2020) highlighted that children tend to imitate the behavior of parents and caregivers by observing their media usage. The same observation was made in the present study, where the more time parents spent watching videos, movies, or programs, the more time their children spent consuming screen content. The focal group's mothers' accounts also supported this result. Both participants reported situations in which their children imitated the parents' behavior, pretending to use computers or smartphones for work, indicating through this playful imitation that children seek to reproduce parental actions, even if they do not fully comprehend the adult context. Additionally, this behavior imitation may partly reflect the children's need to feel connected and included in family activities and their desire to identify with caregivers. The importance of parents as behavioral models for children's development is well established as in Bandura's (2008) social cognitive theory. The author argues that people learn through observation and imitation of significant models, and parents are the primary social models for their children.

The mothers' support network in caring for the children was also an important variable associated with children's screen usage in the present study. While quantitative data exploring this relationship were unavailable, the mothers' accounts in the focal group demonstrated that digital media usage sometimes aimed to compensate for the lack of support in child care, especially during the COVID-19 pandemic. For example, one participant mentioned that, as her entire family lived in another city, she had almost no support network, leading her to offer more screen time to the child to manage her tasks. In contrast, the other participant reported having an extensive and qualified support network, with help from her parents and formal caregivers in child care, allowing her to avoid excessive screen usage since she found support from the people around her. These experiences show how a support network's availability can directly affect how much time children spend in front of screens. In this regard, it is essential to highlight the impact of the pandemic concerning the loss of different types of support in child care. With restrictions and social isolation measures to control COVID-19, 38.9% of the participants in our study reported losing assistance in caring for the children, which was previously provided by family members, friends, daycares, and/or babysitters. This data demonstrates how the pandemic restricted the availability of external support, leaving some mothers with the difficult task of balancing multiple responsibilities without the help they used to have. Consistent with this finding, Hartshorne et al. (2021) showed that the lack of social support is an essential factor in parents' increased screen time allowance for children. Additionally, it is known that the screen time children had during the pandemic provided relief for caregivers, allowing them time to fulfill their tasks and relieve stress (Findley et al., 2022). This partly explains the finding that almost half of the participants in the present study (44.4%) reported an increase in children's media usage compared to the period before the pandemic.

Despite our findings, many questions remain about the use of digital media in childhood. Even though the results available on the topic are not unanimous, there is no doubt that it is a very important topic to be considered. The qualitative results of this chapter show that mothers are concerned about the differential impacts of media usage on their children. They stated they believed there was an impact on various aspects of development, including motor, cognitive, and socio-emotional. While there is still a need for further studies to better understand these impacts, the decision of the World Health Organization and Pediatric Societies to promote more restricted screen use, especially avoiding it in the early years of life, is a guideline backed by the current accumulated knowledge.

The mothers in the sample of this study demonstrated, in general, to have some knowledge about the guidelines and recommendations regarding media use in children, and they showed an active attitude in seeking information, with Instagram and social media being their main allies in this task. However, this is not the reality for everyone. The study by Arantes and de Morais (2022), also conducted in Brazil, showed that 93.1% of the parents and caregivers reported never having received guidance from pediatricians on-screen use for children about health risks and early and excessive use. This difference may reflect socio-cultural disparities in access to information in Brazil. Studies like Kim et al. (2020) have emphasized the importance of parental guidance to ensure that screen usage is balanced and healthy, avoiding potential negative impacts on child development. Public campaigns to inform the population and parental guidance can help minimize possible consequences of accelerated digital media use after the COVID-19 pandemic.

Implications, Future Directions, and Concluding Thoughts

By combining qualitative interviews and quantitative surveys, this chapter provided a comprehensive understanding of digital media use by children and their parents and a preliminary investigation of screen media use and its influences on infant development. Both methodologies contribute to the knowledge in this field and provide insights for appropriate interventions and guidelines on digital media use for this age group. The qualitative data adds context and clinical relevance to the quantitative findings, allowing for a more comprehensive interpretation of the relationships observed and providing some insights into the subjective experiences and perspectives of the participants. Moreover, correlational studies remain valuable for generating hypotheses and exploring associations between variables.

IRaMuTeQ is a relevant tool for extracting valuable insights from textual data. Its ability to discover patterns, key terms, and relationships in textual data supports users in drawing data-driven conclusions and enriching the narrative of this chapter with evidence-based insights. Particularly in this study, it allowed us to explore complex phenomena in depth, providing detailed insights into mother's behaviors, attitudes, motivations, and experiences, such as family dynamics in the context of social isolation. In addition, it has enabled an understanding of the social contexts and complexities of human interactions in specific environments, cultures, or communities, for instance, their concerns about the future implications of screen use in children's lives.

Conversely, it was impossible to establish causation in the quantitative survey, as a correlation between two variables does not prove one causes the other. Hence, experimental research designs are suggested as they allow causal relationships between variables to be established. Correlational studies also suffer from restricted generalizability, as the absence of experimental control and randomization limits their applicability to broader populations or contexts. Lastly, temporal ambiguity in cross-sectional studies makes it difficult to determine the temporal sequence of the observed relationship. Thus, it is recommended to conduct longitudinal studies on the subject.

In conclusion, it is crucial for families to establish clear and consistent rules regarding screen time and digital media usage. This includes limiting screen time daily, especially during meals, bedtime, and family activities, as stated by previous recommendations (AAP, 2016; Canadian Paediatric Society, 2017). Additionally, parents should model healthy media use by demonstrating responsible and balanced media consumption. Engaging in co-viewing and co-playing with their child allows for meaningful discussions and addressing concerns regarding digital content. Encouraging offline interactions through face-to-face communication with family members, friends, and peers is essential for promoting social bonding and emotional well-being. Teaching children emotional literacy and effective online and offline communication about feelings is crucial to their socio-emotional development. Monitoring online activities and social media interactions is necessary to ensure positive and respectful communication and address negative experiences. Furthermore, promoting creative and imaginative activities that do not involve screens fosters emotional expression and cognitive development. Balancing screen time with physical activities, such as outdoor play and sports, contributes to children's overall well-being. Implementing these strategies supports healthy and responsible digital media use among children.

The study also has applications in real-world settings. The association between worse scores in children's development and digital media usage highlights the importance of considering them when conducting psychological evaluations. Psychologists and health workers must be on the lookout for potential developmental delays, concentration problems, and social-emotional problems caused by exposure to digital media. Professionals can better understand a child's development and design interventions and parental counseling that effectively support healthy growth in the digital age by adding these factors into their assessments and involving parents.

References

American Academy of Pediatrics. (2016). Media and young minds. *Pediatrics, 138*(5), e20162591. https://doi.org/10.1542/peds.2016-2591

Arantes, M. C. B., & de Morais, E. A. (2022). Exposição e uso de dispositivo de mídia na primeira infância. *Residência Pediátrica, 212*(4), 10.25060/residpediatr-2022.v12n4-535.

Bellman, M., Byrne, O., & Sege, R. (2013). Developmental assessment of children. *BMJ, 346*, e8687. https://doi.org/10.1136/bmj.e8687

Camargo, B. V., & Justo, A. M. (2013). IRAMUTEQ: Um software gratuito para análise de dados textuais. *Temas em Psicologia, 21*(2), 513–518. https://doi.org/10.9788/TP2013.2-16

Canadian Paediatric Society. (2017). Screen time and young children: Promoting health and development in a digital world. *Paediatric Child Health, 22*(8), 461–477. https://doi.org/10.1093/pch/pxx123

Choi, Y., Lee, D. Y., Lee, S., Park, E.-J., Yoo, H. J., & Shin, Y. (2021). Association between screen overuse and Behavioral and emotional problems in elementary school children. *Journal of the Korean Academy of Child and Adolescent Psychiatry, 32*(4), 154–160. https://doi.org/10.5765/jkacap.210015

Cohen, J. (2016). A power primer. In A. E. Kazdin (Ed.), *Methodological issues and strategies in clinical research* (pp. 279–284). American Psychological Association. https://doi.org/10.1037/14805-018

Common Sense Media. (2013). *Zero to eight: Children's media use in America 2013*. Common Sense Media.

Crespi, L., Noro, D., & Nóbile, M. (2023). Políticas públicas para a primeira infância: fundamentos para a valorização do desenvolvimento neurobiológico infantil. *Educação Online, 18*(42), e231808. https://doi.org/10.36556/eol.v18i42.1422

Domoff, S. E., Borgen, A. L., & Radesky, J. S.. (2020). Interactional theory of childhood problematic media use. *Human Behavior and Emerging Technologies, 2*(4), 343–353. https://doi.org/10.1002/hbe2.217

Durham, K., Wethmar, D., Brandstetter, S., Seelbach-Göbel, B., Apfelbacher, C., Melter, M., et al. (2021). Digital media exposure and predictors for screen time in 12-month-old children: A cross-sectional analysis of data from a German birth cohort. *Frontiers in Psychiatry, 12*, 737178. https://doi.org/10.3389/fpsyt.2021.737178

Findley, E., Labrenz, C. A., Childress, S., Vásquez-Schut, G., & Bowman, K.. (2022). 'I'm not perfect': Navigating screen time among parents of young children during COVID-19. *Child: Care, Health and Development, 48*(6), 1094–1102. https://doi.org/10.1111/cch.13038

Gaudreau, C., King, Y. A., Dore, R. A., Puttre, H., Nichols, D., Hirsh-Pasek, K., & Golinkoff, R. M. (2020). Preschoolers benefit equally from video chat, pseudo-contingent video, and live book Reading: Implications for Storytime during the coronavirus pandemic and beyond. *Frontiers in Psychology, 11*, 2158. https://doi.org/10.3389/fpsyg.2020.02158

Hartshorne, J. K., Huang, Y. T., Lucio Paredes, P. M., Oppenheimer, K., Robbins, P. T., & Velasco, M. D. (2021). Screen time as an index of family distress. *Current Research in Behavioral Sciences, 2*, 100023. https://doi.org/10.1016/j.crbeha.2021.100023

Hatschbach Ourique, M. L., da Costa Lage, L., & Insauriaga Bueno, T. (2020). Infâncias conectadas na pandemia de covid-19: Construções emergente na educação infantil. *Revista De Educação Da Universidade Federal Do Vale Do São Francisco, 10*(22), 600–628. Recuperado de https://www.periodicos.univasf.edu.br/index.php/revasf/article/view/1260

Hosokawa, R., & Katsura, T. (2018). Association between mobile technology use and child adjustment in early elementary school age. *PLoS One, 13*(7), e0199959. https://doi.org/10.1371/journal.pone.0199959

Hua, J., Xie, J., Baker, C., & Du, W. (2022). National prevalence of excessive screen exposure among Chinese Preschoolers. *JAMA Network Open, 5*(7), e2224244. https://doi.org/10.1001/jamanetworkopen.2022.24244

Kim, Y., Han, S., Park, E. J., Yoo, H. J., Park, D., Suh, S., & Shin, Y. M. (2020). The relationship between smartphone overuse and sleep in younger children: A prospective cohort study. *Journal of Clinical Sleep Medicine, 16*(8), 1319–1326. https://doi.org/10.5664/jcsm.8446

Kim, B., Han, S. R., Park, E.-J., Yoo, H., Suh, S., & Shin, Y. (2021). The relationship between mother's smartphone addiction and children's smartphone usage. *Psychiatry Investigation, 18*(2), 126–131. https://doi.org/10.30773/pi.2020.0338

Lin, H.-P., Chen, K.-L., Chou, W., Yuan, K.-S., Yen, S.-Y., Chen, Y.-S., & Chow, J. C. (2020). Prolonged touch screen device usage is associated with emotional and behavioral problems, but not language delay, in toddlers. *Infant Behavior and Development, 58*, 101424. https://doi.org/10.1016/j.infbeh.2020.101424

Nobre, J. N. P., Prat, B. V., Santos, J. N., Santos, L. R., Pereira, L., Guedes, S. C., & Morais, R. L. S. (2019). Quality of interactive media use in early childhood and child development: A multicriteria analysis. *Jornal de Pediatria, 96*(3), 310–317. https://doi.org/10.1016/j.jped.2018.11.015

Nobre, J. N. P., Santos, J. N., Santos, L. R., Guedes, S. D. C., Pereira, L., Costa, J. M., & Morais, R. L. D. S. (2021). Fatores determinantes no tempo de tela de crianças na primeira infância. *Ciência & Saúde Coletiva, 26*(3), 1127–1136. https://doi.org/10.1590/1413-81232021263.00602019

Operto, F. F., Pastorino, G. M. G., Marciano, J., De Simone, V., Volini, A. P., Olivieri, M., Buonaiuto, R., Vetri, L., Viggiano, A., & Coppola, G.. (2020). Digital Devices Use and Language Skills in Children between 8 and 36 Month. *Brain Sciences, 10*(9), 656. https://doi.org/10.3390/brainsci10090656

Owenz, M. B., & Fowers, B. J. (2020). A goal-theoretic framework for parental screen-time monitoring behavior. *Journal of Family Theory & Review, 12*(3), 335–349. https://doi.org/10.1111/jftr.12384

Pedrotti, B. G., Mallmann, M. Y., Almeida, C. R. S., Marques, F. M., Vescovi, G., Riter, H. D. S., et al. (2021). Infants' and toddlers' digital media use and mothers' mental health: A comparative study before and during the COVID-19 pandemic. *Infant Mental Health Journal, 43*(1), 24–35. https://doi.org/10.1002/imhj.21952

Portugal, A. M., Hendry, A., Smith, T. J., & Bedford, R. (2023). Do pre-schoolers with high touchscreen use show executive function differences? *Computers in Human Behavior, 139*, 107553. https://doi.org/10.1016/j.chb.2022.107553

Poulain, T., Ludwig, J., Hiemisch, A., Hilbert, A., & Kiess, W. (2019). Media use of mothers, media use of children, and parent–child interaction are related to behavioral difficulties and strengths of children. *International Journal of Environmental Research and Public Health, 16*(23), 4651. https://doi.org/10.3390/ijerph16234651

Radesky, J. S., Silverstein, M., Zuckerman, B., & Christakis, D. A. (2014). Infant self-regulation and early childhood media exposure. *Pediatrics, 133*(5), e1172–e1178. https://doi.org/10.1542/peds.2013-2367

Ribner, A. D., & McHarg, G. (2021). Screens across the pond: Findings from longitudinal screen time research in the US and UK. *Infant Behavior & Development, 63*, 101551. https://doi.org/10.1016/j.infbeh.2021.101551

Ribner, A. D., Coulanges, L., Friedman, S., Libertus, M. E., Hughes, C., Foley, S., Devine, R., Fink, E., Selby, A., Brocki, K., Frick, M., Badinlou, F., Feng, X., Chan, M., Slaughter, V., Clark, S., Su, Y., Wan, S., Lecce, S., et al. (2021). Screen time in the coronavirus 2019 era: International trends of increasing use among 3- to 7-year-old children. *The Journal of Pediatrics, 239*, 59–66.e1. https://doi.org/10.1016/j.jpeds.2021.08.068

Rocha, B., & Nunes, C. (2020). Benefits and damages of the use of touchscreen devices for the development and behavior of children under 5 years old—A systematic review. *Psicologia: Reflexão E Crítica, 33*(1). https://doi.org/10.1186/s41155-020-00163-8

Rocha, H. A. L., Correia, L. L., Leite, Á. J. M., Machado, M. M. T., Lindsay, A. C., Rocha, S. G. M. O., Campos, J. S., Silva, A. C. E., & Sudfeld, C. R. (2021). Screen time and early childhood development in Ceará, Brazil: A population-based study. *BMC Public Health, 21*(1), 1–8. https://doi.org/10.1186/s12889-021-12136-2

Santos, R. M. S., Mendes, C. G., Marques Miranda, D., & Romano-Silva, M. A. (2022). The association between screen time and attention in children: A systematic review. *Developmental Neuropsychology, 47*(4), 175–192. https://doi.org/10.1080/87565641.2022.2064863

Silva, M. A., de Mendonça, E. J., Filho, & Bandeira, D. R. (2020). *Inventário Dimensional de Avaliação do Desenvolvimento Infantil (IDADI)*. Vetor.

Sociedade Brasileira de Pediatria. (2019). *Manual de Orientação #MenosTelas #MaisSaúde*. Recuperado de https://www.sbp.com.br/fileadmin/user_upload/_22246c-ManOrient_-__MenosTelas__MaisSaude.pdf

Sundqvist, A., Koch, F. S., Birberg Thornberg, U., Barr, R., & Heimann, M. (2021). Growing Up in a Digital World - Digital Media and the Association With the Child's Language Development at Two Years of Age. *Frontiers in Psychology, 12*, 569920. https://doi.org/10.3389/fpsyg.2021.569920

Sweetser, P., Johnson, D., Ozdowska, A., & Wyeth, P. (2012). Active versus passive screen time for young children. *Australasian Journal of Early Childhood, 37*(4), 94–98. https://doi.org/10.1177/183693911203700404

Varadarajan, S., Govindarajan Venguidesvarane, A., Ramaswamy, K. N., Rajamohan, M., Krupa, M., & Winfred Christadoss, S. B. (2021). Prevalence of excessive screen time and its association with developmental delay in children aged <5 years: A population-based cross-sectional study in India. *PLoS One, 16*(7), e0254102. https://doi.org/10.1371/journal.pone.0254102

Viner, R., Davie, M., & Firth, A. (2019). *The health impacts of screen time: A guide for clinicians and parents*. Royal College of Paediatrics and Child Health. Recuperado em https://www.theeducationpeople.org/blog/the-health-impacts-of-screen-time-new-guidance-published-for-parents/

World Health Organization. (2019). *Guidelines on physical activity, sedentary behaviour and sleep for children under 5 years of age*. World Health Organization. https://apps.who.int/iris/handle/10665/311664. Licença: CC BY-NC-SA 3.0 IGO.

Yoo, H. J. (2021). Evolution of digital natives and the new role of research. *Journal of the Korean Academy of Child and Adolescent Psychiatry, 32*(4), 127–128. https://doi.org/10.5765/jkacap.210029

Chapter 12
Preschoolers, Parents, and the Pandemic: Family Media Use During the COVID-19 Crisis and Child Development

Caroline Fitzpatrick, Elizabeth Harvey, Maira Lopes Almeida, Marie-Andrée Binet, Rachelle Wakeham-Lewis, and Gabrielle Garon-Carrier

Children born into the twenty-first century have been referred to as the "digital generation." Owing to the remarkable pace of technological improvements, children today have unprecedented access to traditional (televisions, computers, video game consoles) and newer (smartphones, tablets) media technology (Rideout & Robb, 2020). Screen media has become omnipresent in the ecology of young children. Media and media devices of all types also infiltrate the lives of children at progressively earlier ages (Rideout, 2017; Wartella et al., 2013; Zickuhr, 2013). The popularity of portable device use, in particular, has risen sharply since their market introduction in 2010. For instance, in the United States, the number of children under the age of 8 with access to a smartphone has risen sharply from 38% in 2013 to 84% in 2017 (Rideout, 2017). Currently, 95% of children between the ages of 0 and 8 now have access to a smartphone, and 78% have access to a tablet. Nearly one in two children also possess their own tablet (Rideout & Robb, 2020). Although viewing traditional television programs and movies remains popular, the popularity of YouTube continues to climb among young and older children. Furthermore, the majority of households subscribe to Netflix, Disney +, or other streaming services, which can further multiply viewing occasions (Rideout & Robb, 2020). Marketers

C. Fitzpatrick (✉)
Université de Sherbrooke, Sherbrooke, QC, Canada

University of Johannesburg, Johannesburg, South Africa
e-mail: caroline.fitzpatrick@usherbrooke.ca

E. Harvey
Université Sainte-Anne, Church Point, NS, Canada
e-mail: Elizabeth.harvey@usainteanne.ca

M. Lopes Almeida · M.-A. Binet · R. Wakeham-Lewis · G. Garon-Carrier
Université de Sherbrooke, Sherbrooke, QC, Canada
e-mail: mairaalmeida@ufg.br; marie-andree.binet@usherbrooke.ca; rachelle.wakehamlewis@usherbrooke.ca; gabrielle.garon-carrier@usherbrooke.ca

G. B. Frizzo (ed.), *Digital Media and Early Child Development*,
https://doi.org/10.1007/978-3-031-69224-6_12

also aggressively target families with young children, with 80% of top-selling apps aimed at preschoolers (Takeuchi & Levine, 2014). Finally, parents of young children themselves report spending, on average, a total of 3–4 or more hours per day using screen media outside of work (Bleakley et al., 2014; Madigan et al., 2020).

This trend toward the increased digitization of children's lives has been met with a mix of enthusiasm and concern. Research suggests that too much time spent in front of screens in early childhood can be detrimental to short- and longer-term health and development. Early childhood sedentary behavior can lead to poor cardiometabolic health and fitness and continued sedentariness later in life (Fitzpatrick et al., 2012; Jones et al., 2013). Digital media use by young children has also been linked with neuropsychological risk. Early childhood represents a sensitive time in development because of the rapid pace of environment-dependent brain growth that occurs (Shonkoff, 2016). The development of brain networks that support learning and language depends on children experiencing high-quality stimulation from their caregivers. Indeed, greater screen use and exposure to lower-quality content by preschoolers have been associated with reduced white matter integrity in brain areas that support language and executive functions (Hutton et al., 2020). Spending too much time with screens during the preschool years has also been linked to physical (i.e., fine and gross motor skills), cognitive (i.e., attention, vocabulary), and socioemotional (i.e., empathy, emotion regulation) delays (Madigan et al., 2019; Pagani et al., 2010). These delays appear to translate into lower levels of school readiness (Pagani et al., 2013) especially in more disadvantaged children (Ribner et al., 2017).

Despite evidence linking *screen time* to adverse child outcomes, screen use can contribute to positive socioemotional and cognitive outcomes under the right circumstances. A meta-analysis provides evidence that screen content that is age-appropriate, educational, or prosocial (e.g., *Sesame Street*) can improve cognitive and socioemotional outcomes in young children regardless of socioeconomic status (Mares & Pan, 2013). Similarly, the nature of children's screen use is also likely to influence its impact. The use of video chat technologies (e.g., Skype) that enable interactive, two-way, live exchanges between children and adults can facilitate language learning (Roseberry et al., 2014). The device type is also necessary to consider, as those that employ touch screen technology or those designed for individual use (i.e., smartphones vs. TVs) have been shown to undermine the ability to understand others, attention control, and sleep quality in preschoolers (Cheung et al., 2017; Konok et al., 2021). Finally, the context of use which can include timing (use right before bedtime, at mealtime time), location (bedroom screen use), as well as child using screens alone or with an adult may contribute to additional negative (e.g., disrupted sleep) or positive outcomes (e.g., increased learning opportunities) (Barr et al., 2020; Martinot et al., 2021; Pagani et al., 2019; Sundqvist & Heimann, 2021).

An Unfortunate Historical Event and How We Overcame It

In the March of 2020, the COVID-19 pandemic led to an unprecedented global lockdown. During this time, families found themselves spending an increased amount of time at home. Screens became nearly indispensable in providing families with access to work, learning, social, and leisure activities. A few months prior to the pandemic, my research team and I had received an *Establishment grant* from Nova Scotia Research to study how screen media contributes to the cognitive and social development of preschoolers. Our objective was to gain a more nuanced understanding of the impact of screen media on preschoolers by considering *screen content* (e.g., educational value), *context of use* (e.g., timing of use), and the *nature* (e.g., active vs. passive use, use of videochat) of child screen use, in addition to the more widely used measures of *screen time*. After providing intensive practical training to our research staff to administer child assessments of executive functions and language skills, we began collecting data. A couple of weeks into our study, after having collected data from 11 families, in March of 2020, the pandemic struck. Physical distancing mandates were implemented, and we suspended our study to preserve the safety of our participants, staff, and community.

A few days into the lockdown and after several discussions within our team, we decided that it would be both scientifically and, more importantly, socially beneficial to gain a wider understanding of the pandemic and its collateral impact on the well-being and health of young children. We estimated that it would be possible to collect our data entirely online. Fortunately, our media assessment questionnaire was developed as an online survey. Using an online platform, it would also be possible to program some additional questions in our survey intended to capture child cognitive, social, and physical development. We also added questions related to the family context during the pandemic, including parent transition to remote work, daycare closures, and parenting stress. After a resubmission to the ethics review board of Université Sainte-Anne, and retraining our data collection staff, we were ready to resume our research.

Physical distancing measures complicated our initial recruitment strategy, which included distributing flyers in daycares and family clinics. We opted to purchase on-air radio advertisements, which were then broadcast across the maritime Canadian province of Nova Scotia. Between April and August, we were then able to recruit and collect data from 328 Nova Scotia families. Children were on average 3.5 at this baseline assessment. In the spring-summer of 2021 when children were on average 4.5, we conducted a follow-up with them remotely. At the present date, 3 years after the start of the pandemic, a third measurement time is being completed with our sample, with remote and in-person measures, to better understand child health and development at the time of school entry.

Unhealthy Media Habits: Risk and Protective Factors

As soon as we had finished collecting data from the first assessment by the end of August of 2020, we examined how children and parents used screen media during lockdown. As previously mentioned, a small number of participants in our study completed the online questionnaire prior to the start of the pandemic. Though this sample size is too small to draw any statistical inferences, it was interesting to observe a considerable difference in the screen time of these 11 children. More specifically, during the pandemic, these children spent an additional 45 min per day using screens, according to parents, as can be seen in Fig. 12.1:

When looking exclusively at families surveyed during the pandemic, we found that most children (64%) were exposed to over 2 h of screen time per day, twice the amount of average daily screen time recommended for preschool-aged children (see Fig. 12.2). Furthermore, in our sample, about a quarter of children (23%) exceeded more than 2 h per day of tablet use. We chose a 2-h cut-off because most organisms (e.g., American Academy of Pediatricians, World Health Organization) concerned with the health and well-being of children recommend limiting screen exposure to 1–2 h for children between the ages of 2 and 5. In addition to high levels of overall screen time, we also found that the majority (56%) were exposed to screens within the hour before bedtime (see Fig. 12.3). Exposure to screen media before bedtime is an additional concern because the blue light emitted by screens can interfere with melatonin production and circadian rhythms (Cheung et al., 2017). Finally, parents of preschoolers in our study reported 6.3 h of screen time per day.

An important priority of our study has been to track how children's family ecology, including child, parent, family, and contextual features of the pandemic, was

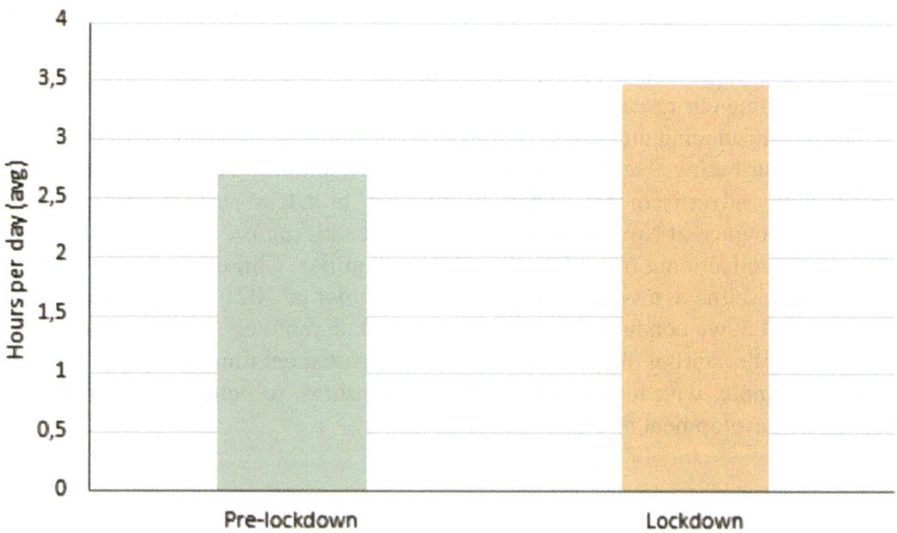

Fig. 12.1 Average amount of screen time used by children per day before and during the pandemic

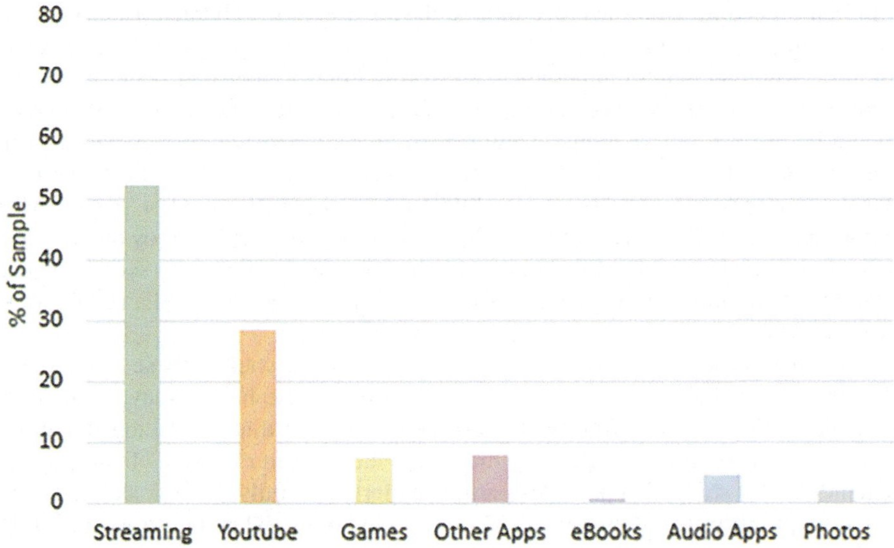

Fig. 12.2 Percentage of children using various types of media on at least a daily basis

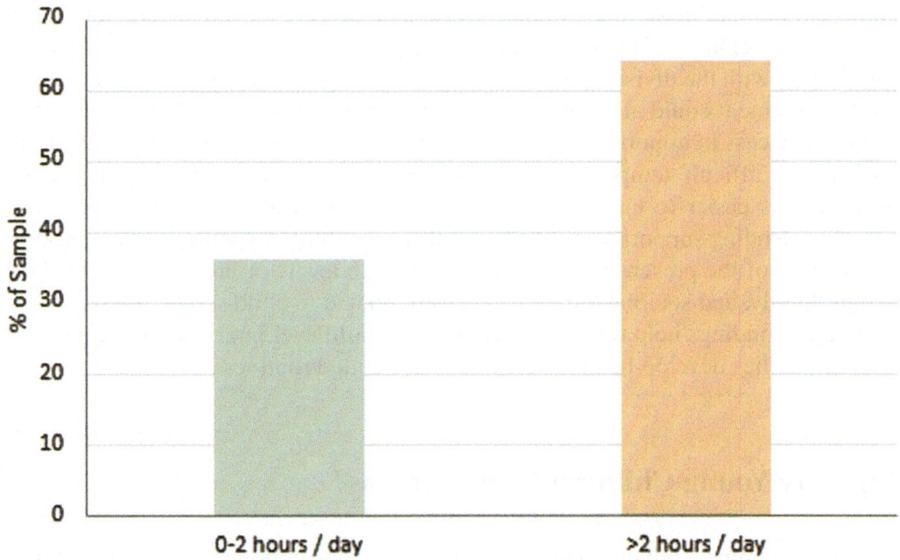

Fig. 12.3 Percentage of children exposed to more than 2 h of screen time per day on average

associated with child screen media use. Parents with a university degree were less likely to report that their child exceeded 2 h of media in the past 24 h. Also parents with higher income and who were more satisfied with the division of childcare between themselves and their partner during lockdown were less likely to have children exceeding 2 h of average mobile device use. Some characteristics of children themselves were associated with their exposure to media. More specifically, children who had better temperamental effortful control, meaning better ability to regulate their emotions, attention, and movement, were less likely to be exposed to media before bedtime. Parents using a *restrictive* supervision style exposed their children to bedtime media less frequently. Restrictive supervision reflects the tendency to set and enforce rules around child screen time use. In contrast, parents who reported more *social co-viewing*, which includes the tendency to enjoy and discuss screen media with children, had children who spent more time with screen media. Finally, having more siblings was associated with less bedtime media (Fitzpatrick et al., 2022a).

Although these findings do not allow us to determine whether these characteristics of children and parents are causes of child media use habits, they do point to potential solutions. For instance, these findings suggest that the establishment of clear and consistent rules regarding media use early on in children's lives may be beneficial. Our study also provides partial support for family distress and differential susceptibility hypotheses of child digital media use (Hartshorne et al., 2021; Valkenburg & Peter, 2013). In particular, lower parental education, income, and satisfaction with the division of childcare, as well as more challenging child temperaments, were all associated with unfavorable preschool media habits. However, child sex, number of siblings, remote work, and daycare closures were not associated with unhealthy preschooler media habits. Lower parental education, a lack of satisfaction with the division of childcare, and having a child with a more challenging temperament could all contribute to higher levels of family distress and a compromised access to important personal and financial resources. In addition, children with more difficult temperaments could illicit more screen time from parents because it is easier to engage them with screen-based activities than with other activities, lending support to the differential susceptibility hypothesis. An important implication of the present findings is that multiple levels of influence at the child, parent, family, and sociohistorical levels were related to child screen use habits. As such, these findings help reinforce the idea that multilevel interventions are needed to help families develop healthy screen use habits and routines.

How Are Young Children Using Screens?

We also examined which media activities were most popular among children. Figure 12.4 shows the most popular screen media activities reported by the parents of preschoolers in our study.

Streaming shows and movies were the most popular with more than half of parents reporting that their child streamed contents on a daily basis. Viewing content on YouTube was also popular with 28% reporting daily YouTube use. In contrast, fewer children reported looking at pictures, reading e-books, and listening to music daily. These findings are consistent with other studies in which video streaming was found

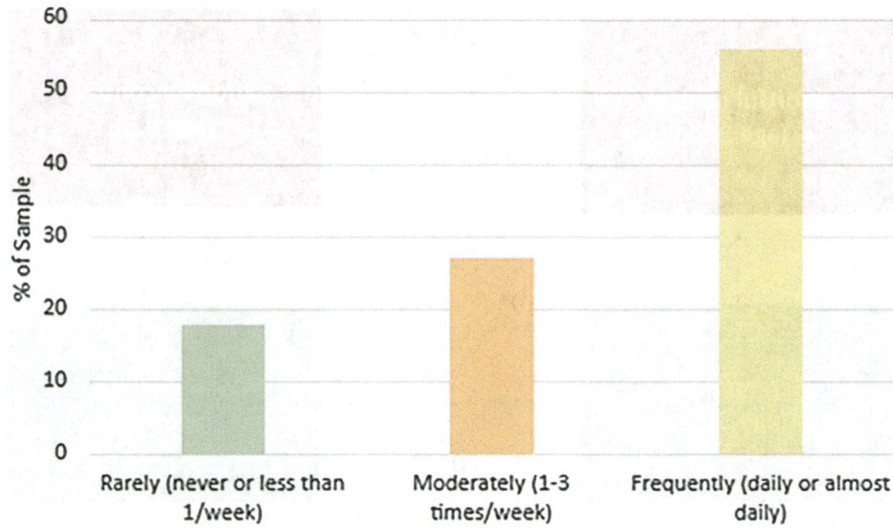

Fig. 12.4 Percentage of children exposed to screen media within an hour before bedtime

to be among the most popular activities among children (Rideout & Robb, 2020). Streaming may be an appealing activity for parents to engage young children in because it allows a continuous supply of content that is appealing to children and capable of maintaining their attention on the screen. As such, parents may feel they benefit from engaging children in these activities as a mean to keep children busy while they complete other tasks. Nevertheless, exposing children to contents that draw attention automatically through salient visual features may harm the development of sustained attention in the long run (Almeida et al., 2023; Christakis et al., 2018).

Little research has examined the prevalence of looking at photos and videos and the consequences of this type of screen use activity on young children. Compared to many contents directed at young children that feature fast pacing and a high frequency of elements designed to capture children's attention, viewing photos and videos may be less harmful to children's developing attentional abilities. As such, future research should seek to understand how this type of activity relates to a child's cognitive development.

Consequences of Child Screen Time During the Pandemic

Given the high levels of screen use by children during the pandemic, we also investigated how these may forecast child developmental outcomes. In a first study, we examined how the amount of time children spend using different devices (e.g., television, computer, mobile phone, tablets) was related to their development of

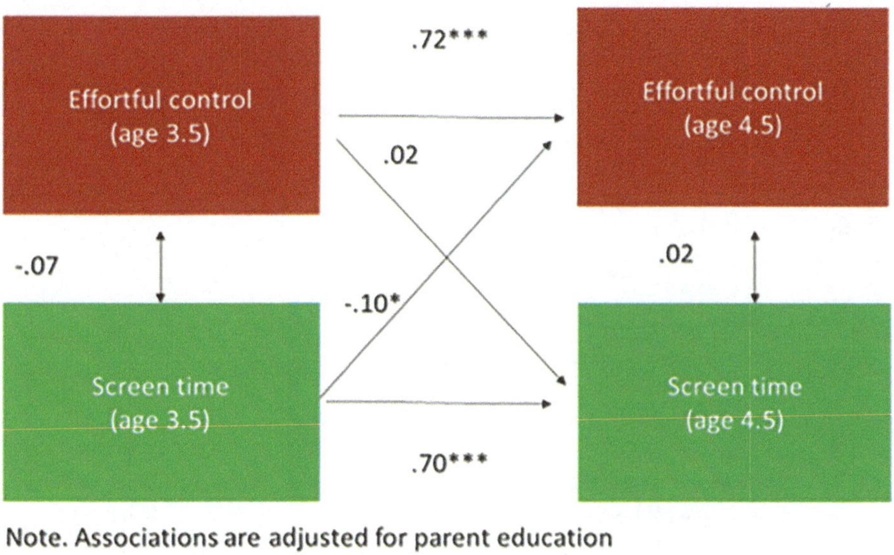

Fig. 12.5 Associations between preschooler screen time and effortful control 1 year later. (Note: Associations are adjusted for parent education)

effortful control. Effortful control is a dimension of temperament that includes attention focusing and cognitive and behavioral control and is considered essential for children to meet their goals and demands of their environments (Rothbart et al., 2006). As a key component of self-regulation, effortful control also plays an important role in helping young children benefit from learning opportunities in formal settings such as daycares and transition to the school environment (Liew, 2012; Merz et al., 2014). Previous work has suggested that children that are less well-regulated are exposed to more screen time (Coyne et al., 2021). Poorly regulated children may also have more difficulty disengaging from screen media (Clifford et al., 2020). Since screen-based activities require less attention focusing from children, it may also require less effort from parents to engage children in screen time than other types of activities (Goodrich et al., 2009). As such, we examined the direction of the association between child screen time and effortful control at 3.5 and these same variables at age 4.5. Results are reproduced in Fig. 12.5. We found that both screen time and effortful control showed continuity between the ages of 3 and 4. In addition, higher levels of child screen time at 3.5 contributed to lower levels of effortful control at 4.5. In contrast, poor effortful control did not contribute to more screen time 1 year later (Fitzpatrick et al., 2022a, b).

Using a similar methodology, we also examined how child screen time contributes to their ability to regulate negative emotions, including frustration and anger. Our analyses, shown in Fig. 12.6, indicated that children who were exposed to more screen time at the age of 3.5 had a tendency to express more negative emotions

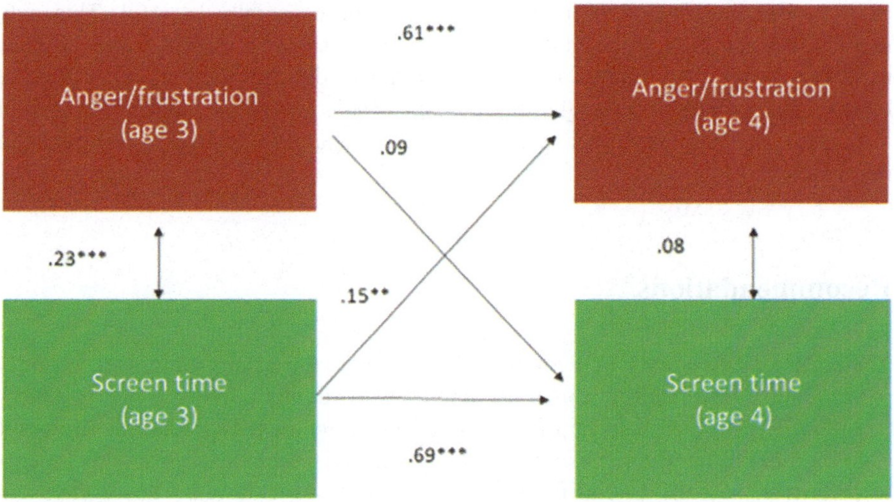

Fig. 12.6 Associations between preschooler screen time and the expression of anger and frustration 1 year later

1 year later. In contrast, children who expressed more negative emotions at 3.5 did not elicit more screen time 1 year later (Fitzpatrick et al., 2023).

Proneness to negative emotions like anger/frustration is an important individual determinant of later personality and the development of socially competent behavior.

Together these results suggest that screen time may take time away from activities that are essential for young children to build their emerging self-regulation skills. In particular, parent scaffolding of self-regulation is essential to help children progress from external means of regulation their thoughts and emotions to the adoption of more personally driven internal strategies of regulation. As such, sufficient time spent engaging with caregivers and other children is important for children to develop the ability to internally regulate thoughts and emotions. In addition, the displacement of physical activity and sleep by screen use may also further interfere with child development of self-regulation skills. Finally, it may also be the case that parents' *digital* emotion regulation, for instance, using screens to calm an upset child, could also be especially detrimental to children's development of internal regulation strategies.

Forthcoming Work

Forthcoming work by our team is currently involved in better understanding how features of child screen use, including content, nature of screen media activities, and context of use, come together to influence preschoolers' screen use *diets* and how they are associated with positive and negative child outcomes. For instance, certain contexts of use, because of their timing, may be especially harmful. This may include use before bedtime, during mealtime or unsupervised screen use. In contrast, the contents and nature of use, and some media use contexts, may provide benefits to children. In particular, highly educational programs, video chatting, and joint media engagement with parents may contribute to positive developmental outcomes.

Recommendations

The American Academy of Pediatrics recommends the establishment of a family plan to help shape healthy screen use habits. In particular, having a clearly articulated family plan may help families establish clear age-based screen time limits for each member of the family, establish which types of screen media use and contents to prioritize, as well as clarify which locations (e.g., children's bedrooms) and moments (e.g., during mealtimes) should be screen free. In addition, adults may also set up *parental controls* to limit content (such as violence) and screen time on apps designed for children. Finally, resources like *Common Sense Media* (Commonsensemedia.org), *Healthy Children* (HealthyChildren.org/Mediauseplan), and the Canadian *Media Smarts* (mediasmarts.ca) and *Pause ton Écran* (pausetonecran.com) can provide useful information about games, programs, and apps that are more likely to provide educational benefits, as well as tips on setting up family plans, guidance on how to substitute screen-based activities for other types of activities, and ways to engage a conversation about screen media with children and youth.

Conclusions

The aim of this chapter was to present our experience conducting research on preschoolers' and their families' screen media use during the pandemic. Our studies revealed high levels of screen media use during lockdown in both parents and young children. We found evidence that greater family adversity and parent screen use habits contributed to children's screen use habits. Finally, we found that preschooler screen time during this sensitive period could forecast worse self-regulation 1 year later. Our research team is currently investigating other aspects of media use, such as nature, content, and context, and their relationships with children's development, in the hope of identifying usage profiles that may minimize harms and maximize benefits to children and families. Finally, we believe that multilevel interventions can be useful for families who have difficulties regulating their media use.

References

Almeida, M. L., Garon-Carrier, G., Cinar, E., Frizzo, G., & Fitzpatrick, C. (2023). Prospective associations between children screen time and inattention symptoms in preschoolers during the COVID-19 pandemic. *Frontiers in Psychology*. https://doi.org/10.3389/fpsyg.2023.1053146

Barr, R., Kirkorian, H., Radesky, J., Coyne, S., Nichols, D., Blanchfield, O., et al. (2020). Beyond screen time: A synergistic approach to a more comprehensive assessment of family media exposure during early childhood. *Frontiers in Psychology, 11*, 1283. https://doi.org/10.3389/fpsyg.2020.01283

Bleakley, A., Vaala, S., Jordan, A. B., & Romer, D. (2014). The Annenberg media environment survey: Media access and use in U.S. homes with children and adolescents. In A. B. Jordan & D. Romer (Eds.), *Media and well-being of children and adolescents* (pp. 1–19). Oxford Press.

Cheung, C. H., Bedford, R., Saez De Urabain, I. R., Karmiloff-Smith, A., & Smith, T. J. (2017). Daily touchscreen use in infants and toddlers is associated with reduced sleep and delayed sleep onset. *Scientific Reports, 7*(1), 1–7. https://doi.org/10.1038/srep46104

Christakis, D. A., Ramirez, J. S. B., Ferguson, S. M., Ravinder, S., & Ramirez, J. M. (2018). How early media exposure may affect cognitive function: A review of results from observations in humans and experiments in mice. *Proceedings of the National Academy of Sciences, 115*(40), 9851–9858. https://doi.org/10.1073/pnas.1711548115

Clifford, S., Doane, L. D., Breitenstein, R., Grimm, K. J., & Lemery-Chalfant, K. (2020). Effortful control moderates the relation between electronic-media use and objective sleep indicators in childhood. *Psychological Science, 31*(7), 822–834. https://doi.org/10.1177/095679762091943

Coyne, S. M., Shawcroft, J., Gale, M., Gentile, D. A., Etherington, J. T., Holmgren, H., & Stockdale, L. (2021). Tantrums, toddlers and technology: Temperament, media emotion regulation, and problematic media use in early childhood. *Computers in Human Behavior, 120*, 106762. https://doi.org/10.1016/j.chb.2021.106762

Fitzpatrick, C., Pagani, L. S., & Barnett, T. A. (2012). Early childhood television viewing predicts explosive leg strength and waist circumference by middle childhood. *International Journal of Behavioral Nutrition and Physical Activity, 9*, 1–6. https://doi.org/10.1186/1479-5868-9-87

Fitzpatrick, C., Almeida, M. L., Harvey, E., Garon-Carrier, G., Berrigan, F., & Asbridge, M. (2022a). An examination of bedtime media and excessive screen time by Canadian preschoolers during the COVID-19 pandemic. *BMC Pediatrics, 22*(1), 1–11. https://doi.org/10.1186/s12887-022-03280-8

Fitzpatrick, C., Harvey, E., Cristini, E., Laurent, A., Lemelin, J. P., & Garon-Carrier, G. (2022b). Is the association between early childhood screen media use and effortful control bidirectional? A prospective study during the COVID-19 pandemic. *Frontiers in Psychology, 13*. https://doi.org/10.3389/fpsyg.2022.918834

Fitzpatrick, C., Binet, M. A., Harvey, E., Barr, R., Couture, M., & Garon-Carrier, G. (2023). Preschooler screen time and temperamental anger/frustration during the COVID-19 pandemic. *Pediatric Research*, 1–6. https://doi.org/10.1038/s41390-023-02485-6

Goodrich, S. A., Pempek, T. A., & Calvert, S. L. (2009). Formal production features of infant and toddler DVDs. *Archives of Pediatrics & Adolescent Medicine, 163*(12), 1151–1156. https://doi.org/10.1001/archpediatrics.2009.201

Hartshorne, J. K., Huang, Y. T., Paredes, P. M. L., Oppenheimer, K., Robbins, P. T., & Velasco, M. D. (2021). Screen time as an index of family distress. *Current Research in Behavioral Sciences, 2*, 100023. https://doi.org/10.1016/j.crbeha.2021.100023

Hutton, J. S., Dudley, J., Horowitz-Kraus, T., DeWitt, T., & Holland, S. K. (2020). Associations between screen-based media use and brain white matter integrity in preschool-aged children. *JAMA Pediatrics, 174*, e193869–e193869. https://doi.org/10.1001/jamapediatrics.2019.3869

Jones, R. A., Hinkley, T., Okely, A. D., & Salmon, J. (2013). Tracking physical activity and sedentary behavior in childhood: A systematic review. *American Journal of Preventive Medicine, 44*(6), 651–658. https://doi.org/10.1016/j.amepre.2013.03.001

Konok, V., Liszkai-Peres, K., Bunford, N., Ferdinandy, B., Jurányi, Z., Ujfalussy, D. J., et al. (2021). Mobile use induces local attentional precedence and is associated with limited socio-cognitive skills in preschoolers. *Computers in Human Behavior, 120*, 106758. https://doi.org/10.1016/j.chb.2021.106758

Liew, J. (2012). Effortful control, executive functions, and education: Bringing self-regulatory and social-emotional competencies to the table. *Child Development Perspectives, 6*(2), 105–111. https://doi.org/10.1111/j.1750-8606.2011.00196.x

Madigan, S., Browne, D., Racine, N., Mori, C., & Tough, S. (2019). Association between screen time and children's performance on a developmental screening test. *JAMA Pediatrics, 173*(3), 244–250. https://doi.org/10.1001/jamapediatrics.2018.5056

Madigan, S., Racine, N., & Tough, S. (2020). Prevalence of preschoolers meeting vs exceeding screen time guidelines. *JAMA Pediatrics, 174*(1), 93–95. https://doi.org/10.1001/jamapediatrics.2019.4495

Mares, M. L., & Pan, Z. (2013). Effects of sesame street: A meta-analysis of children's learning in 15 countries. *Journal of Applied Developmental Psychology, 34*(3), 140–151. https://doi.org/10.1016/j.appdev.2013.01.001

Martinot, P., Bernard, J. Y., Peyre, H., De Agostini, M., Forhan, A., Charles, M. A., et al. (2021). Exposure to screens and children's language development in the EDEN mother–child cohort. *Scientific Reports, 11*(1), 11863. https://doi.org/10.1038/s41598-021-90867-3

Merz, E. C., Landry, S. H., Williams, J. M., Barnes, M. A., Eisenberg, N., Spinrad, T. L., et al. (2014). Associations among parental education, home environment quality, effortful control, and preacademic knowledge. *Journal of Applied Developmental Psychology, 35*, 304–315. https://doi.org/10.1016/j.appdev.2014.04.002

Pagani, L. S., Fitzpatrick, C., Barnett, T. A., & Dubow, E. (2010). Prospective associations between early childhood television exposure and academic, psychosocial, and physical well-being by middle childhood. *Archives of Pediatrics & Adolescent Medicine, 164*(5), 425–431. https://doi.org/10.1001/archpediatrics.2010.50

Pagani, L. S., Fitzpatrick, C., & Barnett, T. A. (2013). Early childhood television viewing and kindergarten entry readiness. *Pediatric Research, 74*(3), 350–355. https://doi.org/10.1038/pr.2013.105

Pagani, L. S., Harbec, M. J., & Barnett, T. A. (2019). Prospective associations between television in the preschool bedroom and later bio-psycho-social risks. *Pediatric Research, 85*(7), 967–973. https://doi.org/10.1038/s41390-018-0265-8

Ribner, A., Fitzpatrick, C., & Blair, C. (2017). Family socioeconomic status moderates associations between television viewing and school readiness skills. *Journal of Developmental & Behavioral Pediatrics, 38*(3), 233–239. https://doi.org/10.1097/DBP.0000000000000425

Rideout, V. (2017). *The Common Sense census: Media use by kids age zero to eight*. Common Sense Media.

Rideout, V., & Robb, M. B. (2020). *The common sense census: Media use by kids age zero to eight, 2020*. Common Sense Media.

Roseberry, S., Hirsh-Pasek, K., & Golinkoff, R. M. (2014). Skype me! Socially contingent interactions help toddlers learn language. *Child Development, 85*(3), 956–970. https://doi.org/10.1111/cdev.12166

Rothbart, M. K., Posner, M. I., & Kieras, J. (2006). Temperament, attention, and the development of self-regulation. In K. McCartney & D. Phillips (Eds.), *Blackwell handbook of early childhood development* (pp. 338–357). Blackwell Publishing. https://doi.org/10.1002/9780470757703.ch17

Shonkoff, J. P. (2016). Capitalizing on advances in science to reduce the health consequences of early childhood adversity. *JAMA Pediatrics, 170*(10), 1003–1007. https://doi.org/10.1001/jamapediatrics.2016.1559

Sundqvist, A., & Heimann, M. (2021). Digital media content and co-viewing amongst Swedish 4-to 6-year-olds during COVID-19 pandemic. *Acta Paediatrica (Oslo, Norway: 1992), 110*(12), 3329. https://doi.org/10.1111/apa.16090

Takeuchi, L. M., & Levine, M. H. (2014). Learning in a Digital Age: Toward a new ecology of human development. In *Media and the well-being of children and adolescents* (pp. 20–33). Oxford Press.

Valkenburg, P. M., & Peter, J. (2013). The differential susceptibility to media effects model. *Journal of Communication, 63*(2), 221–243. https://doi.org/10.1111/jcom.12024

Wartella, E., Rideout, V., Lauricella, A., & Connell, S. (2013). *Parenting in the age of digital technology: A national survey*. Report of the Center on Media and Human Development, School of Communication, Northwestern University.

Zickuhr, K. (2013). *Who's not online and why*. PEW Research center. http://pewinternet.org/Reports/2013/Tablet-Ownership-2013.aspx. Accessed 16 May 2023.

Chapter 13
"It Was a Survival Tool": Parental Perspectives of Preschoolers Media Use During the COVID-19 Pandemic

Maíra Lopes Almeida, Patrícia Santos da Silva, Giana Bitencourt Frizzo, and Caroline Fitzpatrick

Introduction

With more than 180 million cases confirmed worldwide, the COVID-19 pandemic represented a major public health threat. Due to its rapid rate of infection, the pandemic has also given rise to physical distancing and lockdown measures which have significantly disrupted family routines and daily lives (Shafer et al., 2020). In March of 2020, the World Health Organization announced that the COVID-19 virus had lead us into a global pandemic. Although the COVID-19 pandemic no longer represents a global emergency, this historical event continues to have repercussions on those who experienced it. In particular, this pandemic was an important stressor for families, with multiple impacts on parents and children's emotions, attitudes, and behaviors (Taylor, 2022).

Digital media has become an essential resource in this new context, allowing families to work, communicate with relatives and friends, and entertain young children. Not surprisingly, quantitative studies in different countries, such as Canada, Israel, Brazil, and Chile, have indicated a significant increase in the use of digital media by children during the pandemic (Aguilar-Farias et al., 2020; Carroll et al., 2020; Delisle Nyström et al., 2020; Gueron-Sela et al., 2023; Hedderson et al.,

M. Lopes Almeida (✉)
Universidade Federal de Goiás, Goiânia, Goiás, Brazil
e-mail: mairaalmeida@ufg.br

P. S. da Silva · G. B. Frizzo
Universidade Federal do Rio Grande do Sul, Porto Alegre, Rio Grande do Sul, Brazil
e-mail: giana.frizzo@ufrgs.br

C. Fitzpatrick
Université de Sherbrooke, Sherbrooke, QC, Canada

Department of Childhood Education, University of Johannesburg, Johannesburg, South Africa
e-mail: caroline.fitzpatrick@usherbrooke.ca

G. B. Frizzo (ed.), *Digital Media and Early Child Development*,
https://doi.org/10.1007/978-3-031-69224-6_13

2023; Pedrotti et al., 2022). This can be worrisome since excessive screen use can lead to developmental delays (Madigan et al., 2019).

As key gatekeepers of child digital media use, it remains important to better understand parents' experience with digital media during the pandemic. This is especially important given the high levels of digital media use by young children during this time (Pedrotti et al., 2022). Parental beliefs about screen media guide their decisions about limit-setting with preschoolers (Hamilton et al., 2016). Understanding parental experiences during a stressful historical event can therefore be useful for generating hypotheses about the role of family processes in child screen use habits. Furthermore, a better understanding of family processes can be useful for guiding the development of clinical interventions aimed at helping families develop healthy media habits during the pandemic. As such, we address two research questions in the present chapter: (1) What are parents' perceptions of child screen use during the pandemic? And (2) what are parents' perceptions of the harms and benefits of child digital media use? We aim to answer these research questions based on a narrative literature review and an empirical study.

Literature Review

Previous studies have shown that caregivers tend to experience internal conflict and ambivalence regarding their own use of screens (Marques & Frizzo, 2024; Radesky et al., 2016). Amid the crisis of the COVID-19 pandemic, there has been a significant increase in screen time within families. This increase can be attributed to the abrupt increase in family distress occasioned by adapting to remote work and school closures among other stressors. In addition, it is likely that disruptions to family routines and a lack of access to childcare have resulted in increased screen time by children (Hartshorne et al., 2021). In contrast, families with lower childcare needs also reported greater supervision of their children's screen time (Stienwandt et al., 2022).

Existing studies have examined maternal decisions to use screens with children during the pandemic. An in-depth study conducted in North America involved comprehensive interviews with 25 mothers of young children (Findley et al., 2022). The objective was to gain a deeper comprehension of how and why mothers used screens with their children since the onset of the pandemic. Using thematic analysis, the findings revealed that mothers engaged their children with screen media as a coping mechanism to relieve stress and cope with adversities brought about by the pandemic, such as remote work and social isolation. Additionally, they highlighted the positive aspects of screen media usage, including fostering peer interaction, facilitating educational endeavors, and reinforcing connections with extended family members.

In this sense, an additional study delved into parent-reported child screen media usage, both pre-pandemic and during the COVID-19 outbreak (Eales et al., 2021). The responses were grouped into three themes: (a) beliefs and values; (b) practices; and (c) attitudes. In the first theme, before and during the pandemic, parents stated that screen time is easier to manage with one child, when it is not winter and when both parents do not work full time. On the topic of practices, across both years, parents were aware of how they were limiting and monitoring screen content, but post-onset, they were less restrictive with screen time and content. Regarding attitudes, parents also expressed concerns about their child's expected screen media use after COVID-19 considering the high amount of screen time becoming a new norm after the pandemic.

A meta-synthesis of qualitative studies carried out before the pandemic identified three main themes from parental perceptions of child media use (Minges et al., 2015). These themes could be useful during this atypical context too. Parents reported barriers and facilitators to limit screen time. The addictive nature of media and its integration into daily routines pose a significant barrier. On the other side, family resources (e.g., removal of screen-based media from bedrooms, access to a large backyard, dog ownership) and environments (e.g., engagement in extracurricular school-based activities, neighborhood safety) contribute to better child digital media habits.

In light of these findings, certain authors have proposed harm reduction principles for addressing screen time in young children (Vanderloo et al., 2020). A harm reduction approach is pragmatic and acknowledges that some behaviors like drinking and screen use will always exist in society and, as such, proposes using empathy and a nonjudgmental approach to assist parents and their children in managing appropriate screen use during the pandemic. The primary focus shifts to diminishing the potential adverse effects of excessive and low-quality screen use on the child, without condemning the parents for their choices. Several examples of actions within this approach include establishing daily screen use routines, encouraging parents to incorporate screen-free playtime, guiding parents in monitoring screen exposure in the presence of their children, and integrating physical activity during screen engagement, such as live or online workouts.

Families experienced numerous challenges during the COVID-19 pandemic, including remote work, loss of social support, and the closure of childcare facilities. Within this context, children's screen time significantly increased during the pandemic. Therefore, a better understanding of parental perspectives regarding children's screen use is crucial for informing interventions aimed at reducing screen time. The present study aims to address two main questions: (1) What are parents' perceptions of child screen use during the pandemic? And (2) what are parents' perceptions of the harms and benefits of child screen use during the pandemic?

Empirical Evidence

This study employed a qualitative approach to analyze parent responses to the following question: *We would like to know in your own words the role that screen media (*e.g., *watching videos and movies, playing games or using apps, using video chat) has played for you during the COVID-19 crisis. Please describe your experience as a parent, as well as your child's experience with media use during this time.*

You can describe positive experiences, negative experiences, or both. This question was included in a larger online survey of family media use. Prior to completing the assessment, participants completed a brief phone call with a trained research assistant over the course of which they provided consent to participate digitally. The study was approved by the Université Sainte-Anne Institutional Review Board.

In total, 299 participants completed the qualitative component of the questionnaire. Of these, 68% generated responses that were relevant to this study's research questions. Participants were parents with preschool-age children (mean age 3,45; SD = 0,84) who completed an assessment of child screen use during the first wave of the COVID-19 pandemic. Eligibility criteria included being an English-speaking parent and legal guardian of a child 2–4 years. Families were recruited in the Canadian province of Nova Scotia, between April and August of 2020. Schools and daycare centers in this province closed on March 27 and reopened on June 15. Participants were primarily mothers (91.8%), married (82%), born in Canada (91%), and white (90.5%). The child's average age was 3.5 years. The sample was predominantly English-speaking, with 88.1% ($N = 280$).

Only the answers relevant to the selected research questions were coded, resulting in an analytic sample of 202 parents (Braun et al., 2019). For the first research question (*Parents' perceptions of child screen use during the pandemic)*, themes were *increase*, *decrease*, and *no change*. For the second research question (*Parents' perceptions of the harms and benefits of child digital media use?)*, the themes were *benefits* and *harms*.

What Are Parents' Perceptions of Child Screen Use During the Pandemic?

Increase The first theme describes the experience of parents who perceived an increase in screen media use in their homes during the pandemic. This was descriptive of the experiences of a majority of parents in our sample (n = 160) who noticed an increase in their own and their children's media use.

There is more media being used in our household than ever before.—P55
Screen time has increased slightly since COVID-19, because we don't get out to playgrounds and playgroups and with friends as often as before.—P451
I find myself checking my phone more often now.—P414

Parents attributed this increase to several factors, including a loss of social support ($n = 44$), increased video chatting with family ($n = 40$), and the need to entertain children on rainy days ($n = 5$). However, the most cited factors were the closure of daycare centers and the need to keep children busy while parents worked from home.

> The kids watch tv in the morning now since preschool and daycare are not happening for the remainder of the summer. Rain days we are on devices more.—P362

> At times, watching YouTube videos on the iPad or phone has helped in the sense that it has calmed her down or kept her busy when days were rainy and we had run out of things to do.—P245

> I have been letting my kids watch more TV and movies because I have been working more and working from home so I feel torn. It's also been hard to not have access to friends, daycare, and outdoor spaces (for the beginning of the pandemic).—P421

> My child has definitely been using more media during the COVID-19 crisis. Although, we've found more ways to use media when we weren't able to get out and play with other people. My child has used media for physical activity as well by playing just dance and participating in yoga for kids videos.—P389

Parents cited several negative feelings such as guilt and disappointment when discussing an increase in screen media use:

> I feel very guilty though about her screen use and hope that I have not caused permanent damage to her by allowing her to watch so much television.—P354

No Change A minority of parents ($n = 30$) reported having noticed neither an increase nor a decrease in their child's screen time during the pandemic.

> My child's screen usage has remained the same during COVID-19. In the beginning, I was hopeful that it wouldn't last long so I stuck to our regular schedule so that it would be easy to go back to "normal." As time went on, it was clear that things were going to be different for an extended period of time and my husband and I felt it was even more important to keep our children on the schedule that works for us.—P103

Parents who reported no change in family media use also reported that they restricted their child's screen time prior to the start of the pandemic and that they were able to maintain their family routines during lockdown. Other parents indicated that they were able to maintain pre-pandemic media habits because their routines were not significantly altered by public health measures. This stands in contrast to the parents who reported an increase in screen media use because of the changes they experienced as a result of daycare closures and changes to their work situation.

> Screen media has not played a role for us during the COVID-19 crisis. We have always been a limited screen time household.—P36

> We were a screen-time free house (with the exception of a weekly Skype with grandparents in Ontario) before COVID and remained that way through COVID. We view screen time as a lazy excuse for parenting and a way to waste your kid's time.—P368

Decrease Some caregivers perceived a reduction in their child's screen time during the pandemic. Even though they were a small minority ($n = 6$), these parents reported that the lockdown and increased time at home allowed them to spend more leisure time with their children.

> Since being home, I had to go on pandemic leave, so screen media is playing less of a babysitting role. I have increased physical play dramatically now that I am off work, so media time has decreased because of this.—P275

> On a positive note, since the COVID-19 crisis, we have intentionally tried to reduce screen time and direct him into various other activities. So, even though I am not very satisfied with his "screen-free" time, it's a huge cut-down. That shows better behavior too.—P45

> Being home during this situation has allowed me to keep up to date with household chores so I find myself relying a lot less on screen time to keep my son occupied while I clean. I'm able to accomplish more with his help like laundry and picking up toys. I find he is less interested in tv and phone use than ever before and he has rediscovered his love for his toys.—P158

What Are Parents' Perceptions of the Harms and Benefits of Child Digital Media Use?

In addition to the amount of time children spent with screen media, caregivers also described their perceptions of the harms and benefits of their family's digital media use on children.

Perceived Benefits Parents indicated that screen media played several positive roles during the pandemic ($n = 202$). These include the opportunity to use video chat to remain connected with relatives and friends during quarantine ($n = 103$) and keep their child occupied while doing household chores or working remotely ($n = 88$). Parents also viewed media as a means to educate and increase learning opportunities for their children.

> We used it some days as a survival tool, especially on rainy days where we couldn't get outside and play as much as we could have liked. It was used as a tool to allow us parents to be able to get housework and other things done that was normally done while they were in preschool.—P87

> It has given us the opportunity to explore new learning programs and online books/storytelling videos. I have also introduced video games in the goal of introducing new problem solving techniques.—P74

> It has helped to create a great bond with his extended family who lives far away. He calls them everyday now and they both love the connection/communication.—P65

Parents also perceived screen media use as beneficial to their mental health ($n = 67$). In particular, they viewed media as providing relief and in helping them cope with the challenges of the pandemic.

> And sometimes when I just needed a break from them for my own sanity (…) I am truly thankful for the access we had to different types of media during that time (and now). Who am I kidding? Some days still feel like survival mode where the tv goes on and I hide from the kids for a few minutes of peace!—P444

> Honestly, as the sole care provider, during COVID, the use of a TV show here and there has provided me with a break and helped to maintain my sanity.—P345

Harms Participants also noticed that their child's screen media use (n = 107) was related to a number of negative consequences. The main harms were related to their child's behavior (n = 77) and regulation of their screen media use (n = 56). In particular, parents reported perceiving their children as more irritated and angry following screen media use (n = 54). Parents also reported experiencing difficulties setting limits on their child's screen media use and dealing with their child's reaction when trying to limit digital media use.

> I also notice that his behaviour is usually worse on the days he gets more screen time.—P364

> Because of the increase in screen time our son's mood/response will sometimes be a bit more dramatic when we deny or turn off screen time. He has also started asking for it more or wakes up asking for it immediately.—P304

Unexpectedly, four parents reported harms associated with the use of video chat technology. More specifically, these parents reported that engaging in video calls was emotionally disturbing to their children because it reminded them of the impossibility of meeting with relatives and friends in person.

> It's also difficult that she facetimes family and friends and that makes her remember that she can't see people.—P56

> Using video chat has been mostly positive, however, also negative because [Child's name] has gotten upset because we can't just go see our family members.—P315

Discussion

The present study allowed us to describe parents' experiences with screen media during the COVID-19 pandemic. In particular, we explored parents' perceptions of child screen use during the pandemic and their parents' perceptions of the harms and benefits of child screen use.

In terms of parent perceptions of child screen use during the pandemic, the majority (80.1%) noticed an increase in this use during the pandemic. This finding is consistent with previous quantitative studies conducted in Canada, Brazil, Chile, and Sweden, which also revealed a significant increase in media usage among children following the onset of the COVID-19 pandemic (Aguilar-Farias et al., 2020; Carroll et al., 2020; Delisle Nyström et al., 2020; Pedrotti et al., 2022). Our results are in line with these previous studies which compared the time spent in digital media use before and during the pandemic. Furthermore, the findings that parents perceived an increase in media use by their children is of interest since perceptions of problematic behavior in children (e.g., excessive media use, disruptive behavior) are a key determinant of help-seeking behavior by parents (Hamilton et al., 2016) and may therefore open avenues for intervention research.

Parents reported an increase not only in their children but also in their own screen media use. According to qualitative research conducted with American parents using focus groups, participants also observed an increase in screen time for both parents and children (Hammons et al., 2021). Prior to the pandemic, research had noted a strong association between child and parent screen time (Domoff et al., 2020). Furthermore, research suggests that excessive screen media use by parents can lead to technoference and the interference of technology in parent-child relationships, which can reduce parental sensitivity and availability toward children (McDaniel & Radesky, 2018).

Parents who perceived an increase in their child's screen use during the pandemic, as noted in previous studies (Calvano et al., 2022; Vescovi et al., 2021), reported certain recurring challenges resulting from COVID-19 related public health measures. These challenges included a loss of social support due to physical distancing regulations, which may have contributed to the rise in screen time during this period. Reduced social support and the increased need to work while home in this scenario are therefore likely to have increased tension and stress for parents. In a German study, parents of children under the age of 17 identified similar sources of stress during the pandemic, including physical distancing and restrictions on healthcare, shopping, leisure, and childcare.

In our study, parents who reported no change or a decrease in their child's screen time also reported less pandemic-related disruption to their daily routines and more flexible work arrangements. In this sense, working parents, especially those lacking flexible work arrangements, often found it challenging to allocate dedicated playtime with their children and were more likely to allow screen time (Hu et al., 2018). Conversely, some other participants perceived their time at home as an opportunity to decrease screen time and involve their children in alternative activities, such as involving them in household chores. A survey completed by 459 Polish parents revealed that some families had more positive experiences in this period, enjoying the moments with more closeness and affection (Woźniak-Prus et al., 2023). This Polish study showed that social support was an important predictor of positive caregiver-child experiences during the pandemic. This result is similar to the data found in the present study in which parents who needed to work at home and do household chores reported an increase in children's media use. As such, families with lower levels of social support may have been especially reliant on screen media to help them keep their children busy.

Considering the descriptions of the perceived benefits and harms of using digital media during the pandemic, parents reported several benefits of child screen use during the pandemic. These include remaining close to relatives and friends through video chatting, keeping children occupied while doing household chores or working from home, and providing educational experiences for children, and as a resource to cope with the pandemic. For example, one participant defined media as a *survival tool*. Research has demonstrated that media could have served as a "survival tool" during lockdown, as it provided parents with a means to take a break when other options were limited, engage in self-care, find moments of quiet, and maintain their well-being (Findley et al., 2022). This description echoes previous research in which parents reported using media as a *babysitter*. According to a meta-synthesis, it is common for parents to report that media plays the role of babysitter, allowing them to keep their child occupied while doing chores (Mallmann & Frizzo, 2019; Minges et al., 2015). Our own data is consistent with this idea and further suggests that digital media is used to provide parents with relief, especially in periods of strain.

An interesting finding in our study was that most of the benefits listed by parents of child screen use were related to parents' own needs. For instance, they referred to the usefulness of screens for keeping their child occupied. This finding is in line with previous studies conducted pre- and post-pandemic (Mallmann & Frizzo, 2019; Pedrotti et al., 2022). However, parents tended to formulate the harms of digital media in terms of consequences for their child's behavior and development. The harms reported in our study include children tending to become more irritable and angrier after screen use and parents facing increased difficulty in both monitoring screen usage and managing their children's reactions when attempting to set limits. Consistent with another study, parents also noted impairments in children's behavior, especially social skills, and focus abilities, after child screen use (Rideout & Robb, 2020).

One novel finding that emerged from our study was with regard to the use of video chatting technology. More specifically, some parents reported that engaging in video calls was an emotionally disturbing experience for their children. Parents also explained that this was the case because it reminded their children that they could not meet in person with the person on camera. Video chat technology can be used to reduce feelings of loneliness and to minimize the negative impact of a loss of contact with others. However, our results suggest that some young children may experience emotional distress as a result of being reminded of their separation from those who appear through the video chat.

Taken together, our data, combined with studies conducted before the pandemic, provide a basis for hypothesizing that digital media use during the pandemic increased parental fear and guilt. This is worrisome since the chronic and repeated experience of negative emotions is a risk factor for the development of poor mental health and mental disorders. In contrast, parent and child media use during lockdown provided relief and helped parents cope with stressors related to the public health measures that accompanied the pandemic. As such, in certain situations media use may represent a strategy for avoiding parental burnout. Parental burnout is characterized by intense exhaustion and occurs when parenting stress is severe, chronic, and overwhelms parents' ability to cope. Research has shown that parental burnout can result from potentially traumatic situations, such as the pandemic and measures of social distance (Mikocka-Walus et al., 2021). Parental burnout can then have a negative impact on parenting practices and child development (Mikolajczak et al., 2018). A study of 995 Portuguese parents found high rates of parental burnout during the pandemic, with mothers especially at risk (Aguiar et al., 2021). Similarly, an American study found that concerns about COVID-19 predicted parental burnout (Prikhidko et al., 2020). These studies further highlight the need to identify resources and strategies to help parents cope with stress during the pandemic. According to our results, the moderate use of digital media might have contributed to parental coping during the pandemic.

Our chapter presents several strengths and limitations and has several implications for future interventions and research. Although most studies conducted during the pandemic have been quantitative, our qualitative approach brought some additional insights on parental perspectives on child screen use. Several parents of preschoolers have provided valuable insights into their perspectives on child screen use in this atypical context. Parental perspectives serve as crucial gateways to better inform interventions. As a limitation, our large sample size prevented us from conducting in-depth interviews. Future studies may seek to answer these research questions in populations showing diversity on the basis of their race/ethnicity, gender, socioeconomic status, and COVID-19 experience (job losses, deaths, virus infection, time in social isolation, and others). Qualitative interviews with parents who identified decreased or no changes in screen time to identify parental mediation strategies may be useful for clinical guidance.

Conclusion

The outbreak of the COVID-19 pandemic has considerably changed the lives of families. As a result, it remains important to consider this historical event's psychological and health impact on parents and children, as consequences are likely to persist. Our study suggests that digital media provides relief for parents. In contrast, parents also reported fear and guilt of using digital media with their children. However, some families have found positive ways to spend that period playing more with the children and including them in household chores. The various parental perspectives on child screen use in this study suggest that screen media use is embedded in a complex system that should be considered when planning family interventions or clinical guidance on the use of family media.

References

Aguiar, J., Matias, M., Braz, A. C., César, F., Coimbra, S., Gaspar, M. F., & Fontaine, A. M. (2021). Parental burnout and the COVID-19 pandemic: How Portuguese parents experienced lockdown measures. *Family Relations, 70*(4), 927–938. https://doi.org/10.1111/fare.12558

Aguilar-Farias, N., Toledo-Vargas, M., Miranda-Marquez, S., Cortinez-O'Ryan, A., Cristi-Montero, C., Rodriguez-Rodriguez, F., Martino-Fuentealba, P., Okely, A. D., & Del Pozo Cruz, B. (2020). Sociodemographic predictors of changes in physical activity, screen time, and sleep among toddlers and preschoolers in Chile during the COVID-19 pandemic. *International Journal of Environmental Research and Public Health, 18*(1), 176. https://doi.org/10.3390/ijerph18010176

Braun, V., Clarke, V., Hayfield, N., & Terry, G. (2019). Thematic analysis. In P. Liamputtong (Org.), *Handbook of research methods in health social sciences* (1st ed., pp. 843–860). Springer Nature.

Calvano, C., Engelke, L., Di Bella, J., Kindermann, J., Renneberg, B., & Winter, S. M. (2022). Families in the COVID-19 pandemic: Parental stress, parent mental health and the occurrence of adverse childhood experiences—Results of a representative survey in Germany. *European Child & Adolescent Psychiatry, 31*(7), 1–13. https://doi.org/10.1007/s00787-021-01739-0

Carroll, N., Sadowski, A., Laila, A., Hruska, V., Nixon, M., Ma, D., Haines, J., & on behalf of the Guelph Family Health Study. (2020). The impact of COVID-19 on Health behavior, stress, financial and food security among middle to high income Canadian families with young children. *Nutrients, 12*(8), 2352. https://doi.org/10.3390/nu12082352

Delisle Nyström, C., Alexandrou, C., Henström, M., Nilsson, E., Okely, A. D., Wehbe El Masri, S., & Löf, M. (2020). International Study of Movement Behaviors in the Early Years (SUNRISE): Results from SUNRISE Sweden's pilot and COVID-19 study. *International Journal of Environmental Research and Public Health, 17*(22), 8491. https://doi.org/10.3390/ijerph17228491

Domoff, S. E., Borgen, A. L., & Radesky, J. S. (2020). Interactional theory of childhood problematic media use. *Human Behavior and Emerging Technologies, 2*(4), 343–353. https://doi.org/10.1002/hbe2.217

Eales, L., Gillespie, S., Alstat, R. A., Ferguson, G. M., & Carlson, S. M. (2021). Children's screen and problematic media use in the United States before and during the COVID-19 pandemic. *Child Development, 92*(5), e866. https://doi.org/10.1111/cdev.13652

Findley, E., LaBrenz, C. A., Childress, S., Vásquez-Schut, G., & Bowman, K. (2022). 'I'm not perfect': Navigating screen time among parents of young children during COVID-19. *Child: Care, Health and Development, 48*(6), 1094–1102. https://doi.org/10.1111/cch.13038

Gueron-Sela, N., Shalev, I., Gordon-Hacker, A., Egotubov, A., & Barr, R. (2023). Screen media exposure and behavioral adjustment in early childhood during and after COVID-19 home lockdown periods. *Computers in Human Behavior, 140*, 107572. https://doi.org/10.1016/j.chb.2022.107572

Hartshorne, J. K., Huang, Y. T., Lucio Paredes, P. M., Oppenheimer, K., Robbins, P. T., & Velasco, M. D. (2021). Screen time as an index of family distress. *Current Research in Behavioral Sciences, 2*, 100023. https://doi.org/10.1016/j.crbeha.2021.100023

Hamilton, K., Spinks, T., White, K. M., Kavanagh, D. J., & Walsh, A. M. (2016). A psychosocial analysis of parents' decisions for limiting their young child's screen time: An examination of attitudes, social norms and roles, and control perceptions. *British Journal of Health Psychology, 21*(2), 285–301. https://doi.org/10.1111/bjhp.12168

Hammons, A. J., Villegas, E., & Robart, R. (2021). "It's been negative for us just all the way across the board": Focus group study exploring parent perceptions of Child screen time during the COVID-19 pandemic. *JMIR Pediatrics and Parenting, 4*(2), e29411. https://doi.org/10.2196/29411

Hedderson, M. M., Bekelman, T. A., Li, M., Knapp, E. A., Palmore, M., Dong, Y., Elliott, A. J., Friedman, C., Galarce, M., Gilbert-Diamond, D., Glueck, D., Hockett, C. W., Lucchini, M., McDonald, J., Sauder, K., Zhu, Y., Karagas, M. R., Dabelea, D., Ferrara, A., & Environmental Influences on Child Health Outcomes Program. (2023). Trends in screen time use among children during the COVID-19 pandemic, July 2019 through August 2021. *JAMA Network Open, 6*(2), e2256157. https://doi.org/10.1001/jamanetworkopen.2022.56157

Hu, B. Y., Johnson, G. K., & Wu, H. (2018). Screen time relationship of Chinese parents and their children. *Children and Youth Services Review, 94*, 659–669. https://doi.org/10.1016/j.childyouth.2018.09.008

Madigan, S., Browne, D., Racine, N., Mori, C., & Tough, S. (2019). Association between screen time and children's performance on a developmental screening test. *JAMA Pediatrics, 173*(3), 244. https://doi.org/10.1001/jamapediatrics.2018.5056

Marques F. M., & Frizzo, G. B. (2024) Mídias Digitais na primeira infância: uma análise qualitativa e longitudinal dos fundamentos das práticas maternas. *Psicologia Argumento, 42*(116), 99–130. https://doi.org/10.7213/psicolargum.42.116.AO05

Mallmann, M. Y., & Frizzo, G. B. (2019). O uso das novas tecnologias em famílias com bebês: um mal necessário? *Revista Cocar, 7*, 26–46. https://periodicos.uepa.br/index.php/cocar/article/view/2789

McDaniel, B. T., & Radesky, J. S. (2018). Technoference: Parent distraction with technology and associations with Child behavior problems. *Child Development, 89*(1), 100–109. https://doi.org/10.1111/cdev.12822

Mikocka-Walus, A., Stokes, M., Evans, S., Olive, L., & Westrupp, E. (2021). Finding the power within and without: How can we strengthen resilience against symptoms of stress, anxiety, and depression in Australian parents during the COVID-19 pandemic? *Journal of Psychosomatic Research, 145*, 110433. https://doi.org/10.1016/j.jpsychores.2021.110433

Mikolajczak, M., Raes, M.-E., Avalosse, H., & Roskam, I. (2018). Exhausted parents: Sociodemographic, child-related, parent-related, parenting and family-functioning correlates of parental burnout. *Journal of Child and Family Studies, 27*(2), 602–614. https://doi.org/10.1007/s10826-017-0892-4

Minges, K. E., Owen, N., Salmon, J., Chao, A., Dunstan, D. W., & Whittemore, R. (2015). Reducing youth screen time: Qualitative meta-synthesis of findings on barriers and facilitators. *Health Psychology, 34*(4), 381–397. https://doi.org/10.1037/hea0000172

Pedrotti, B. G., Mallmann, M. Y., Almeida, C. R. S., Marques, F. M., Vescovi, G., Riter, H. D. S., Almeida, M. L., Pieta, M. A. M., & Frizzo, G. B. (2022). Infants' and toddlers' digital media use and mothers' mental health: A comparative study before and during the COVID-19 pandemic. *Infant Mental Health Journal, 43*(1), 24–35. https://doi.org/10.1002/imhj.21952

Prikhidko, A., Long, H., & Wheaton, M. G. (2020). The effect of concerns about COVID-19 on anxiety, stress, parental burnout, and emotion regulation: The role of susceptibility to digital emotion contagion. *Frontiers in Public Health, 8*, 567250. https://doi.org/10.3389/fpubh.2020.567250

Radesky, J. S., Kistin, C., Eisenberg, S., Gross, J., Block, G., Zuckerman, B., & Silverstein, M. (2016). Parent perspectives on their Mobile technology use: The excitement and exhaustion of parenting while connected. *Journal of Developmental & Behavioral Pediatrics, 37*(9), 694–701. https://doi.org/10.1097/DBP.0000000000000357

Rideout, V., & Robb, M.B. (2020). *The Common Sense census: Media use by kids age zero to eight*. https://www.commonsensemedia.org/sites/default/files/uploads/research/2020_zero_to_eight_census_final_web.pdf

Shafer, K., Scheibling, C., & Milkie, M. A. (2020). The division of domestic labor before and during the COVID-19 pandemic in Canada: Stagnation versus shifts in fathers' contributions. *Canadian Review of Sociology/Revue Canadienne de Sociologie, 57*(4), 523–549. https://doi.org/10.1111/cars.12315

Stienwandt, S., Cameron, E. E., Soderstrom, M., Casar, M., Le, C., & Roos, L. E. (2022). Family factors associated with hands-on play and screen time during the COVID-19 pandemic. *Child & Youth Care Forum, 51*(6), 1091–1115. https://doi.org/10.1007/s10566-021-09668-4

Taylor, S. (2022). The psychology of pandemics: Lessons learned for the future. *Canadian Psychology/Psychologie canadienne, 63*(2), 233–246. https://doi.org/10.1037/cap0000303

Vanderloo, L. M., Carsley, S., Aglipay, M., Cost, K. T., Maguire, J., & Birken, C. S. (2020). Applying Harm Reduction Principles to Address Screen Time in Young Children Amidst the COVID-19 Pandemic. *Journal of developmental and behavioral pediatrics : JDBP, 41*(5), 335–336. https://doi.org/10.1097/DBP.0000000000000825

Vescovi, G., Riter, H. D. S., Azevedo, E. C., Pedrotti, B. G., & Frizzo, G. B. (2021). Parenting, mental health, and Covid-19: A rapid systematic review. *Psicologia – Teoria e Prática, 23*(1). https://doi.org/10.5935/1980-6906/ePTPC1913554

Woźniak-Prus, M., Gambin, M., Sękowski, M., Cudo, A., Pisula, E., Kiepura-Nawrocka, E., Boruszak-Kiziukiewicz, J., & Kmita, G. (2023). Positive experiences in the parent-child relationship during the COVID-19 lockdown in Poland: The role of emotion regulation, empathy, parenting self-efficacy, and social support. *Family Process, 63*, 443. https://doi.org/10.1111/famp.12856

Chapter 14
Technoference: How Digital Media May Interfere with Family Interactions

Maíra Lopes Almeida, Manoela Yustas Mallmann, Sofia Sebben, Caroline Fitzpatrick, and Giana Bitencourt Frizzo

Introduction

Nowadays, people are embedded in a digital world, where digital media are ubiquitous in everyday life and social interactions. A recent study shows that 95% of American households have at least one smartphone (Rideout, 2017). In this sense, mobile device ownership provides the possibility for full-time connectivity to Internet content and others through instant messaging or social media (Kildare & Middlemiss, 2017; McDaniel & Radesky, 2018b; Rideout, 2017; Rideout & Robb, 2020; Stockdale et al., 2018). Furthermore, the increased popularity of mobile devices forecasts important changes in how we communicate and interact with others.

According to the latest Common Sense Media, over the last 9 years, media use patterns in children have remained stable (Rideout & Robb, 2020). Most screen time is spent watching TV and videos. In 2020, screen time among children aged

M. L. Almeida
Faculty of Education, Universidade Federal de Goiás, Goiânia, Goiás, Brazil

Psychology Postgraduation Program, Universidade Federal do Rio Grande do Sul, Porto Alegre, Rio Grande do Sul, Brazil
e-mail: mairaalmeida@ufg.br

M. Y. Mallmann · S. Sebben · G. B. Frizzo (✉)
Psychology Postgraduation Program, Universidade Federal do Rio Grande do Sul, Porto Alegre, Rio Grande do Sul, Brazil
e-mail: sofia.colognese@ufrgs.br; giana.frizzo@ufrgs.br

C. Fitzpatrick
University of Sherbrooke, Sherbrooke, Quebec, Canada

Department of Childhood Education, University of Johannesburg, Porto Alegre, Rio Grande do Sul, Brazil
e-mail: caroline.fitzpatrick@usherbrooke.ca

G. B. Frizzo (ed.), *Digital Media and Early Child Development*,
https://doi.org/10.1007/978-3-031-69224-6_14

0–8 was 2 h and 24 min a day. Furthermore, parental factors, such as family income and education, were also associated with children's media use.

The use of digital media can afford users some benefits. For instance, it can increase social support, facilitate interaction with relatives who live in other areas, enable individuals to work from home, and even bring information and enjoyable moments to individuals, couples, and families (McDaniel & Coyne, 2016). However, excessive or poorly regulated use of digital media can also harm interpersonal relationships. The extent to which technology use interferes with the quality of interpersonal relationships has been named *technoference* (McDaniel & Coyne, 2016; McDaniel & Radesky, 2018a; Stockdale et al., 2018). Past research brought attention to not only considering screen time but the entire context of media use (Barr, 2019; Barr et al., 2020). In this sense, technoference may be a phenomenon of interest to better understand how digital devices might interfere with personal interaction.

Technoference may occur in various interpersonal relationships, with initial studies exploring this concept among couples (McDaniel & Coyne, 2016; McDaniel & Drouin, 2019). Researchers have also examined the possible effects of technoference in other types of relationships, such as parent-child interaction (Lemish et al., 2019) and child behavior (McDaniel & Radesky, 2018b). In families with young children, parents' use of technology is frequently associated with less parent-infant interaction and child externalizing behavior (McDaniel & Radesky, 2018b). Given the increase in studies regarding technoference and its possible effects on individuals and family relationships, what would be its effects on individuals and family relationships? Moreover, how do studies consider and measure technoference? In this chapter, we aim to address these two questions.

Measurement of Technoference

The *Technology Device Interference Scale* (TDIS) has been one of the most used measures of technoference. This scale involves participants rating how frequently digital media get in the way of or interrupt interactions with their partners or family members. The TDIS is a six-point Likert-type scale that people can rate their perceptions on: 0 (never), 1 (rarely), 2 (sometimes), 3 (often), 4 (very often), and 5 (all the time). There are adaptations of the TDIS to parent-child relationships (McDaniel & Radesky, 2018a; Stockdale et al., 2018) and Spanish idiom (González-Rivera & Hernández-Gato, 2018). Regarding its psychometric properties, this scale shows moderate internal reliability (Cronbach's alpha was .67), with some evidence of construct validity.

Another instrument that is most used (25%) is the *Technology Interference in Life Examples Scale* (TILES). The TILES also aims to assess participant's perceptions of how frequently technology interferes in their daily relationships. Examples of items include the following: "During a typical lunch that my partner and I spend together, my couple uses and checks their cell phone or mobile device." Participants rate five items on an eight-point scale: 0 (never) to 7 (10 or more times a day).

Cronbach's alpha was .85; furthermore, the principal components analysis revealed one factor, supporting its construct validity.

Other examples of scales used to evaluate the construct are Parent Problematic Digital Technology Use (McDaniel & Radesky, 2018a), Parental Phubbing Scale (Wang et al., 2020), and Technology Interference with parenting (Newsham et al., 2018). The first one is a three-item self-report instrument: (1) "When my mobile phone alerts me to indicate new messages, I cannot resist checking them." (2) "I often think about calls or messages I might receive on my mobile phone." (3) "I feel like I use my mobile phone too much." Participants should rate a 6-point scale ranging from 1 (strongly disagree) to 6 (strongly agree). Higher scores indicate more problematic use; Cronbach's alpha was .74 for mothers and .78 for fathers. The second one is an adapted version of the Partner Phubbing Scale (Roberts & David, 2016). It has nine items, such as "My parents' glance at his/her cell phone when talking to me." They rated each item on a five-point scale ranging from 1 (never) to 5 (always), and Cronbach's alpha was .82. The third one, participants answered how many minutes per day they engaged in 11 activities, such as mealtime and bathing, which were reported as individual scores as well as a combined *Time in all activities score* (Cronbach's alpha = .73). Participants were then asked how often they felt technology interfered with each of the 11 activities on a 6-point Likert scale (1 = never, 6 = always). The authors created a composite variable by calculating the mean for all the parenting domains *Technoference in all activities* (Cronbach's alpha = 0.94).

Impacts of Technoference on Family Relationships

The central aim of the studies on technoference and parent-child relationships was to determine the associations between technoference and parent technology use, child behavior, parenting stress, maternal representations of their children, media use of children, parent-child interaction, prosocial behavior, self-esteem, depressive symptoms, perceived social support, and maternal depression. To summarize, we can understand the impact of technoference on family relationships based on two main aspects: the impact of technoference on parent-child interaction and technoference and its impact on child developmental outcomes.

Parents' Technoference and Its Implications for Parent-Child Interaction

Lemish et al. (2019) found that parents' mobile phone use was related to parents' disengagement from their children. Although mobile use was not the only distractor, compared to others, it was highly observed during playground visits. McDaniel and Radesky (2018b) found a similar result once their study showed that increased technoference due to parent's use predicted their perceptions of interruptions in parent-child interaction, especially regarding mobile phones. Technoference can also negatively affect family relationship dynamics, such as the coparenting relationship, which can be harmful even for the child (McDaniel et al., 2018).

Radesky et al. (2018) found positive associations between the use of mobile phones during family meals and the mother's perception of her child as difficult, which was associated with less sensitivity to child emotions and needs, suggesting poorer parent-child interactions (Radesky et al., 2018). On the other hand, no significant association was found between parents and child media use and the amount of parent-child interaction (Poulain et al., 2019). The authors hypothesize that this result may be due to the study design, as it was impossible to assess shared activities' frequency, quality, and duration. A recent study also evaluated the social media use, parental stress, technoference, and perceptions of reduced family time among 183 caregivers of a young child. The results showed that there is more likely to occur greater interference from phone use in family interactions when parents are stressed (McDaniel et al., 2024).

A North American study examined, with a sample of 80 mothers and their elementary-aged children, the extent to which technoference correlated with their attachment (Zayia et al., 2021). It was found that frequent technoference might not significantly impact a mother's attachment to her child, but it does affect the child's attachment to the mother. Increased technoference frequency was linked to mothers giving lower ratings of their child's social-emotional functioning. Moreover, maternal attachment played a moderating role in the relationship between technoference and child externalizing behaviors, with a stronger attachment acting as a protective factor against the negative effects of technoference on child externalizing behaviors.

Parental Technoference: Child Behavior and Development Outcomes

Parents' technoference and child development outcomes are frequently associated in the scientific literature. Lemish et al. (2019) observed parents and their children in playgrounds and suggested that when parents were using their mobile devices, they paid less attention to their children, which could lead to health risks and a lack of sensitivity of parents to correspond appropriately to child's bid for attention, stressful situations, or the impossibility to share positive situations and feelings. These situations can be potentially detrimental to child development in the long term.

Most selected studies that addressed development outcomes investigated child behavior. In a longitudinal study, McDaniel and Radesky (2018a) suggest a bidirectional relation between young children (0–5), higher externalizing behavior, higher rates of technoference, and parenting stress. The results found associations with internalizing child behavior weaker and more related to child withdrawal. The authors also found similar results in a cross-sectional study (McDaniel & Radesky, 2018b). A study in the same field reported that higher media use by children and parents is associated with more difficulties and less prosocial behavior (Poulain et al., 2019). They also found that parent-child interaction was associated with fewer child behavioral difficulties. Only one study has reported attachment anxiety and gender as the main predictors of technoference, with women perceiving more conflict and problematic use of technology, both in their own and in their partners' behavior (McDaniel et al., 2018).

The study by Sundqvist et al. (2020) examined parental perceptions of technoference and the behavior of 4- and 5-year-old children through parental self-reporting. The results revealed that parents reported experiencing daily technology interference from both their own use of digital media and their children's use. Furthermore, parents' perceived technoference significantly explains child behavior problems. These studies above show that parental technoference has been linked to adverse developmental and behavioral outcomes in childhood. However, only a minority of studies have explored technoference related to children's media use, which could be an important avenue for future research.

Discussion

The present study aimed to review the scientific literature on technoference, especially its possible effects on individuals and family relationships. The selected publications support the fact that research on this construct has been increasing. Technologies and digital media are widely used, especially by younger generations, and offer both health benefits and risks for users (Chassiakos et al., 2016). Thus, studies must focus on technoference and its effects since this phenomenon seems definitive.

Although two articles used Principal Component Analysis (PCA) to extract factors, PCA generates components, not factors (Damásio, 2012) offering a simplified representation of the data. Therefore, Exploratory Factor Analysis would be more appropriate to provide valid evidence based on these instruments' internal content. In the search for reliable tools to assess technoference, the main instruments used were TDIS and TILES. The methodological procedures used in instrument development were not described in any article. In this respect, the authors do not report evidence of content validity or evidence based on the internal structure of the instruments.

Overall, almost all revised articles used quantitative methods and were cross-sectional. More longitudinal studies are needed to observe the effects of technoference on child development and family relationships. Besides, qualitative studies can provide new information about the motivations behind technoference and how this phenomenon occurs in families. Previous research identified significant benefits in longitudinal qualitative studies, especially in observing emotions and aspects of the experience involved in some topics (Lohani et al., 2018).

Concerning participants, the findings indicate that just a few articles included fathers' perceptions in addition to mothers (McDaniel et al., 2018; McDaniel &

Radesky, 2018a, b). Including the male perspective can be an improvement in technoference studies since, according to a systematic review, men and women have different perceptions of marital satisfaction (Zaheri et al., 2016). This can be considered a methodological advance since paternal involvement can significantly influence the child's developmental outcomes (Barker et al., 2017; Rempel et al., 2017).

Notably, the average age of adult participants in all articles is 33.4, mostly Caucasian and non-Hispanic. Future research should increase racial, ethnic, and socioeconomic diversity in their samples. Furthermore, it is important to highlight which type of digital media was considered in the studies, as each digital media can generate a different individual reaction. For example, a meta-analysis showed that phone calls and SMS messages increase psychological well-being while social media and online gaming decrease (Liu et al., 2019).

In the context of family relationships, it was observed that technoference is frequently investigated in families with young children. The current review outlines a critical role for this concept by suggesting that technoference can be detrimental to parent-child interactions once they find parents being less sensitive (Radesky et al., 2018) and engaged with the child (Lemish et al., 2019) due to technology as a distractor (McDaniel & Radesky, 2018b).

This result aligns with scientific literature about technology use in families with young children, which investigates the motivations for use and possible consequences of the ubiquitous presence of digital media in family routines (Domoff et al., 2019; Hinkley et al., 2017; Kildare & Middlemiss, 2017; Mallmann & Frizzo, 2019; Radesky et al., 2016). These studies indicate a relationship between excessive parental technology use and parents' difficulties, such as turning to technology to escape from conflicts, needing time to relax or do some household tasks, which may lead to a decreased interaction among family members. Another important finding is that parental technology use is commonly associated with more technology use and digital media exposure among children (Domoff et al., 2019; Pedrotti et al., 2022).

On the other hand, Poulain et al. (2019) offers a counterpoint once they found no significant association between greater technology use and parent-child interaction. According to the authors, these findings suggest that media use does not necessarily displace parent-child interaction. Moreover, it highlights the importance of considering that technology can also be one tool to promote parent-child interaction when it is used to improve shared moments and activities. In this sense, researchers should promote healthy ways to introduce technology in family relationships, not only excluding it from daily routines (Coyne et al., 2017; McDaniel et al., 2018; Radesky & Christakis, 2016). Notably, studies usually investigated parent-infant interactions and possible consequences for child development in the same studies. One possible reason is that they can influence each other and create a bidirectional dynamic over time (McDaniel & Radesky, 2018a). In this sense, some studies found that when technoference and higher media exposure distance parents from their children, the most common predicted outcome is increased externalizing behavior in children (Radesky et al., 2014).

Overall, regarding children's development outcomes, the studies stated that technoference is associated primarily with child behavior problems (McDaniel & Radesky, 2018a, b; Poulain et al., 2019). Children with self-regulation problems can be considered more challenging and be more exposed to digital media, as a coping mechanism for parents to deal with conflict and stress in their relationship with the child (McDaniel & Radesky, 2018a, b; Poulain et al., 2019; Radesky et al., 2014, 2018).

Besides, Lemish et al. (2019) also found a significant association with parents' technoference, which is safety and emotional concerns as possible consequences for the child. The first is related to the risk of accidents in the playground, for example, when parents are distracted using their mobile devices. The second refers to consequences, especially in the long term, when parents are disengaged from the interaction with his or her children due to technology and respond less to the child's bids for attention, to the child's difficulties, and even miss decisive moments. This context can be detrimental not only to child development but also to family relationships and cohesion (McDaniel et al., 2018). All the aforementioned possible development outcomes associated with technoference and extensive technology use raise attention to the need to help families to cope with difficulties and manage family media use (Radesky et al., 2014).

Several reports have also shown associations between parents' increased digital media use, parenting stress, more conflicts over digital media use with children, and child externalizing behaviors (McDaniel & Radesky, 2018b; Poulain et al., 2019; Reus & Mosley, 2019). Other factors are positive parental beliefs about screen exposure and parents' use, which predicted an increase in young children's screen exposure (Reus & Mosley, 2019). The scientific literature about technoference also shows that depression (Newsham et al., 2018), anxiety, and relationship satisfaction are factors also related to more significant measures of technoference (González-Rivera & Hernández-Gato, 2018).

Final Considerations

This review points out that despite being a new concept, studies on technoference are increasing. Further research is needed to study the concept with different samples and methodological designs. Another suggestion is to conduct psychometric studies with the instruments to assess technoference.

The findings showed that technoference was associated with adverse effects on parental relationships. No study has pointed out the benefits of these relationships until now. As technoference is a new concept, we identified interesting data and reflections regarding technoference in interpersonal relationships. We raised additional possibilities for research by identifying concerns, especially in the family dynamic, which may help develop future interventions.

References

Barker, B., Iles, J. E., & Ramchandani, P. G. (2017). Fathers, fathering, and child psychopathology. *Current Opinion in Psychology, 15*, 87–92. https://doi.org/10.1016/j.copsyc.2017.02.015

Barr, R. (2019). Growing up in the digital age: Early learning and family media ecology. *Current Directions in Psychological Science, 28*(4), 341–346. https://doi.org/10.1177/0963721419838245

Barr, R., Kirkorian, H., Radesky, J., Coyne, S., Nichols, D., Blanchfield, O., et al. (2020). Beyond screen time: A synergistic approach to a more comprehensive assessment of family media exposure during early childhood. *Frontiers in Psychology, 11*, 1283. https://doi.org/10.3389/fpsyg.2020.01283

Chassiakos, Y., Radesky, J., Christakis, D., Moreno, M. A., Cross, C., & Council on Communications and Media. (2016). Children and adolescents and digital media. *Pediatrics, 138*(5), e20162593. https://doi.org/10.1542/peds.2016-2593

Coyne, S. M., Radesky, J., Collier, K. M., Gentile, D. A., Linder, J. R., Nathanson, A. I., et al. (2017). Parenting and digital media. *Pediatrics, 140*(Supplement 2), S112–S116. https://doi.org/10.1542/peds.2016-1758N

Damásio, B. F. (2012). Uses of exploratory factorial analysis in psychology. *Avaliação Psicológica, 11*(2), 213–228. http://pepsic.bvsalud.org/scielo.php?script=sci_arttext&pid=S1677-04712012000200007&lng=pt&tlng=

Domoff, S. E., Radesky, J. S., Harrison, K., Riley, H., Lumeng, J. C., & Miller, A. L. (2019). A naturalistic study of child and family screen media and mobile device use. *Journal of Child and Family Studies, 28*(2), 401–410. https://doi.org/10.1007/s10826-018-1275-1

González-Rivera, J. A., & Hernández-Gato, I. (2018). Conflicts in romantic relationships over Facebook use: Validation and psychometric study. *Behavioral Sciences, 9*(2), 18. https://doi.org/10.3390/bs9020018

Hinkley, T., Carson, V., Kalomakaefu, K., & Brown, H. (2017). What mums think matters: A mediating model of maternal perceptions of the impact of screen time on preschoolers' actual screen time. *Preventive Medicine Reports, 6*, 339–345. https://doi.org/10.1016/j.pmedr.2017.04.015

Kildare, C. A., & Middlemiss, W. (2017). Impact of parents mobile device use on parent-child interaction: A literature review. *Computers in Human Behavior, 75*, 579–593. https://doi.org/10.1016/j.chb.2017.06.003

Lemish, D., Elias, N., & Floegel, D. (2019). "Look at me!" Parental use of mobile phones at the playground. *Mobile Media & Communication*. https://doi.org/10.1177/2050157919846916

Liu, D., Baumeister, R. F., Yang, C., & Hu, B. (2019). Digital communication media use and psychological well-being: A meta-analysis. *Journal of Computer-Mediated Communication, 24*(5), 259–273. https://doi.org/10.1093/jcmc/zmz013

Lohani, M., Hendershot, K. A., Pelletier, W., Stegenga, K., Dixon, M., Hinds, P., et al. (2018). Potential benefits to families, children, and adolescents, enrolled in longitudinal qualitative research. *IRB: Ethics & Human Research, 40*(4), 1–7. https://doi.org/10.1002/eahr.404001

Mallmann, M. Y., & Frizzo, G. B. (2019). O uso das novas tecnologias em famílias com bebês: Um mal necessário? [The use of new technologies in families with babies: A necessary evil?]. *Revista Cocar, 7*, 26–46. https://periodicos.uepa.br/index.php/cocar/article/view/2789

McDaniel, B. T., & Coyne, S. M. (2016). "Technoference": The interference of technology in couple relationships and implications for women's personal and relational well-being. *Psychology of Popular Media Culture, 5*(1), 85–98. https://doi.org/10.1037/ppm0000065

McDaniel, B. T., & Drouin, M. (2019). Daily technology interruptions and emotional and relational well-being. *Computers in Human Behavior, 99*, 1–8. https://doi.org/10.1016/j.chb.2019.04.027

McDaniel, B. T., & Radesky, J. S. (2018a). Technoference: Parent distraction with technology and associations with child behavior problems. *Child Development, 89*(1), 100–109. https://doi.org/10.1111/cdev.12822

McDaniel, B. T., & Radesky, J. S. (2018b). Technoference: Longitudinal associations between parent technology use, parenting stress, and child behavior problems. *Pediatric Research, 84*(2), 210–218. https://doi.org/10.1038/s41390-018-0052-6

McDaniel, B. T., Galovan, A. M., Cravens, J. D., & Drouin, M. (2018). "Technoference" and implications for mothers' and fathers' couple and coparenting relationship quality. *Computers in Human Behavior, 80*, 303–313. https://doi.org/10.1016/j.chb.2017.11.019

McDaniel, B. T., Ventura, A. K., & Drouin, M. (2024). Parent social media use and gaming on mobile phones, technoference in family time, and parenting stress. *Psychology of Popular Media*. Advance online publication. https://doi.org/10.1037/ppm0000539

Newsham, G., Drouin, M., & McDaniel, B. T. (2018). Problematic phone use, depression, and technology interference among mothers. *Psychology of Popular Media Culture*. https://doi.org/10.1037/ppm0000220

Pedrotti, B. G., Mallmann, M. Y., Santos Almeida, C. R., Marques, F. M., Vescovi, G., Riter, S., Almeida, M. L., Pieta, M. A. M., & Frizzo, G. B. (2022). Infants' and toddlers' digital media use and mothers' mental health: A comparative study before and during the COVID-19 pandemic. *Infant Mental Health Journal, 43*(1), 24–35. https://doi.org/10.1002/imhj.21952

Poulain, T., Ludwig, J., Hiemisch, A., Hilbert, A., & Kiess, W. (2019). Media use of mothers, media use of children, and parent–child interaction are related to behavioral difficulties and strengths of children. *International Journal of Environmental Research and Public Health, 16*(23), 4651. https://doi.org/10.3390/ijerph16234651

Radesky, J. S., & Christakis, D. A. (2016). Increased screen time: Implications for early childhood development and behavior. *Pediatric Clinics of North America, 63*(5), 827–839. https://doi.org/10.1016/j.pcl.2016.06.006

Radesky, J. S., Silverstein, M., Zuckerman, B., & Christakis, D. A. (2014). Infant self- regulation and early childhood media exposure. *Pediatrics, 133*(5), e1172–e1178. https://doi.org/10.1542/peds.2013-2367

Radesky, J., Kistin, C., Eisenberg, S., Gross, J., Block, G., Zuckerman, B., & Silverstein, M. (2016). Parent perspectives on their mobile technology use: The excitement and exhaustion of parenting while connected. *Journal of Developmental & Behavioral Pediatrics, 37*(9), 694–701. https://doi.org/10.1097/DBP.0000000000000357

Radesky, J., Leung, C., Appugliese, D., Miller, A. L., Lumeng, J. C., & Rosenblum, K. L. (2018). Maternal mental representations of the child and mobile phone use during parent-child mealtimes. *Journal of Developmental & Behavioral Pediatrics, 39*(4), 310–317. https://doi.org/10.1097/DBP.0000000000000556

Rempel, L. A., Rempel, J. K., Khuc, T. N., & Vui, L. T. (2017). Influence of father–infant relationship on infant development: A father-involvement intervention in Vietnam. *Developmental Psychology, 53*(10), 1844–1858. https://doi.org/10.1037/dev0000390

Reus, E. J., & Mosley, I. T. (2019). The health and development correlates of screen media exposure in children 0-5yrs: An integrative literature review. *Australian Journal of Child and Family Health Nursing, 15*(2), 12–21. https://doi.org/10.3316/informit.192484297913792

Rideout, V. (2017). *The Common Sense census: Media use by kids age zero to eight*. https://www.commonsensemedia.org/sites/default/files/uploads/research/2020_zero_to_eight_census_final_web.pdf

Rideout, V., & Robb, M. B. (2020). *The Common Sense census: Media use by kids age zero to eight, 2020*. https://www.commonsensemedia.org/sites/default/files/uploads/research/2020_zero_to_eight_census_final_web.pdf

Roberts, J. A., & David, M. E. (2016). My life has become a major distraction from my cell phone: Partner phubbing and relationship satisfaction among romantic partners. *Computers in Human Behavior, 54*, 134–141. https://doi.org/10.1016/j.chb.2015.07.058

Stockdale, L. A., Coyne, S. M., & Padilla-Walker, L. M. (2018). Parent and child Technoference and socioemotional behavioral outcomes: A nationally representative study of 10- to 20-year-Old adolescents. *Computers in Human Behavior, 88*, 219–226. https://doi.org/10.1016/j.chb.2018.06.034

Sundqvist, A., Heimann, M., & Koch, F.-S. (2020). Relationship between family Technoference and behavior problems in children aged 4–5 years. *Cyberpsychology, Behavior, and Social Networking, 23*(6), 371–376. https://doi.org/10.1089/cyber.2019.0512

Wang, X., Gao, L., Yang, J., Zhao, F., & Wang, P. (2020). Parental phubbing and adolescents' depressive symptoms: Self-esteem and perceived social support as moderators. *Journal of Youth and Adolescence, 49*(2), 427–437. https://doi.org/10.1007/s10964-019-01185-x

Zaheri, F., Dolatian, M., Shariati, M., Simbar, M., Ebadi, A., & Hasanpoor Azghadi, S. B. (2016). Effective factors in marital satisfaction in perspective of Iranian women and men: A systematic review. *Electronic Physician, 8*(12), 3369–3377. https://doi.org/10.19082/3369

Zayia, D., Parris, L., McDaniel, B., Braswell, G., & Zimmerman, C. (2021). Social learning in the digital age: Associations between technoference, mother-child attachment, and child social skills. *Journal of School Psychology, 87*, 64–81. https://doi.org/10.1016/j.jsp.2021.06.002

Chapter 15
How Do Coparenting and Maternal Support Networks Influence Infants' Digital Media Use?

Laura Canani da Rosa, Bruna Gabriella Pedrotti, Manoela Yustas Mallmann, and Giana Bitencourt Frizzo

Introduction

It is common to observe babies and small children using smartphones and tablets in public places and mainly on television within their homes. Scientific studies have also reported this phenomenon (Chassiakos et al., 2016; Radesky & Christakis, 2016; Domingues-Montanari, 2017; Elias et al., 2019). There has been a significant increase in the use of these digital media by babies and small children, including babies under 2 years old (Chassiakos et al., 2016; Nevski & Siibak, 2016). A study conducted in the United States identified an increase in the frequency of children using tablets and smartphones up to 2 years old, from 10% in 2011 to 46% in 2017 (Common Sense Media, 2017).

A worrying fact raised by a Brazilian study (Nobre et al., 2019) conducted with 104 children between 12 and 24 months is that, despite the median time of screen exposure being 45 min daily, there were cases where this time reached 8 h a day. It is important to remember that the Brazilian Society of Pediatrics recommends that children between 2 and 5 years old use screens for a maximum of 1 h daily and babies up to 2 years old should not be exposed to digital media due to possible risks to development, such as problems with sleep, vision, and learning associated with this use (SBP, 2019).

The use of digital media by this population has been done in various ways, such as during leisure and entertainment times, as an educational resource, and also so that parents can carry out household tasks (Nevski & Siibak, 2016; Nobre et al., 2019; Rideout & Robb, 2020). In the Brazilian context, the needs of mothers are a strong motivator for providing digital media to babies, for example, when they need to occupy them to perform some task (Mallmann & Frizzo, 2019). Another parental

L. C. da Rosa · B. G. Pedrotti · M. Y. Mallmann · G. B. Frizzo (✉)
Universidade Federal do Rio Grande do Sul, Porto Alegre, Brazil
e-mail: laura.canani@ufrgs.br; giana.frizzo@ufrgs.br

G. B. Frizzo (ed.), *Digital Media and Early Child Development*,
https://doi.org/10.1007/978-3-031-69224-6_15

motivator is to use this tool to calm and distract babies in times of difficulty (Radesky et al., 2016) or to assist in the behavioral regulation of the young child (Nevski & Siibak, 2016; Nobre et al., 2019), such as in tantrum situations, but this practice can be considered somewhat problematic.

Studies conducted in Brazil mainly focus on the maternal figure and her perspective on using and offering digital media to babies (Mallmann & Frizzo, 2019; Pedrotti, 2019). Mothers often play the role of primary caregiver of the child, assuming more roles in baby care than fathers. However, there may be differences between their perceptions and agreements regarding media (Connell et al., 2015). Thus, it is interesting to think about the processes of coparenting and their possible associations with the use of digital media in families. Coparenting is a concept that deals with how partners work together to perform the parental function (Feinberg, 2003; Frizzo et al., 2005; McDaniel & Coyne, 2016). It is a predictor for various factors such as marital satisfaction, parental quality (McDaniel & Coyne, 2016; Schoppe-Sullivan et al., 2004), as well as the behaviors and emotional security of the child (McDaniel & Coyne, 2016; Teubert & Pinquart, 2010). Also, coparenting has proven important in how digital media use occurs in families with children (Brown & Smolenaers, 2018).

Moments of positive use of digital media must prevail, in which they contribute to family dynamics, such as by providing moments of connection and support for parents and children through joint use, and that care is taken with situations in which they interrupt interactions both between parents and children, as well as between the parental couple (McDaniel & Coyne, 2016), it is essential to understand how parents have organized to include digital media in the family routine. It is noteworthy that baby care is not restricted only to the parental couple. Many children spend a significant part of their time under the care of other relatives, such as grandparents, so using digital media in this context should also be investigated (Elias et al., 2019).

The role of other family members beyond the nuclear family is referred to here as the support network. These ties are extremely important for maintaining individual health, especially during significant changes and difficulties (Juliano & Yunes, 2014). Support networks can perform different functions, such as emotional support (expressions of care and comfort), informational (guidance and information), or instrumental (provision of resources, services, and problem-solving) (Rapoport & Piccinini, 2006). In the context of motherhood, the social support that the woman receives constitutes a protective factor in times of stress and significantly influences her well-being, facilitating responsive mothering (Rapoport & Piccinini, 2006) and also influencing child development.

In the globalized world, geographical distance significantly aggravates the support networks, especially the instrumental ones (Rapoport & Piccinini, 2006). In this context, digital media has begun to be seen as allies in child care for busy mothers and fathers, providing distractions in a safe environment so caregivers can perform other activities (Pinto et al., 2016). However, the support network can be considered an alternative to offering screens to babies at these times for parents who can count on the help of other family members in the care of their children (Lampard et al., 2013). A study in the United States identified family factors as the most important characteristics of restricting children's screen time. Screen time was lower in families that received more social support (Lampard et al., 2013). However, this idea is not a consensus. A recent study that investigated the use of media by children aged 2 to 7 when they were under the care of their grandparents showed that the children spent about half of the time under the care of their grandparents using media (Elias et al., 2019). From this, it is understood that aspects related to family dynamics can influence the supply and demand of digital media use by parents and their babies. With this in mind, the objectives of this study were to investigate the processes of co-parenting and the configuration of the support networks of mothers who use digital media in their routine with their babies and those who do not, as well as their possible influences on babies' access to digital media.

Getting in Touch with Mothers

To learn more about this, we gathered seven mothers who offered screens to their babies in a focus group to explore how this use was and in which contexts it happened openly and flexibly. We also interviewed eight mothers who did not offer screens to their babies, with whom we explored the adults' use of technology, what their opinions on the topic were, what motivations led them to avoid the use of technologies by their babies, as well as what strategies they used as a substitute. When analyzing the mothers' reports through thematic analysis (Braun et al., 2019), three main themes were identified: "The role of the father," "Grandparents as the main support network," and "Screens as babysitters." The first theme encompasses two sub-themes: "Parental consensus in the decision to offer screens" and "Participation in the care and play with the baby."

The first theme, "The role of the father," deals with the father's involvement in the family dynamics, precisely considering the importance of parental support and co-parenting processes for babies' use of digital media. Regarding the first sub-theme, it was identified that mothers who chose not to use digital media in their routine with their children reported more frequently that there was consensus between the parental couple in this decision. This can be observed through the report of P1G2: "Yes... Actually, [partner's name], he has the same line, like, very much... rescuing the natural and such then... it was something that we, when we talked, it was already a common opinion, it was never like: 'Ah, but I want them to watch...,' like, we always agreed on this." On the other hand, mothers who used digital media with their children reported greater disagreements on the topic, as can be seen in the speech of P1G1: "I just wish my husband had the same awareness that I do because I have to... like, he doesn't, he does not get mad or anything, but I have to say like [...] then he puts away his cell phone, you know, but if not, girl...."

Regarding the sub-theme "Participation in the Care and Play with the Baby," it was decided to divide the type of paternal participation into "more interactive" and "less interactive" based on the mothers' reports. It was found that mothers who did not offer digital media to their babies portrayed their children's fathers as more involved in their care and interaction, mainly in games. Thus, when mothers wanted to rest, fathers said they would care for the baby, carrying out activities with traditional toys and musical instruments. For example:

> It is a consensus between us; we divide a lot, too. When he [P2G2's husband] comes home, I am not working, right? However, he, when he is at home, he spends much time with her [the baby] and… our idea is really to play with her, is to be there for her, to offer stimuli, right, we already have, like, some games that we play with her, with animals, with colors, with sounds, right, he plays, she likes to see him playing the guitar… (P2G2)

Meanwhile, mothers who chose to offer digital media to their children reported that the babies' fathers interacted less in care, opting to distract them with digital media:

> […]he [P4G1's husband] allows more than I do, in the sense of giving the cell phone or putting them on TV. He leaves her [the baby] with "Galinha Pintadinha[1]" and goes to do his things. […] But he doesn't use the toy resource. He grabs them, booms, sits her in the chair, and turns on "Galinha Pintadinha." Then I get up, "No, let's turn off the chicken; we're not going to put on "Galinha Pintadinha." Leave that for when nothing else works, right. So that's something I notice, that he allows more than I do… (P4G1)

On the other hand, in the same group of mothers who offered screens to their children, Participant 6 from Group 1 reported that the baby's father participated in the child's care in a "more interactive" way, which reduced her screen exposure time:

> At home it is a bit different. My husband likes to sit and play with the children more. Or make them use toys like that. So much so that he instituted that the TV is not turned on at mealtime. Moreover, some other things, not that I don't care, I do, but he is more emphatic about playing, not using.

Regarding the second theme, "Grandparents as the main support network," it was identified that most mothers from both groups rely on grandparents as their main support network, who mainly provide operational help, such as taking care of the child at a time when neither the mother nor the father was available. It is observed in the speeches: "[…]who has been helping a lot is my mother. She picks him up from… she picks him up from daycare" (P4G2) and "[…]when I went back to work, for example, my mother stayed with her, so, when she was 5 months old, and my mother stayed with her" (P1G1).

An important point highlighted by most mothers was the fact that grandparents, especially the maternal grandmother, were the main source of children's screen exposure, even in cases where mothers chose not to offer screens to them, even becoming a cause of family conflict:

> […]any whim that she [the baby] makes my mother "oh come here," she already pulls out the cell phone and starts to show her own videos, that she records and goes there… but then, like, I usually don't do that. […] Then my mother, man, anything she stays, then when my mother is there, my daughter gets much more glued [to the cell phone], like that. And then, for example, when the mother wants to see something, okay, it's over, my daughter starts… then she gets mad because she wants more, then she starts to hunt for the cell phone. Then I said, no, it doesn't work. Then when I'm at home and see my mother doing this, I say: "Mom, don't keep showing, giving her the cell phone all the time." (P3G1)

[1] Galinha Pintadinha is a very popular character of music videos for children in Brazil, she sings a lot of very popular Brazilian songs that parents used to hear when they were a child.

The third and last theme, "Screens as babysitters," dealt with the relevance of digital media as an extra component of the maternal support network in caring for their children. This happened because they were offered to the babies by the mothers as a way to distract the children in moments of their own need when they could not attentively participate in the baby's care:

> Yes, to be able to cook, to be able to make her dinner, those things right... it's exactly what happens at home [...]I think it's... it's a way out... Bah, these days... I remembered I had to go to my hairdresser. "Just do a strand test, like, for an hour and a half, and I didn't have anyone to leave [baby's name] with... she goes along, right." Then she wanted to walk around, and she was touching the manicurists' nail polishes... this won't end well. I said: "Daughter, come here." And then she didn't want to, she wanted to stir things up, right, stir things up, I don't know what... and then I said: "Okay. Sit here." Look, I think it must have been almost an hour, right here. And then the phone, when I started to see that the battery would die... (P3G1)

Beyond that, digital media were accepted by mothers who did not offer media to their babies as a legitimate resource at certain times, as reported below: "Ah, I, um... no... no condemn, like, right. No... I think... each one... knows what is necessary at that moment. Right, we sometimes, as a mother, hear so much... so much advice, so much stuff, right, but nobody is living what we are living at that moment. I do not use this artifice; there are other things that I use..." (P4G2).

Through these vignettes, it was possible to investigate nuances of the co-parenting process and the configuration of the support network in families that use digital media in their routine with their babies and in families that do not use it. It should be noted that in the families participating in the research, the mothers were the main caregivers of the babies, according to their report. It was noticed that there was a prior agreement on the use of digital media, as well as good communication and consensus of the parental couple regarding the theme (Brown & Smolenaers, 2018). In families that did not offer digital media to children, this decision seems to have been made from a consensus of the couple, being a possible positive indicator of co-parenting (Frizzo et al., 2005). In the group of mothers who offered digital media, some reported difficulties or even the absence of dialogue on the subject.

Through the mothers' reports, the couples' consensus on offering or not offering digital media to their babies seems to be related to a more cooperative performance of co-parenting. Furthermore, since such consensus was more evident in families that do not offer digital media to babies, it may also be related to the parent's own use. As pointed out by McDaniel and Coyne (2016), there is an association between a worse ability to perform cooperative co-parenting in couples and a relationship more permeated by interruptions of digital media, a phenomenon known as technointerference.

The term mentioned above has been widely studied in the literature and refers to interruptions in various types of relationships, having been initially much studied in the conjugal sphere. However, these interferences can also extend to the parent-baby relationship (McDaniel & Radesky, 2018) and parent-child, contributing to the reduction of interaction in moments of baby care (Canadian Paediatrics Society,

2017), to the lesser quantity and quality of family interaction and even to behavior problems in children (McDaniel & Radesky, 2018).

This finding points to the relevance of parents receiving help and greater openness from health professionals to talk about the topic (Brown & Smolenaers, 2018). The more parents reflect on the use of digital media and its role within families' routines, the more space is opened for media not to be idealized nor rejected but used in the best possible way within the family (Nevski & Siibak, 2016). Having more knowledge about the risks and benefits of using digital media, parents can make more conscious choices concerning the construction of habits related to the family's decision to incorporate or not incorporate digital media into the household routine, which should be based on reliable information and not just on common sense (Brown & Smolenaers, 2018).

For this, another important point identified in the study concerns the way media is offered to babies. For example, according to the mothers' reports, how parents offer media to babies seemed related to the father's availability to take care of the baby. In this sense, mothers who considered the father's participation as "more interactive" identified that the partner used more play than media when caring for the baby. Therefore, even though digital media were considered a valid resource in these families, other activities were prioritized during parent-baby interaction times. According to the mothers' reports, it can be thought that the fathers in this study seem to engage in more active and agitated play with their children, with greater physical involvement (Waldman-Levi, 2021). This reality may encourage them to create more play with their children as alternatives to media use. However, it should be noted that, in addition to playing, it is important that there is an appropriate division of care within the family environment involving the various types of demands that the baby requires so that no parent feels overwhelmed, as tends to be the role of women in today's society, who are usually the main caregivers for the baby (Frizzo et al., 2019).

To seek the best possible use of digital media within the family, it is also important to consider the role of other members who are important caregivers for the children. Due to different family configurations and the participation of both men and women in the labor market, grandparents have a significant presence as caregivers of grandchildren and even in the economic functions of the home (Kaptijn et al., 2010).

In the present study sample, grandparents were mentioned as the main components of the support network. In addition, the help offered to families by grandparents is configured as an instrumental support network (Rapoport & Piccinini, 2006). Even so, a surprising and very relevant result of the present study was that grandparents were considered the main source of exposure of babies to digital media. This reality becomes a challenge for mothers and fathers who seek, precisely, to count on parents or in-laws to take care of their children to avoid their exposure to digital media. Considering that, according to the reality of many families, this is often the only option for parents, it may be even more difficult to follow the recommendations of experts regarding screen time (Beck et al., 2015).

Elias et al. (2019) found results aligned with those of the present study, identifying that children under the care of grandparents used digital media about half the time they were with them. Seeking to better understand the findings, the authors raised pertinent questions that can also be considered in our research. One of them concerns the greater tendency of grandparents to be more permissive with their grandchildren, offering screens even when their parents told them not to do so with the grandchildren (Elias et al., 2019). Another hypothesis raised is that, just as parents' exposure to digital media can occur at times when parents need to rest or are less available to entertain and play with their children (Mallmann & Frizzo, 2019; Pedrotti et al., 2021), the same can occur with grandparents, using this resource when they are tired. Also, it highlights how grandparents' care for their grandchildren has changed. Due to the increasing inclusion of the elderly in the digital world, they master the use of media much more, incorporating them into their routine. Nowadays, for example, many of them make video calls to interact with their grandchildren, talking, playing, and telling stories (Azambuja & Ramos, 2019).

The changes brought by the current technological world in moments when mothers do not have a member of their support network to assist in caring for babies also reflect the complex interplay of contemporary families and their decisions and possibilities about media usage. According to reports from mothers who offer media to their babies, media actually function as "nannies" (Brown & Smolenaers, 2018; Pinto et al., 2016).

It was possible to identify, as pointed out in the literature, that often the offer of digital media to babies, made by both parents and grandparents, occurred as a resource in times of need (Mallmann & Frizzo, 2019; Pedrotti et al., 2021). In light of this, when considering the reasons for using digital media in families with babies, it is necessary to consider caregivers' possible difficulties regarding the demands required in caring for a baby, which are many and often challenging, making caregivers feel tired. It can be hypothesized that guilt, a feeling that permeates motherhood in various aspects (Souza, 2018), is intensified by the ambivalence of feelings and the lack of information regarding media use (Mallmann & Frizzo, 2019).

Therefore, it is necessary to look at the caregivers' care. Also, especially when calming the baby, digital media cannot replace human interaction (Canadian Paediatrics Society, 2017; Raman et al., 2017). In this sense, the importance of coparenting becomes evident when it is satisfactory within the family environment—that is, when there is support and shared responsibility between parents (Frizzo et al., 2019; Schoppe-Sullivan & Mangelsdorf, 2013)—it is more likely that parents can count on mutual support in difficult times, such as calming the baby, without having to resort to digital media.

In light of this, we believe that parents' knowledge about the use of digital media and the importance of quality moments and affective exchanges with their babies can contribute to digital media being used beneficially within the family routine. It is also noted that this knowledge should be shared with all the people who make up the baby's support network and nuclear family, and the recommendations and guidelines on the subject should involve not only the parents but all the people involved in caring for a baby.

Final Considerations

This study aimed to investigate the processes of co-parenting and the configuration of the support networks of mothers who use digital media in their routine with their babies and those who do not. The importance of practicing cooperative co-parenting was highlighted, in which both mother and father actively engage with the child's care and seek to discuss arrangements regarding the child's care, aiming for better communication and consensus on parental decisions. Furthermore, even though some families choose not to offer digital media to babies, it is necessary to consider the insertion of digital media as a new component of family support networks in modernity (Brown & Smolenaers, 2018; Pinto et al., 2016; Rappoport & Piccinini, 2006).

Regarding the particularities of the studied population, differences were identified between the groups in the co-parenting processes and the paternal figure's participation in caring for the baby. From the mothers' reports, it can be thought that in a configuration in which the woman does not become overwhelmed and with the greatest load in the division of care and tasks in the family environment, there is a tendency for the father not to resort as much to the use of digital media in caring for the baby. The importance of dividing work and parental care is emphasized, considering that in a positive and satisfactory co-parenting for both parents, the division does not need to be necessarily divided equally but in a truly suitable way for both (Frizzo et al., 2019). On the other hand, similarities were perceived between the groups regarding the role of grandparents as important components of support networks and as a source of babies' access to screens. Therefore, although the support network is commonly associated with an alternative to screen use, it is configured as another source of access to technologies by babies.

The present study reinforces the relevance of thinking about the support network when exploring the use of digital media in families with babies, not only in the motivations and difficulties parents face. Furthermore, when thinking about strategies for the best possible use of digital media in the routine of families, as well as the reduction of use, when necessary, interventions that promote co-parenting are also suggested due to its influence on the process of choosing to offer digital media to babies and children.

Acknowledgments The original version of this chapter was written in Portuguese and translated into English with the help of artificial intelligence. A subsequent human revision was done primarily in terms of content.

Part of this work is published in the format of an article in the journal Rosa, L.C., Pedrotti, B.G., Mallmann, M.Y., and Frizzo, G.B. (2020). O Papel da coparentalidade e da rede de apoio materna no uso de mídias digitais por bebê. Contextos Clínicos, 13(3), 786-806. Available at: http://pepsic.bvsalud.org/scielo.php?script=sci_arttext&pid=S1983-34822020000300005&lng=pt&tlng=pt.

The editor has authorized the partial reproduction of the content for this chapter.

References

Azambuja, R. M. M., & Ramos, M. N. P. (2019). Avós e netos face às tecnologias de informação e comunicação. In E. P. Rabinovich et al. (Orgs.), *Envelhecimento & intergeracionalidade [Em linha]: Olhares Interdisciplinares* (Vol. 2, pp. 307–322). https://doi.org/10.248224/978854443065.1

Beck, A. L., Takayama, J., Badiner, N., & Halpern-Felsher, B. (2015). Latino parents' beliefs about television viewing by infants and toddlers. *Journal of Health Care for the Poor and Underserved, 26*(2), 463–474. https://doi.org/10.1353/hpu.2015.0037

Braun, V., Clarke, V., Hayfield, N., & Terry, G. (2019). Thematic analysis. In P. Liamputtong (Ed.), *Handbook of research methods in health social sciences* (pp. 843–860). Springer.

Brown, A., & Smolenaers, E. (2018). Parents' interpretations of screen time recommendations for children younger than 2 years. *Journal of Family Issues, 39*(2), 406–429. https://doi.org/10.1177/0192513X16646595

Canadian Paediatrics Society. (2017). *Paediatrics & child health* (pp. 461–468). Canadian Paediatrics Society. https://doi.org/10.1093/pch/pxx123

Chassiakos, Y. L. R., Radesky, J., Christakis, D., Moreno, M. A., & Cross, C. (2016). Children and adolescents and digital media. *Pediatrics, 138*(5), e20162593. https://doi.org/10.1542/peds.2016-2593

Common Sense Media. (2017). *The Common Sense Census: Media use by kids age zero to eight.* Common Sense Media.

Connell, S. L., Lauricella, A. R., & Wartella, E. (2015). Parents co-use of media technology with their young children in the USA. *Journal of Children and Media, 9*(1), 5–21. https://doi.org/10.1080/17482798.2015.997440

Domingues-Montanari, S. (2017). Clinical and psychological effects of excessive screen time on children. *Journal of Paediatrics and Child Health, 53*(4), 333–338. https://doi.org/10.1111/jpc.13462

Elias, N., Nimrod, G., & Lemish, D. (2019). The ultimate threat? Young Israeli children's media use under their grandparents' care. *Journal of Children and Media, 13*(4), 472–483. https://doi.org/10.1080/17482798.2019.1627228

Feinberg, M. E. (2003). The internal structure and ecological context of coparenting: A framework for research and intervention. *Parenting: Science and Practice, 3*(2), 95–131. https://doi.org/10.1207/S15327922PAR0302_01

Frizzo, G. B., Kreutz, C. M., Schmidt, C., Piccinini, C. A., & Bosa, C. A. (2005). O conceito de coparentalidade e suas implicações para a pesquisa e para a clínica. *Revista Brasileira Crescimento e Desenvolvimento Humano, 15*(3), 84–94. Retrieved from http://pepsic.bvsalud.org/scielo.php?script=sci_arttext&pid=S0104-12822005000300010.

Frizzo, G. B., Schmidt, B., Vargas, V., & Piccinini, C. A. (2019). Coparentalidade no Contexto de Depressão Pós-parto: um estudo qualitativo. *Revista Psico-USF, 24*(1), 85–96. https://doi.org/10.1590/1413-82712019240107

Juliano, M. C. C., & Yunes, M. A. M. (2014). Reflexões sobre rede de apoio social como mecanismo de proteção e promoção de resiliência. *Ambiente e Sociedade, 17*, 135–154. Retrieved from http://www.scielo.br/pdf/asoc/v17n3/v17n3a09.pdf

Kaptijn, R., Thomese, F., van Tilburg, T. G., & Liefbroer, A. C. (2010). How grandparents matter. *Human Nature, 21*, 393–405. https://doi.org/10.1007/s12110-010-9098-9

Lampard, A. M., Jurkowski, J. M., & Davison, K. K. (2013). The family context of low-income parents who restrict child screen time. *Childhood Obesity, 9*(5), 386–392. https://doi.org/10.1089/chi.2013.0043

Mallmann, M. Y., & Frizzo, G. B. (2019). O uso das novas tecnologias em famílias com bebês: um mal necessário? *Revista Cocar, 7*, 26–46. Retrieved from: https://paginas.uepa.br/seer/index.php/cocar/article/view/2789/1229

McDaniel, B. T., & Coyne, S. (2016). Technology interference in the parenting of young children: Implications for mother's perceptions of coparenting. *The Social Science Journal, 53*(4), 435–443. https://doi.org/10.1016/j.soscij.2016.04.010

McDaniel, B. T. & Radesky, J. S. (2018). Technoference: Parent distraction with technology and associations with child behavior problems. *Child Development, 89*(1), 100–109. https://doi.org/10.1111/cdev.12822

Nevski, E., & Siibak, A. (2016). The role of parents and parental mediation on 0–3-year olds' digital play with smart devices: Estonian parents' attitudes and practices. *Early Years, 36*(3), 227–241. https://doi.org/10.1080/09575146.2016.1161601

Nobre, J. N. P., Prat, B. V., Santos, J. N., Santos, L. R., Pereira, L., Guedes, S. C., & Morais, R. L. S. (2019). Quality of interactive media use in early childhood and child development: a multicriteria analysis. *Jornal de Pediatria, 96*(3), 310–317. https://doi.org/10.1016/j.jped.2018.11.015

Pedrotti, B. G. (2019). *Como prescindir das novas tecnologias no cuidado e na interação com os bebês?* Dissertação de Mestrado, Universidade Federal do Rio Grande do Sul, Porto Alegre, RS, Brasil.

Pedrotti, B. G., Mallmann, M. Y., Almeida, C. R. S., Marques, F. M., Vescovi, G., Riter, H. S., Almeida, M. L., Pieta, M. A. M., & Frizzo, G. B. (2021). Infants' and toddlers' digital media use and mothers' mental health: A comparative study before and during the COVID-19 pandemic. *Infant Mental Health Journal, 43*(1), 24–35. https://doi.org/10.1002/imhj.21952

Pinto, M. B., Jales, R. D., Andrade, L. D. F., & Santos, N. C. C. B. (2016). O brinquedo e o brincar: Infância e mudanças relacionais na modernidade líquida. *Revista de Enfermagem UFPE On Line, 10*, 3183–3189. https://doi.org/10.5205/reuol.9571-83638-1-SM1009201601

Radesky, J. S., & Christakis, D. A. (2016). Increased screen time: Implications for early childhood development and behavior. *Pediatric Clinics of North America, 63*(5), 827–839. https://doi.org/10.1016/j.pcl.2016.06.006

Radesky, J., Peacock-Chambers, E., Zuckerman, B., & Silverstein, M. (2016). Use of mobile technology to calm upset children: Associations with social-emotional development. *JAMA Pediatrics, 170*(4), 397–399. https://doi.org/10.1001/jamapediatrics.2015.4260

Raman, S., Guerrero-Duby, S., McCullough, J. L., Brown, M., Ostrowski-Delahanty, S., Langkamp, D., & Duby, J. C. (2017). Screen exposure during daily routines and a young child's risk for having social-emotional delay. *Clinical Pediatrics, 56*(13), 1244–1253. https://doi.org/10.1177/0009922816684

Rapoport, A., & Piccinini, C. A. (2006). Apoio social e experiência da maternidade. *Revista Brasileira de Crescimento e Desenvolvimento Humano, 16*(1), 85–96. https://doi.org/10.7322/jhgd.19783

Rideout, V., & Robb, M. B. (2020). *The Common Sense Census, Common Sense Media, 65*. https://pubmed.ncbi.nlm.nih.gov/28493400/

Schoppe-Sullivan, S. J., & Mangelsdorf, S. C. (2013). Parent characteristics and early coparenting behavior at the transition to parenthood. *Social Development, 22*, 363–383. https://doi.org/10.1111/sode.12014

Schoppe-Sullivan, S. J., Mangelsdorf, S. C., Frosch, C. A., & McHale, J. L. (2004). Associations between coparenting and marital behavior from infancy to the preschool years. *Journal of Family Psychology, 18*(1), 194–207. https://doi.org/10.1037/0893-3200.18.1.194

Sociedade Brasileira de Pediatria. (2019). *Menos telas, mais saúde*. Manual de Orientação, Grupo de Trabalho e Saúde na Era Digital. Retrieved from https://www.sbp.com.br/fileadmin/user_upload/_22246c-ManOrient_-__MenosTelas__MaisSaude.pdf

Souza, A. L. F. (2018). Maternidade, culpa e ruminação em tempos digitais. *Revista Ártemis, 25*(1), 89–112. https://doi.org/10.22478/ufpb.1807-8214.2018v25n1.37640

Teubert, D., & Pinquart, M. (2010). The association between coparenting and child adjustment: A meta-analysis. *Parenting: Science and Practice, 10*(4), 286–307. https://doi.org/10.1080/15295192.2010.492040

Waldman-Levi, A. (2021). Differences in how mothers and fathers support children playfulness. *Infant and Child Development, 30*(5), 1–10. https://doi.org/10.1002/icd.2257

Chapter 16
What Do Mothers Think About Toddlers' Digital Media Use?

Bruna Gabriella Pedrotti, Manoela Yustas Mallmann, and Giana Bitencourt Frizzo

Introduction

The use of digital media is increasingly frequent in today's society (Azevedo et al., 2022; Pedrotti et al., 2021; Rideout & Robb, 2020; Rocha et al., 2021). Thus, it is very difficult to imagine life and current relationships without the use of these devices. In the routines of families with children, digital media are also a constant presence, allowing caregivers and children to always be connected to the virtual world. Moreover, it is worth noting that the current generation of children is the first to be born immersed in a fully digital world, thus being exposed to these devices from an increasingly early age (Azevedo et al., 2022; Rideout & Robb, 2020).

Thus, parent-child relationships, so important in the first years of life, are currently permeated by digital media (Frizzo et al., 2020; Pempek & Lauricella, 2017). Child development is highly dependent on the environment in which the child develops (Bronfenbrenner, 2002). The first years of life are not only crucial for healthy development but also for establishing fundamental habits and relationships that will serve as a basis for adult life (Winnicott, 1987/2006). This occurs because the stimuli from the environment, as well as the relationships and bonds developed in the family environment, directly influence the way the child perceives the world and their own emotions, as well as acquires knowledge (Andrade et al., 2005; Navarro & Tudge, 2022; Neto & Gonçalves, 2019; Pempek & Lauricella, 2017; Vygotsky, 1989). In fact, the child learns not only through didactic explanations about how things work but mainly through models. By observing adults performing basic daily tasks, interacting with each other and with the child themselves, the child learns about how the world works, from a micro perspective (within their family environment), and later expands their acquired knowledge to other environments

B. G. Pedrotti (✉) · M. Y. Mallmann · G. B. Frizzo
Universidade Federal do Rio Grande do Sul (UFRGS), Porto Alegre, Brazil
e-mail: giana.frizzo@ufrgs.br

G. B. Frizzo (ed.), *Digital Media and Early Child Development*,
https://doi.org/10.1007/978-3-031-69224-6_16

in which they are inserted (Navarro & Tudge, 2022; Vygotsky, 1989). In this context, it is extremely relevant to investigate the use of digital media in families with infants and toddlers, understanding how it is utilized and what parents' views and motivations to offer or not digital media to their children.

In general, pediatric societies discourage the use of digital media for children up to 2 years old and recommend that usage between 2 and 5 years old be limited to up to 1 hour per day (AAP, 2016; Brazilian Pediatric Society, 2019). However, many studies suggest that this does not reflect the reality of most families. The literature points out that digital media use increases with children's age, even within the first 2 years of life (Goh et al., 2016). For example, the study by Goh et al. (2016) identified that by the age of 6 months, 29% of infants were already exposed to screens daily. Between 18 and 24 months of age, daily activities involving screens were part of the routine for 88.2% of toddlers, according to parental reports (Goh et al., 2016).

Also, a study conducted in the United States with 350 parents of children aged 6 months to 4 years investigated various aspects, including the circumstances under which parents allowed their children to use a mobile media device (Kabali et al., 2015). The results showed that 24.4% of 1-year-old infants already had access to mobile devices, and by the age of 2, most children were using mobile devices daily and spending a considerable amount of time in front of screens (TV and smartphones). In addition, most parents allowed their children to play with smartphones while they attended to their own tasks (70%) and to keep the child calm in public places (65%).

A study conducted through interviews with 26 Latino parents of children up to 2 years old highlighted that only four of the interviewed parents stated that children under 2 years old should not watch TV. However, only one parent reported that their child did not watch television. This sheds light on the fact that some parents offer digital media to their children, even though they understand that they should not use these technologies for certain reasons (Beck et al., 2015).

Seeking to rethink the way families use digital media, the *Royal College of Paediatrics and Child Health* (2019) in the United Kingdom took a position on the use of technologies by young children. Unlike previous recommendations, the institution proposed some questions about how families use digital media so that they could identify whether they are making good use of it, regardless of specific screen time limits. The four guiding questions they present are as follows: Is screen use in your home controlled? Does screen use interfere with what your family wants to do? Does screen use interfere with sleep? Do you control snack consumption during screen use (Royal College of Paediatrics and Child Health, 2019)?

Although they are flexible, the current guidelines continue to discourage the use of digital media by children up to 2 years old. Consequently, despite the constant and irreversible use of digital media in today's world, concerns persist regarding its usage, especially in excess, in families with infants. There are questions about how it might interfere with interactions and in child development. Specifically, regarding the use and exposure of young children (0–3 years old), this topic generates controversies, particularly considering the potential risks and benefits of digital media use by infants and toddlers.

The benefits are related to the possibility of connecting with distant family members through video calls, providing moments of leisure and entertainment for the family. It can also be an opportunity for exchange and learning, especially for children over 2 years old, with the assistance of a caregiver who helps them make sense of the content they are exposed to (AAP, 2016; Coyner et al., 2017). There is also greater learning through screens when the child does it in interaction with an important adult for them (Radesky et al., 2016). In this sense, the literature points out that digital media use can enhance family interactions and children's development as long as there is mediation from parents/guardians during its use (Coyner et al., 2017).

The risks pointed out in the literature are related to damages in developing self-regulation, language skills, cognition, and attention (Radesky et al., 2014), as well as behavioral difficulties (McDaniel & Radesky, 2018). Excessive media use by children is also associated with obesity, a sedentary lifestyle (AAP, 2016; Domingues-Montanari, 2017), and sleep problems (Cheung et al., 2017). Faced with these risks, many families do not know if and how to insert digital media into their children's routines. In practice, to make decisions regarding this matter, they rely on common sense and their own subjectivity (Brown & Smolenaers, 2018). From this reality, one of the main objectives of our research group was to understand how digital media use occurs in the daily routine of families with children up to 3 years old and to explore mothers' perspectives on this topic.

Understanding Mothers—Usage or Not of Digital Media with Their Babies and Toddlers

Two studies were conducted to understand mothers' motivations for offering and avoiding the use of digital media by their children under 2 years of age. In the first study (Mallmann & Frizzo, 2019), two focus groups were conducted with seven mothers who reported using digital media in their family routines with their babies. The groups aimed to provide a space for listening and exchange for these mothers, as well as to gain deeper insight into how digital media use occurred in each of their realities. On the other hand, we conducted another study to understand mothers' motivations for avoiding screen media use by their children (Pedrotti, 2019). The study included eight mothers of babies under 2 years old who stated they did not offer digital media to their children, as recommended by pediatric societies (AAP, 2016; Brazilian Society of Pediatrics, 2019) and the WHO (World Health Organization, 2019). In this study, semi-structured interviews were conducted with the mothers, exploring maternal beliefs on the subject, family routines, guidance received from professionals regarding infants' and toddlers' digital media use, support networks, and alternatives to offering digital media to their children.

Main Results

In the first study (Mallmann & Frizzo, 2019), themes were constructed from the content generated in the focus groups. The themes identified through thematic analysis (Braun et al., 2019) were the following: mothers' perspectives on the use of digital media, reasons for using digital media, adult use of digital media, and limitations regarding the use of digital media. Concerning the first theme, most mothers expressed a positive view of digital media, emphasizing its potential for children's learning and even mentioning the fear that children might "fall behind" compared to peers who were already proficient with contemporary technologies. However, fears also emerged related to the effects of use, especially when it is excessive. This fear appeared to be associated with concerns about the extent to which children become "hypnotized" while watching videos.

The theme concerning the reasons for using digital media yielded interesting results. The primary reason for exposing children up to 24 months to digital media is related to the caregivers' needs and not necessarily for the child's immediate benefit. This highlights the importance of focusing on the caregivers, who may possibly be overwhelmed and/or facing difficulties in the care and management of their children.

The theme of adults "use of digital media highlighted mothers" concerns about their own usage habits. For example, they acknowledge that they often spend much more time than they desire in front of their smartphones, which ends up interfering with their relationship with their children and serving as a model that they can follow. The theme related to the limits of digital media use pointed out the ambivalence of mothers who, while recognizing the positive aspects of its use, also consider it important to limit. They express concerns about the potential effects of digital media on children's development, as well as a resource that, when used without moderation, can distance family members. On the other hand, despite considering limiting the use, most of them admitted that, in practice, this does not occur; there is often no prior agreement between parents and/or caregivers regarding screen time. Consequently, usage remains uncontrolled and often becomes excessive, according to their opinion.

From the results of this study, the ambivalence of mothers becomes evident, and, consequently, the difficulty in "dosing" the use of digital media in their families' routines. Another noteworthy point is that, according to the mothers' report, the vast majority of them did not receive guidance from their child's pediatrician regarding exposure to digital media. As a result, many caregivers feel lost and even guilty about their children's use and exposure to digital media. Rather than simply advising that the use should be avoided, there is a clear need to support these families to ensure that digital media is utilized in the most beneficial manner possible. Space should be opened for reflection at these moments, focusing on promoting strategies to prevent negative interference in family interactions and/or children's development.

In the second study (Pedrotti, 2019), three themes were identified through thematic analysis (Braun et al., 2019): motivations to avoid digital media use, professional guidelines on digital media use, and alternatives to digital media use. The first theme refers to the motivations of mothers to avoid offering screens to their children during moments of care and interaction. Within this theme, maternal beliefs were identified, including their beliefs about the importance of early childhood, their perception of the priorities of motherhood, their understanding of the quality of initial interactions, and their perception of children who use these technologies. All participants, except one, stated that the choice not to offer screens to their children was a consensus reached between themselves and their partners. However, regarding agreements with other caregivers, such as grandparents, mothers reported encountering difficulties. This occurred because the support network relies on digital media to entertain children and also because mothers were afraid to demand family members to follow this guidance when they were already offering help in baby care.

Furthermore, all mothers expressed in their discourse that children's use of digital media is necessary for parents/adults rather than for the children themselves. The participants reported that they observed children becoming "hypnotized" when using screens. Moreover, according to the mothers' understanding, while digital media may assist adults in engaging in other activities while children are occupied, it may also hinder children from responding and being attentive to stimuli outside the screen. Even so, the report that digital media can be a positive resource was also present in the mothers' speech, with the caveat that this resource would become positive at other stages of development, but in the first 2 years, there would be other activities more beneficial for babies.

In order to delve into the study of children's needs in early childhood and base their practices in motherhood, many participants in this study sought scientific knowledge by reading articles and materials prepared by health and education professionals. For these mothers, reading scientific articles about children's digital media use was fundamental in their decision not to offer screens to their children. Moreover, the fact that studies present results that supported their choices reinforced their attitudes. This knowledge was indeed shared with other family members, primarily to ensure that everyone would be aware of the advantages of not offering digital media to babies, as well as the disadvantages of doing so.

In addition to associating the use of digital media by babies as a benefit for adults, the participants did not report other advantages in digital media use for infants and toddlers. Instead, the mothers emphasized the advantages of not offering screens to babies, including the development of creativity, the ability to perceive other interesting resources and stimuli in the environment, as well as the ability to play, be alone, and maintain focus on a specific activity. The disadvantages of offering digital media to infants and toddlers, from the mothers' perspective, included the reduction of interaction with others, damage to the development of creativity due to excessive stimuli from media, resources that would not allow symbolic play by children, fast-paced and minimally educational content, as well as potential harm to children's vision due to screen light and proximity.

Even with these mothers' scientifically based understanding, the majority of participants did not receive guidance from health or education professionals on how to proceed regarding infants' and toddlers' digital media use. Only two participants received guidance from their child's pediatrician without having to ask about the subject, and one participant was guided after questioning the pediatrician about the subject. The guidance provided to the mothers aligned with their beliefs as reported during the interviews, either emphasizing the potential damages of children's digital media use for the development of creativity, interaction, and attention capacity or highlighting the multitude of stimuli already available in the child's environment.

The participants of this study understood that early childhood is a crucial time when personal interactions are paramount for children's development. This understanding led them to seek alternatives to the use of screens, which constitutes the third theme identified in the thematic analysis of this study. Mothers attributed a playful connotation when describing the routines of caring for their babies, including toys and games related to the task (mealtime, diaper changing, or sleeping) so that the child engages in the activity and interacts with the adult. Additionally, some mothers mentioned the child's autonomy in exploring the entire environment during playtime and engaging in activities that did not require adult involvement but required supervision to ensure the baby's safety. Others described moments when babies demanded interaction with their mothers during playtime or when they shared such moments even without actively engaging in the game, which also required mothers' attention and presence at the child's playtime.

Nevertheless, mothers also mentioned toys that entertained their children during individual activities, which did not require the mother's direct participation in play, such as stacking blocks, puzzles, and fitting toys. They emphasized the importance of following the child's interest in certain toys and having these resources available to offer them during times when they should play alone. Even when unable to interact with their children because they needed to do other tasks, such as cooking, working, or taking a bath, most mothers offered objects related to the task they were performing or even toys to keep the child entertained nearby. The support of older children to entertain the baby was also mentioned as an alternative. Indeed, the maternal support network proved fundamental for mothers to carry out specific tasks, such as bathing. Almost half of the mothers reported only taking a bath when another caregiver was present in the house to attend to the baby. During situations like car trips, where the baby needs to be accommodated in the safety seat, mothers mentioned using toys and books to distract the child. However, this moment was also described as quite challenging for some mothers, as evidenced by one mother who chose to remove the baby from the car seat to calm and distract him on her lap instead of opting for other alternatives with less risk. Thus, the primary resources used by mothers to calm their babies consisted of holding them in their laps, engaging in conversation, and breastfeeding.

The participants also associated children's digital media use with the needs of adults rather than those of the children themselves. The decision not to offer screens to babies was related to the mothers' understanding that, at this development stage, screens are not indicated for them and that other resources can be more beneficial. Despite the majority of mothers not receiving professional guidance on the use of screens by infants and toddlers, access to scientific knowledge on the subject influenced some mothers' decision not to offer screens to their children. Thus, it was not the recommendations of pediatric societies themselves that were decisive in this choice, but rather the personal characteristics of the mothers. From the participants' reports, it was noticed the mothers' availability to meet their babies' demands, so they prioritized interaction with them over carrying out their own tasks.

What Can Be Concluded About Mothers' Choice to Expose or Not Their Children to Digital Media?

Some studies problematize the choice of mobile devices and television as a means to occupy children based on the availability of the father and mother to the child during the time they spend together (Santos & Barros, 2017). However, many parents spend the majority of their day involved with work so that children are under the care of others. When they are together, commonly at the end of the day, mothers and fathers are tired and seek refuge in digital media so that they can relax from their worries (Pedrotti et al., 2021; Radesky et al., 2016) and so that their children do not demand so much attention from them and can eventually carry out other tasks.

The interviewed mothers who declared not to offer digital media to their babies positioned themselves against offering screens to distract their children so that they could carry out other activities. These mothers seemed to prioritize their children's needs at first, leaving to fulfill other tasks when possible. Thus, they chose to seek alternatives to distract or calm their children, which did not involve the use of screens. However, they reported difficulty in balancing basic tasks such as taking a bath, traveling in cars, and performing work tasks in the absence of other caregivers. On the other hand, mothers who did offer screens to their babies reported feelings of guilt for doing so, once again highlighting the misalignment between the needs of families and the existing recommendations on this theme (Straker et al., 2018).

The studies conducted by Bentley et al. (2016) and Brown and Smolenaers (2018) found similar results, identifying that parents used digital media as a resource to distract their children when they needed to attend to other activities, desired rest, or during childcare tasks such as diaper changing and feeding. Even though the participants who offered digital media to their children reported the use of screens as a tool in these moments, they positioned themselves against the practice, stating that they would prefer to focus on their baby's needs over their own.

Furthermore, the majority of mothers expressed concerns about children's isolation from the environment when they use screens. Similarly, the study conducted by Bentley et al. (2016) pointed out that mothers perceived the use of mobile devices as a solitary and negative activity for the development of children's sociability, even though they allowed their children to use digital media, with some reluctance, because they understood that mobile devices are a necessary and inevitable part of life, just like the mothers who declared offering screens to their children in our study.

Even though some mothers who opted not to offer screens to their babies thought that digital media could potentially have positive aspects, they expressed a preference for their children to play with other things at this stage of development. They also prioritized family interaction and closeness. In this regard, the study by McCloskey et al. (2018) points out that some parents opted against exposing their children to digital media more frequently because they believed there were better ways for their children to play. Another factor that refers to the results of this study is that parents with higher levels of education were more likely to provide this type of answer (McCloskey et al., 2018), a characteristic similar to the sample of participants in this study, whose level of education corresponds to higher education or postgraduate studies. Furthermore, even among the mothers who reported offering screens to their babies, critical thinking was observed regarding the time, content, and manner in which children used digital media.

The critical thinking of mothers about this subject, as well as their interest in acquiring knowledge about this theme, can be related to the high level of education of the participants. However, the literature presents contrasting data regarding the relationship between the parent's education and the use of mobile devices and television by infants and toddlers. According to McCloskey et al. (2018), beliefs about digital media use and the reasons for its use varied according to ethnicity and parents' level of education, although there were no significant differences in relation to the family's socioeconomic level. However, other authors (Goh et al., 2016) did not observe significant associations between parents' education and the use of screens by children.

In the mothers' opinion, the main advantages of infants and toddlers not using digital media were related to the development of creativity and the ability to concentrate and focus on activities and moments of family interaction. Similarly, mothers who offered screens to their babies also expressed concern about the amount of time they spent in front of screens, the difficulty of limiting their babies' screen time, and the potential reduction in family interaction resulting from this. Primarily, parents' media use influences the child's screen use within the family microsystem (Domoff et al., 2020). Amid the numerous demands of motherhood, work, and other routine demands, added to the expectations outlined by pediatric societies' recommendations that may not align well with the realities of families with young children, mothers turn to screens both as a form of refuge and as a means to share their overload with other women who may be experiencing similar feelings (Pesce et al., 2023).

The concerns that motivate mothers not to offer these devices to their babies were intrinsically related to their children social well-being and the potential reduction in family interaction within this context (Hinkley et al., 2017; Peres et al., 2012; Radesky et al., 2016). Nevertheless, the mothers in this study who did offer screens to their children perceived it as advantageous for their children's cognitive development, a perspective also identified in other studies due to the educational value attributed to these devices (Beck et al., 2015; Bentley et al., 2016; Brown & Smolenaers, 2018; Ebbeck et al., 2016).

This is an advantage pointed out by several parents of infants and toddlers (Brown & Smolenaers, 2018; Domingues-Montanari, 2017). However, for learning to be possible, many cognitive functions are involved, such as attention, memory, language, and executive functions, among others. The context in which information is processed and the means by which it is accessed can significantly influence these mental processes (Barr & Linebarger, 2017). The impact of digital media on the development of children under 3 years old is complex and seems to be related to the amount of exposure, the content of the program, the context, and the manner in which the exposure occurs (Anderson & Subrahmanyam, 2017; Guellai et al., 2022; Swider-Cios et al., 2023). These data are important because they highlight the relevance of considering other factors besides screen time to understand the possible positive and negative impacts of screens in childhood. Moreover, during the first 3 years of life, the brain develops most rapidly, making this period one of heightened receptivity and vulnerability to environmental stimuli. Therefore, for healthy cognitive development to occur, it is crucial that the child's environment is verbally stimulating and permeated by positive interactions between the child and caregivers (Neto & Gonçalves, 2019).

However, up to this point, there are few studies that explore the effectiveness and adherence to guidelines set forth by pediatric societies regarding digital media use by infants and toddlers worldwide (Brown & Smolenaers, 2018). Consequently, questions arise about the feasibility of implementing these guidelines, whether they are achieving the desired impact, and what obstacles parents face in following them (Brown & Smolenaers, 2018). A very small proportion of parents with children in this age group are aware of the existence of these guidelines (Beck et al., 2015; Brown & Smolenaers, 2018; Goh et al., 2016). In both samples of participants in this study, receiving guidance on how to use digital media in families with infants was an exception. Findings from the study by Howe et al. (2017) indicate that parental awareness of these guidelines influences their practices regarding their children's screen use, as children whose parents were unaware of the guidelines used digital media more frequently compared to children whose parents were aware of the recommendations.

The results of these studies point to a common topic: the importance of considering the needs of mothers when developing realistic parameters regarding the use of digital media in families with infants and toddlers (Pedrotti et al., 2021). There is a need to discuss how to reconcile the demands of motherhood, which are often multifaceted and include various responsibilities and tasks, with creating an environment that offers adequate stimuli and safety for healthy child development. To achieve this, it is essential to approach digital media in a non-polarized way, viewing it not as inherently good or bad but rather promoting the use of these devices in the best possible way for both the mother and the child.

Acknowledgments The original version of this chapter was written in Portuguese and translated into English with the help of artificial intelligence. A subsequent human revision was done primarily in terms of content.

Part of this work is published in the format of an article in the journal: Mallmann, M.Y & Frizzo, G.B. (2019). O uso das novas tecnologias em famílias com bebês: um mal necessário? Revista Cocar, 7, 26–46. Available at https://periodicos.uepa.br/index.php/cocar/article/view/2789

The editor has authorized the partial reproduction of the content for this chapter.

References

American Academy of Pediatrics, Council on Communications and Media. (2016). Media and young minds. *Pediatrics, 138*(5), 1–8. https://doi.org/10.1542/peds.2016-2591

Anderson, D. R., & Subrahmanyam, K. (2017). Digital screen media and cognitive development. *Pediatrics, 140*(s2), e20161758. https://doi.org/10.1542/peds.2016-1758C

Andrade, S. A., Santos, D. N., Bastos, A. C., Pedromônico, M. R. M., Almeida-Filho, N., & Barreto, M. L. (2005). Family environment and child cognitive development: An epidemiological approach. *Public Health Journal, 39*(4), 606–611. https://doi.org/10.1590/S0034-89102005000400014

Azevedo, E. C., Riter, H. S., Pieta, M. A. M., & Frizzo, G. B. (2022). Digital media use on interactions between mother and child: Differences in infants' early years. *Paidéia (Ribeirão Preto), 32*. https://doi.org/10.1590/1982-4327e3210

Barr, R., & Linebarger, D. N. (2017). The new blooming, buzzing confusion: Introduction to media exposure during infancy and early childhood. In R. Barr & D. N. Linebarger, Orgs (Eds.), *Media exposure during infancy and early childhood: The effects of content and context on learning and development* (pp. XI–XVI). Springer.

Beck, A. L., Takayama, J., Badiner, N., & Halpern-Felsher, B. (2015). Latino parents' beliefs about television viewing by infants and toddlers. *Journal of Health Care for the Poor and Underserved, 26*(2), 463–474. https://doi.org/10.1353/hpu.2015.0037

Bentley, G. F., Turner, K. M., & Jago, R. (2016). Mothers' views of their preschool child's screen-viewing behaviour: A qualitative study. *BMC Public Health, 16*(718), 1–11. https://doi.org/10.1186/s12889-016-3440-z

Braun, V., Clarke, V., Hayfield, N., & Terry, G. (2019). Thematic analysis. In P. Liamputtong (Ed.), *Handbook of research methods in health social sciences* (pp. 843–860). Springer.

Brazilian Society of Pediatrics. (2019). *Less screens, more health*. Guidance Manual, Working Group and Health in the Digital Age. https://www.sbp.com.br/fileadmin/user_upload/_22246c-ManOrient_-__MenosTelas__MaisSaude.pdf

Bronfenbrenner, U. (2002). *The ecology of human development: Natural and planned experiments*. Medical Arts. (Original work published 1996).

Brown, A., & Smolenaers, E. (2018). Parent's interpretations of screen time recommendations for children younger than 2 years. *Journal of Family Issues, 39*(2), 1–24. https://doi.org/10.1177/0192513X16646595

Cheung, C. H. M., Bedford, R., Saez de Urabain, I. R., Karmiloff-Smith, A., & Smith, T. J. (2017). Daily touchscreen use in infants and toddlers is associated with reduced sleep and delayed sleep onset. *Scientific Reports, 7*(46104), 1–7. https://doi.org/10.1038/srep46104

Coyner, S. M., Radesky, J., Collier, K. M., Gentile, D. A., Linder, J. R., Nathanson, A. I., Rasmussen, E. E., Reich, S. M., & Rogers, J. (2017). Parenting and digital media. *Pediatrics, 140*(2), 112–116. https://doi.org/10.1542/peds.2016-1758N

Domingues-Montanari, S. (2017). Clinical and psychological effects of excessive screen time on children. *Journal of Paediatrics and Child Health, 53*, 333–338. https://doi.org/10.1111/jpc.13462

Domoff, S. E., Borgen, A. L., & Radesky, J. S. (2020). Interactional theory of childhood problematic media use. *Human Behavior and Emerging Technologies, 2*, 343–353. https://doi.org/10.1002/hbe2.217

Ebbeck, M., Yim, H. Y. B., Chan, Y., & Goh, M. (2016). Singaporean parents' views of their young children's access and use of technological devices. *Early Childhood Education Journal, 44*, 127–134. https://doi.org/10.1007/s10643-015-0695-4

Frizzo, G. B., Azevedo, E. C., Mallmann, M. Y., Pedrotti, B. G., & Pieta, M. A. M. (2020). Parenting in the digital age. In M. Benincasa, A. N. Romagnolo, & M. G. V. Heleno (Orgs.) (Eds.), *Motherhood, parenthood and conjugality: New perspectives in perinatal psychology* (pp. 293–311). CRV Publishing.

Goh, S. N., Teh, L. H., Tay, W. R., Anantharaman, S., Dam, R. M. V., Tan, C. S., et al. (2016). Sociodemographic, home environment and parental influences on total and device-specific screen viewing in children aged 2 years and below: An observational study. *BMJ Open*, 1–12. https://doi.org/10.1136/bmjopen-2015-009113

Guellai, B., Somogyi, E., Esseily, R., & Chopin, A. (2022). Effects of screen exposure on young children's cognitive development: A review. *Frontiers in Psychology, 13*(923370). https://doi.org/10.3389/fpsyg.2022.923370

Hinkley, T., Carson, V., Kalomakaefu, K., & Brown, H. (2017). What mums think matters: A mediating model of maternal perceptions of the impact of screen time on preschoolers' actual screen time. *Preventive Medicine Reports, 6*, 339–345. https://doi.org/10.1016/j.pmedr.2017.04.015

Howe, A. S., Heath, A. M., Lawrence, J., Galland, B. C., Gray, A. R., Taylor, B. J., … Taylor, R. W. (2017). Parenting style and family type, but not child temperament, are associated with television viewing time in children at two years of age. *PLoS ONE, 12*(12). https://doi.org/10.1371/journal.pone.0188558

Kabali, H. K., Irigoyen, M. M., Nunez-Davis, R., Budacki, J. G., Mohanty, S. H., Leister, K. P., & Bonner, R. L. (2015). Exposure and use of mobile media devices by young children. *Pediatrics, 136*(6), 1044–1050. https://doi.org/10.1542/peds.2015-2151

Mallmann, M. Y., & Frizzo, G. B. (2019). *O uso das novas tecnologias em famílias com bebês: um mal necessário? Revista Cocar, 7*, 26–46. Retrieved from: https://periodicos.uepa.br/index.php/cocar/article/view/2789

McCloskey, M., Johnson, S. L., Benz, C., Thompson, D. A., Chamberlin, B., Clark, L., & Bellows, L. L. (2018). Parent perceptions of mobile device use among preschool-aged children in rural head start centers. *Journal of Nutrition Education and Behavior, 50*(1), 83–89. https://doi.org/10.1016/j.jneb.2017.03.006

McDaniel, B. T., & Radesky, J. S. (2018). Technoference: Parent distraction with technology and associations with child behavior problems. *Child Development, 89*(1), 100–109. https://doi.org/10.1111/cdev.12822

Navarro, J. L., & Tudge, J. R. H. (2022). Technologizing Bronfenbrenner: Neo-ecological theory. *Current Psychology.*, 1. https://doi.org/10.1007/s12144-022-02738-3

Neto, R., & Gonçalves, D. D. (2019). Effects of exposure to digital devices on language development in preschool age. *Gazeta Médica, 6*(3), 154–162. https://orcid.org/0000-0001-9473-4563

Pedrotti, B. G. (2019). *Como prescindir das novas tecnologias no cuidado e na interação com os bebês?* [Master's thesis, Universidade Federal do Rio Grande do Sul, Porto Alegre, RS, Brazil].

Pedrotti, B. G., Mallmann, M. Y., Almeida, C. R. S., Marques, F. M., Vescovi, G., Riter, H. S., Almeida, M. L., Pieta, M. A. M., & Frizzo, G. B. (2021). Infants' and toddlers' digital media use and mothers' mental health: A comparative study before and during the COVID-19 pandemic. *Infant Mental Health Journal, 43*(1), 24–35. https://doi.org/10.1002/imhj.21952

Pempek, T. A., & Lauricella, A. R. (2017). The effects of parent-child interaction and media use on cognitive development in infants, toddlers, and preschoolers. In F. C. Blumberg & P. J. Brooks (Eds.), *Cognitive development in digital contexts* (pp. 53–74). Academic Press. https://doi.org/10.1016/B978-0-12-809481-5.00003-1

Peres, J., Dias, A. C. S., Suassuna, A. M. V., Almeida, M. A., Guedes, S. A., & Sanches, G. P. (2012). Technological culture and vulnerability to psychic trauma. *The World of Health, 36*(2), 303–310. http://pesquisa.bvsalud.org/bvsvs/resource/pt/lil-757719

Pesce, L. R., Pedrotti, B. G., Frizzo, G. B., & Lopes, R. C. S. (2023). Sharing experiences or prescribing guidelines? A study from blogs about motherhood. *Psycho, 54*(1), 1–12. https://doi.org/10.15448/1980-8623.2023.1.38081

Radesky, J. S., Silverstein, M., Zuckerman, B., & Christakis, D. A. (2014). Infant self-regulation and early childhood media exposure. *Pediatrics, 133*(5), 1172–1178. https://doi.org/10.1542/peds.2013-2367

Radesky, J. S., Kistin, C., Eisenberg, S., Gross, J., Block, G., Zuckerman, B., & Silverstein, M. D. (2016). Parent perspectives on their mobile technology use: The excitement and exhaustion of parenting while connected. *Journal of Developmental & Behavioral Pediatrics, 37*(9), 694–701. https://doi.org/10.1097/DBP.0000000000000357

Rideout, V. & Robb, M. B. (2020). *The common sense census: Media use by kids age zero to eight.* Retrieved from: https://www.commonsensemedia.org/sites/default/files/research/report/2020_zero_to_eight_census_final_web.pdf

Rocha, H. A. L., Correia, L. L., Leite, A. J. M., Machado, M. M. T., Lindsay, A. C., Rocha, S. G. M. O., Campos, J. S., Silva, A. C., & Sudfeld, C. R. (2021). Screen time and early childhood development in Ceará, Brazil: A population based study. *BMC Public Health, 21*(2072), 2072. https://doi.org/10.1186/s12889-021-12136-2

Royal College of Paediatrics and Child Health. (2019). *The health impacts of screen time: A guide for clinicians and parents.* Retrieved from https://www.rcpch.ac.uk/resources/health-impacts-screen-time-guide-clinicians-parents

Santos, C. C., & Barros, J. F. (2017). *Effects of the use of new information and communication technologies for child emotional development: A psychoanalytic understanding* (pp. 1–25). Psicologia. http://www.psicologia.pt/artigos/ver_artigo_licenciatura.php?efeitos-do-uso-das-novas-tecnologias-da-informacao-e-comunicacao-para-o-desenvolvimento-emocional-infantil-uma-compreensao-psicanalitica&codigo=TL0435&area=D4A

Straker, L., Zabatiero, J., Danby, S., Thorpe, K., & Edwards, S. (2018). Conflicting guidelines on young children's screen time and use of digital technology create policy and practice dilemmas. *The Journal of Pediatrics, 202*, 300–303. https://doi.org/10.1016/j.jpeds.2018.07.019

Swider-Cios, E., Vermeij, A., & Sitskoorn, M. M. (2023). Young children and screen-based media: The impact on cognitive and socioemotional development and the importance of parental mediation. *Cognitive Development, 66*(101319), 101319. https://doi.org/10.1016/j.cogdev.2023.101319

Vygotsky, L. S. (1989). *The social formation of the mind.* Martins Fontes.

Winnicott, D. W. (2006). *Babies and their mothers.* Martins Fontes. (Originally published in 1987).

World Health Organization. (2019). *Guidelines on physical activity, sedentary behaviour and sleep for children under 5 years of age.* World Health Organization. Retrieved from http://www.who.int/iris/handle/10665/311664

Chapter 17
Parenting and Problematic Internet Use

Fernanda Saraiva Almeida, Bruna Cardoso Gerhardt, and Adriane Xavier Arteche

Problematic Internet Use in Adults

The use of the Internet has grown over the past two decades, and today we live in a hyperconnected society (Sánchez-Fernández & Borda-Mas, 2022). The Internet is a tool that provides numerous benefits, conveniences, and entertainment opportunities and is now considered one of the primary leisure activities for adults in many cultures (Zhou et al., 2014). Particularly during the COVID-19 pandemic, due to the implementation of social isolation measures, Internet usage has increased, and digital media has become part of everyday life as it was the only safe way to communicate, seek information, perform work functions, and study during lockdown (Lopes et al., 2022). Despite the advantages offered by the Internet, there is a growing concern regarding individuals who exhibit a dysfunctional pattern of Internet use, which leads to negative impacts on mental health and well-being. This phenomenon is referred to as problematic Internet use, defined as the use of the Internet that causes harm to the individual, whether it be emotional, social, or occupational in nature (Caplan, 2010; Davis, 2001).

The emotional impairments caused by problematic Internet use in adults are being studied, and research has shown a relationship between problematic Internet use and symptoms of anxiety, stress, depression, social anxiety, and loneliness (Elhai et al., 2021; Faghani et al., 2020). Davis (2001) and Caplan (2010) were the first researchers to define problematic Internet use from a cognitive-behavioral therapy perspective, understanding that this phenomenon arises as a consequence of preexisting emotional symptoms associated with dysfunctional beliefs regarding Internet use. Due to a scarcity of longitudinal studies, causal relationships between emotional problems and problematic Internet use cannot be inferred definitively, but

F. S. Almeida · B. C. Gerhardt · A. X. Arteche (✉)
Pontifical Catholic University of Rio Grande do Sul (PUCRS), Porto Alegre, Brazil
e-mail: bruna.gerhardt@edu.pucrs.br; adriane.arteche@pucrs.br

G. B. Frizzo (ed.), *Digital Media and Early Child Development*,
https://doi.org/10.1007/978-3-031-69224-6_17

the relationship appears to be bidirectional: individuals with emotional issues seek the Internet more, as well as Internet use can exacerbate emotional symptoms (Lopes et al., 2022).

The central aspects of problematic Internet use in adults include compulsive use and difficulty in interrupting Internet use, experiencing negative outcomes due to Internet use, concerns about being constantly connected, using the Internet for mood regulation, and a preference for online interactions over face-to-face interactions (Davis et al., 2001; Caplan, 2010). The number of hours spent browsing the Internet per day is not the central underlying mechanism of problematic Internet use (Griffiths & Mamun, 2020). In a hyperconnected society where many rely on the Internet for work and study purposes, solely judging the amount of time spent online is not a reliable measure to determine dysfunctionality. We need to go beyond this one element and assess the individual's relationship with the Internet, the emotions it triggers, the role it assumes, and whether there are impairments in well-being or functionality.

One aspect associated with problematic Internet use in adults is a deficit in emotional regulation skills (Pettorrusso et al., 2020; Faghani et al., 2020). Individuals who struggle with handling their emotions tend to seek strategies for immediate emotional relief and emotional suppression, and the Internet can serve as a means to achieve that goal (Yen et al., 2018). The Internet offers multiple entertainment activities and can be used as a way to alleviate negative emotions, which may explain the association between stress and problematic Internet use (Gong et al., 2021). We can engage in numerous online activities, many of which provide immediate well-being and allow individuals to disconnect from daily problems and concerns. Adults lacking emotional regulation strategies may use the Internet to alleviate the negative emotional state caused by responsibilities, problems, and daily tasks. Online gaming, for example, represents a leisure and entertainment activity that can be sought by individuals who want to disconnect from their emotions and routine (Yen et al., 2018). Online gaming has been cited as one of the online activities with the highest potential for addiction, as it offers immediate gratification, serves as an escape from reality, and provides an outlet from daily problems (Starcevic, 2013; Demirtas, 2021).

The use of social media is also associated with symptoms of emotional distress: individuals who are experiencing distress tend to use social media more, and consuming social media content can worsen symptoms of anxiety, depression, and stress (Lopes et al., 2022). Social media platforms foster social comparison; trigger feelings of envy, loneliness, and frustration; and can activate beliefs of inferiority or failure (Boer et al., 2021; Lopes et al., 2022; Lup et al., 2015). More vulnerable individuals may harm themselves using social media if they are unable to filter what they consume and understand that people only share a small fraction of their reality on social media, keeping their vulnerabilities and weaknesses offline (Lopes et al., 2022). Problematic social media use is an emerging issue that is associated with negative impacts on well-being and mental health.

Another central aspect of problematic Internet use is the difficulty in interrupting usage, even when the individual recognizes that the amount of time spent online is causing harm (Caplan, 2010; Davis, 2001). The inability to go offline, turn off the computer, stop playing a game, or cease scrolling through social media feeds is a symptom that indicates an unhealthy relationship with the Internet. Being able to manage online time is a skill that needs to be developed to prevent negative outcomes associated with problematic Internet use. Controlling online time can be even more challenging for individuals diagnosed with attention deficit hyperactivity disorder (ADHD), as difficulties in impulse control and self-management are central symptoms of the disorder. Individuals with ADHD are more vulnerable to developing problematic Internet use, considering that online activities offer numerous stimuli and immediate rewards (Tsai et al., 2020; Wang et al., 2017). Individuals diagnosed with ADHD need to be constantly vigilant about their relationship with the Internet and the difficulty in interrupting its use.

Problematic Internet use is also associated with individual characteristics and traits, although findings are inconclusive. Adults with social anxiety, perceived low social skills, shyness, low self-esteem, social isolation, and negative self-beliefs are susceptible to experiencing problematic Internet use (Davis, 2001; Caplan, 2010; Odaci, 2013). In these cases, the Internet is seen as a less threatening way to interact, communicate, create, and strengthen social ties (Caplan, 2010; Davis, 2001). The relationship between personality traits and problematic Internet use is still not a consensus in the literature, so it is not possible to determine if there is a specific profile that is more susceptible to developing problematic use. The Internet offers multiple leisure and entertainment activities, with options that cater to all types of personalities and different individual characteristics. Identifying at-risk groups is a challenge for the scientific community, and further studies are needed.

Just as there is no consensus regarding the individual characteristics that make individuals vulnerable to problematic Internet use, there is also no unanimity in the findings regarding sex effects. Some studies (Andrade et al., 2020; Sechi et al., 2021; Peterka-Bonetta et al., 2019) support the idea that men and women are equally affected by problematic Internet use. On the other hand, a systematic review by Anderson et al. (2017) found that problematic Internet use is higher in men, and the authors discuss that this may be due to a preference for online gaming and a higher prevalence of impulsive behaviors. Andreassen et al. (2016) also found that men engage more in online gaming, while women tend to use social media more. Men and women may have different preferences when it comes to Internet browsing, but both are susceptible to developing problematic Internet use since the phenomenon encompasses multiple forms of Internet usage.

Parenthood and Problematic Internet Use

As discussed in the previous section, adults are experiencing difficulties related to problematic Internet use, often harming their well-being, quality of life, and mental health. The challenges become even more prominent when it comes to individuals who have not yet completed their process of brain and emotional development: children and adolescents. There is a growing concern in society, and the scientific community regarding the impact of Internet and screen use on neurodevelopment (Piteo & Ward 2020), and parents are primarily responsible for mediating the relationship with the Internet and establishing healthy boundaries and ways of dealing with screens. For parents who struggle with managing their own online time and have difficulty controlling their Internet use, establishing such limits for their children can be extremely challenging.

Children and adolescents, born into a digitalized and hyperconnected society, use the Internet from an early age for various purposes: playing games, watching videos, learning, and communicating with family and friends (Nakayama et al., 2020; Piteo & Ward 2020). Nowadays, it is difficult for parents to prevent their children from using screens and connecting to the Internet (a total ban would not be advantageous for children, considering they will need to adapt to a digital society). However, it is important for parents to be able to control the use and mediate the relationship with the Internet from the early years of development. The age at which a child begins to use the Internet regularly in their daily routine can influence how they relate to the Internet (Nakayama et al., 2020). The study by Nakayama et al. (2020) found that boys who started daily Internet use earlier (before the age of 5) exhibited more problematic Internet use after the age of 12, highlighting the importance of managing online time in the early years of childhood.

The American Academy of Pediatrics recommends that children under 2 years of age have no exposure to screens whatsoever (Rosen et al., 2014). After reaching that age, controlled and supervised use is allowed. However, when it comes to teenagers, there are no specific guidelines or directions regarding the number of hours of screen time, leaving it up to parents to decide how to limit their access. Consequently, many parents feel lost and unsure about how to establish these rules. There is a lack of sufficient guidance, and the rapidly evolving nature of social media platforms further complicates matters. For instance, Instagram, a popular social media platform among children and teenagers, was only launched in 2010 (Lopes et al., 2022). The unfamiliarity of parents with these technologies and digital platforms can contribute to challenges in effectively controlling and mediating their children's Internet usage (Chou et al., 2015). Therefore, it is recommended that parents strive to become familiar with the digital media platforms their children use. The issue of social media usage is relatively new, and more studies and definitive guidelines are needed to assist parents and families in navigating this complex landscape.

The relationship between parents and children can either be protective or detrimental to the development of problematic Internet use in children and adolescents. A longitudinal study conducted with 12-year-old children by Lukavská et al. (2020) found that parenting styles play an important role in their children's problematic Internet use, with the authoritative style (high demands and high responsiveness) being the most protective in preventing such outcomes. The results also revealed that the highest prevalence of problematic Internet use was found among young individuals whose mothers exhibited authoritative behavior while their fathers displayed neglectful behavior (Lukavská et al., 2020).

Establishing a good relationship with children and implementing an authoritative parenting style should be goals for parents concerned about protecting their children from problematic Internet use. Low perceived parental care was associated with excessive Internet use in a sample of Spanish adolescents aged 14–18 (Casaló & Escario, 2019). Family relationships and the existence of conflicts among family members also interfere with children's problematic Internet use (van Dijk et al., 2021). The study by Chou et al. (2015) found that low satisfaction with family relationships was the strongest predictor associated with problematic Internet use among adolescents. Adolescents who are dissatisfied with family interactions may resist parental attempts to control Internet use, putting them at greater risk of developing problematic Internet use (Chou et al., 2015). The study by Milani et al. (2020) evaluated children and adolescents who play online games, and the authors discuss that when young individuals feel lonely, isolated from others, and fearful of social interactions, they may turn to online games to disconnect from these problems and seek emotional relief, thereby increasing vulnerability to developing problematic Internet use. This finding aligns with previous research indicating that online games are often used as a means of emotional disconnection, avoidance, and suppression (Yen et al., 2018).

The quality of the parent-child relationship is a variable that influences how young individuals engage with the Internet (Chou et al., 2015; Li et al., 2020). Parents should be concerned about monitoring and establishing boundaries for their children's online time and activities, but they should also prioritize building a strong bond of affection and trust with their children. It is a parenting challenge to balance controlling their children's internet use with respecting their privacy and individuality, especially when it comes to adolescents. Restricting access to digital media does not seem to be the solution, and in fact, this approach can have negative impacts on both adolescents and the family bond. The study by Liu, (2020) found that parental Internet restriction (controlling usage time, consumed content, and accessed platforms) is perceived by adolescents as an invasion of privacy. Individuals who feel their personal boundaries are violated may experience negative outcomes such as emotional distress, irritability, defensiveness, reactive responses toward their parents, and problematic Internet use. Moreover, restrictive mediation measures can lead to defensive strategies by children, such as using the Internet in secret, deleting conversations, lying, or withholding information about their online activities, thus increasing vulnerability to problematic Internet use (Liu, 2020). However, it is important to note that this finding remains controversial in the literature. The controversy in the research findings and perspectives reflects the difficulty in defining the best approach for parents to handle their children's Internet use. It is expected that specific guidelines and recommendations will be developed soon to assist parents in finding the best way to mediate their children's Internet use, ensuring that they do not feel violated or disrespected in their privacy, while also being protected and well-informed about Internet use. Currently, the strategy that has shown the most benefits and advantages for fostering a strong parent-child bond seems to be an open and honest dialogue about digital media use, where parents can provide non-judgmental active listening and guidance through a conversation about Internet use (Liu, 2020).

Mothers and Fathers Online

The use of social media is one of the primary online activities that people engage in. When it comes to mothers and fathers, accessing the Internet through these platforms serves various purposes, with mothers being the primary users (Djafarova & Trofimenko, 2017). However, the issue of problematic Internet use among mothers and fathers is underexplored in the literature, as most studies focus on childhood, adolescence, young adults, and university students. Therefore, more research is needed to investigate the online activities that parents of children and adolescents engage in, their motivations for use, the consequences for their relationship with their children, the association with problematic internet use, and the impact on mental health.

It is common for mothers to use social media to connect with their support network, follow other mothers' social media accounts, consume content from motherhood influencers, alleviate feelings of loneliness, gather tips and information about parenting, share photos and videos of their children, and seek entertainment and leisure (Djafarova & Trofimenko, 2017). This type of use can offer both benefits and drawbacks to well-being. On the one hand, social media provides knowledge, information about parenting, a sense of belonging, and exchanges with people going through the same phase. On the other hand, social media can represent a space for criticism, judgment, competition, comparison with other mothers, and pressure to portray a perfect image of motherhood and also contribute to the spread of false or unscientific information about child care (Chee et al., 2023). It is important to caution mothers and fathers to filter the content consumed on social media and verify the validity of information with healthcare professionals committed to science and child development.

Furthermore, it is widely recognized that the early years of a child's life are marked by multiple changes, challenges, and a reorganization of roles in parents' lives. These transformations create a period of extreme vulnerability for the onset or exacerbation of emotional difficulties and mental disorders in mothers (Cantwell, 2021). A significant proportion of them are affected by symptoms of postpartum depression and anxiety, and studies indicate that these symptoms are related to greater difficulties in emotional regulation (Marques et al., 2018). Therefore, the association between psychopathological symptoms, ineffective strategies of emotional regulation, and increased problematic Internet use highlights the need to pay attention to the possibility of excessive social media use in parenthood. This understanding is based on the assumption that parents, especially mothers, who experience an increase in psychopathological symptoms during this period and face greater difficulties in emotional regulation may end up resorting to excessive use of social media as a way to avoid and suppress emotions. Despite the overwhelming demands of tasks and childcare, it is understood that the use of electronic devices can be a form of disconnection utilized by parents (Fig. 17.1).

However, the literature on this topic remains limited. Studies examining parents' problematic Internet use have primarily focused on understanding its consequences

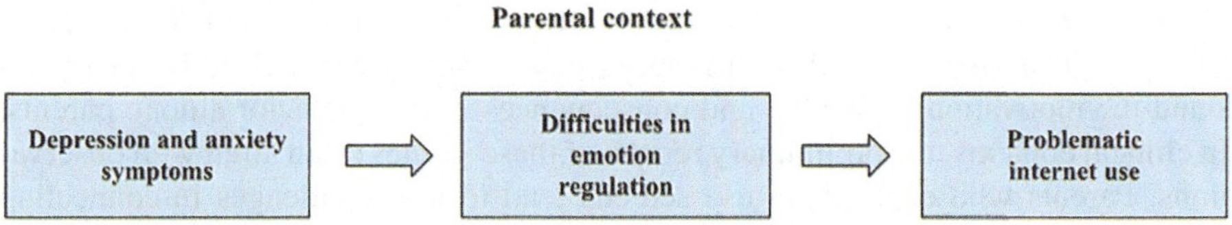

Fig. 17.1 Hypothetical model regarding parenthood and problematic Internet use

rather than exploring its underlying causes. As a result, the lack of data regarding parents' motivations and patterns of electronic device usage complicates the development of effective interventions aimed at mitigating this phenomenon's negative repercussions. Nevertheless, research on the impact of parental Internet use has already highlighted the necessity of involving parents in interventions targeting children's problematic Internet use and preventive measures.

The findings from these initial studies suggest that problematic Internet use among mothers of young children is linked to lower quality in the mother-child relationship (Nourozi et al., 2021), as well as to reduced dedicated quality time spent with their children (Kushlev & Dunn, 2019). Both of these indicators are recognized as significant predictors of emotional and behavioral outcomes throughout child development. Mother-infant interaction plays a pivotal role in language, cognition, motor, and social development during the first year of life (Rocha et al., 2020), and it is inversely associated with the presence of lifelong psychopathological symptoms (Erickson et al., 2019). Therefore, the problematic Internet use by caregivers may underlie the diminished quality of relationships with their children, thereby triggering a series of adversities.

According to Kushlev and Dunn's (2019) research, increased smartphone usage by parents has been linked to a higher perceived sense of distraction during interactions with their children, thereby hindering the formation of emotional connections. Studies by Farajdonyavi (2022) and Nourozi et al., (2021) suggest that problematic Internet use by mothers predicts greater behavioral problems in children. In terms of physical health, mothers with problematic Internet use were found to have higher levels of underweight in male children at 4 months or 1.5 years of age (Sakakihara et al., 2019). Moreover, Sakakihara et al.'s (2019) study revealed that mothers with indications of problematic Internet use reported a higher potential for child abuse at multiple stages of childhood (4 months, 1.5 years, and 3 years). The authors discuss these findings, highlighting that the more mothers are engaged in Internet use, the greater the likelihood of neglect and difficulty in managing stressful situations related to their children. During adolescence, this pattern becomes even more evident, indicating not only more pronounced negative emotional outcomes in children resulting from parents' problematic Internet use but also a higher likelihood of adolescents developing problematic Internet use themselves (Lam & Wong, 2015; Mun & Lee, 2021). Thus, it is understood that modeling, an important aspect of learning, may play a role in shaping children's relationship with social media.

In summary, while the literature does not consistently provide a comprehensive understanding of problematic Internet use in parents, the initial research findings highlight the significance of this issue. Excessive Internet use has been linked to various indicators of mental health, necessitating further research to better understand the motivations, patterns, and consequences of this behavior among parents. In clinical contexts, the preliminary results of these studies often align with observations. Parents who excessively use screens tend to face challenges in connecting with their children and may adopt neglectful or authoritarian parenting styles. Additionally, there is often a correlation between problematic Internet use by parents and similar behavior in their children.

The absence of problematic Internet use by parents does not guarantee that their children will not face such issues. As mentioned earlier, a set of assertive parenting practices is crucial for fostering a healthier relationship between children and electronic devices. Conversely, problematic Internet use by parents appears to be a significant predictor of the same complication in their children. It is important to note that this relationship is not exclusive, as other factors may also contribute to the association between these aspects. Nevertheless, it serves as a valuable indicator of potential challenges that may arise in the parent-child relationship and impact the emotional and behavioral well-being of children.

In light of this, it is crucial to invest in interventions involving parents when their children exhibit excessive screen use, particularly when caregivers themselves face this problem. Including parents in the treatment process emerges as a significant approach to mitigate the adverse effects of problematic Internet use on both parents and children. However, it is important to acknowledge that addressing this issue can present additional challenges. Therefore, within a clinical setting, conducting individual sessions with parents becomes essential to grasp the motivations and underlying reasons behind problematic Internet use. Subsequently, collaborative strategies can be developed to establish a healthier relationship with electronic devices, incorporating techniques such as emotional regulation and mindfulness (Augner et al., 2022). Concurrently, empowering caregivers with more assertive parenting practices becomes crucial, aiming to reduce behavioral problems in children and enhance the quality of the parent-child relationship (Lukavská et al., 2020). Parents need to be well-informed about the detrimental effects of excessive Internet use, including its association with psychopathological symptoms and interpersonal difficulties.

Stay Up to Date with the Latest Findings!

In a research study on problematic Internet use conducted by the Affective Neuroscience and Transgenerationality Research Group at the Pontifical Catholic University of Rio Grande do Sul (PUCRS) in 2022, we compared data from parents and non-parents regarding their Internet usage. The study employed a cross-sectional, quantitative, observational, and descriptive design. The final sample consisted of 294 Brazilian individuals who provided sociodemographic information and completed at least one instrument (144 men/149 women/1 preferred not to mention), aged between 18 and 55 years ($M = 29.31$, $SD = 7.99$). Participants completed the Informed Consent Form, Sociodemographic Data Sheet, and Internet Usage Type (a questionnaire developed by the researchers), as well as the Generalized Problematic Internet Use Scale (GPIUS-2; Caplan, 2010), Online Cognition Scale (OCS; Davis, 2002), Depression Anxiety Stress Scale-21 (DASS-21; Lovibond & Lovibond, 1995), and the Difficulties in Emotion Regulation Scale (DERS; Gratz & Roemer, 2004). The research was approved by the Research Ethics Committee of the Pontifical Catholic University of Rio Grande do Sul, under registration number CAAE: 56281222.7.0000.5336. Data collection took place between June and September 2022, using the Qualtrics digital platform. The data were analyzed using SPSS statistical software version 25.0, with a significance level set at 5%. Descriptive frequency analyses and multiple regression analysis were conducted.

Based on the data gathered from the questionnaire on Internet usage patterns, we were able to identify the average daily online time during weekdays (Monday to Friday) and weekends (Saturday and Sunday), excluding time allocated to professional activities like work or study. Among participants with children, the weekday average stood at 2.88 h, dropping slightly to 2.73 h on weekends. Conversely, for those without children, the weekday average was slightly higher at 3.19 h, with weekends averaging at 3.11 h. Despite the marginally elevated figures observed among participants without children, this difference was not statistically significant.

Furthermore, an investigation was conducted to ascertain whether the participants' occupation or professional activities were solely reliant on the Internet. Among those with children, 43.9% indicated that their work activities depended on the Internet, whereas 50.6% of those without children relied on Internet usage for professional purposes.

Figure 17.2 presents an overview of Internet usage types among participants, comparing parents and non-parents. The most frequent activities in this sample were information searching and watching videos or movies, reaching nearly 100% of the participants. Upon analyzing these data, it can be observed that the Internet usage type was similar between parents and non-parents. Significant differences were observed regarding online gaming and the use of dating websites and applications—activities significantly more frequent among non-parents.

Figure 17.3 presents the results regarding the Online Cognition Scale, which aims to assess the beliefs and cognitions associated with problematic Internet use. Some examples of items included in this scale are statements such as "I feel safer when I am on the internet," "I cannot imagine my life without the internet for a long time," and "Sometimes, I use the internet to postpone other responsibilities." Again, as seen in Fig. 17.3, results indicated that there were few differences in the dimensions between parents and non-parents. Although the average scores observed in parents were slightly lower than those observed in non-parents in all subscales, this difference was not statistically significant. Therefore, it can be hypothesized that both parents and non-parents present similar beliefs and thoughts regarding problematic Internet use, despite their different life demands.

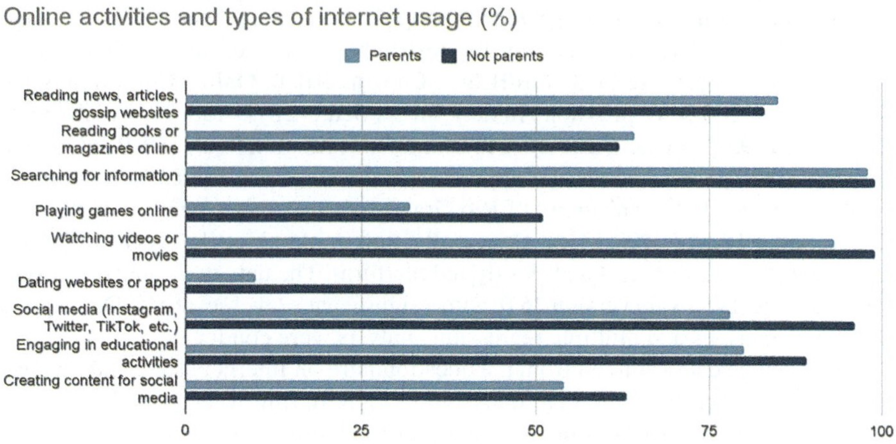

Fig. 17.2 Percentage results regarding online activities and types of Internet usage

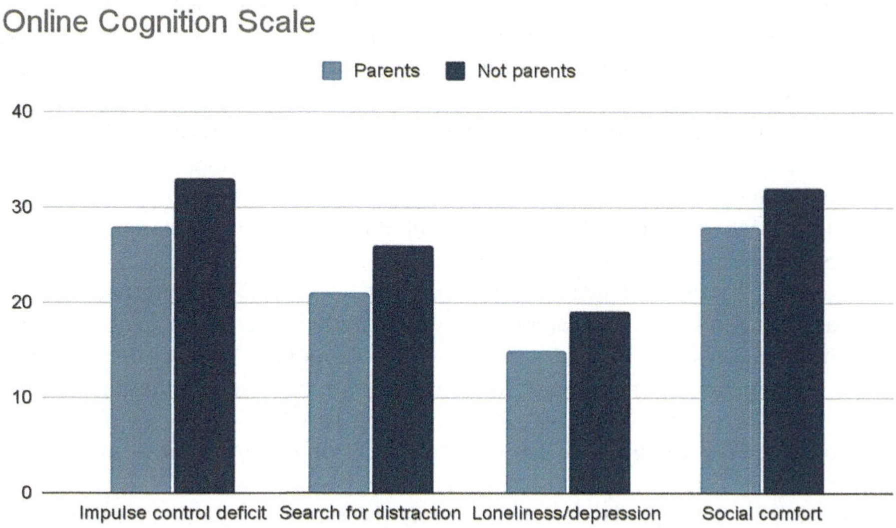

Fig. 17.3 Results of the online cognition scale

Figure 17.4 presents the results for the GPIUS-2 subscales. Noteworthy that the subscales mood regulation and cognitive preoccupation with being online, albeit not significantly different, parents showed an important tendency of lower scores.

Finally, in the results of a regression analysis having the total score of the GPIUS-2 scale as dependent variable and age, sex, and being a parent as predictors, being a parent was not a significant factor in determining differences in average scores of problematic Internet use (Fig. 17.5). These results suggest that there may be other factors, such as age (being young), that play a more significant role in this matter, irrespective of parenthood.

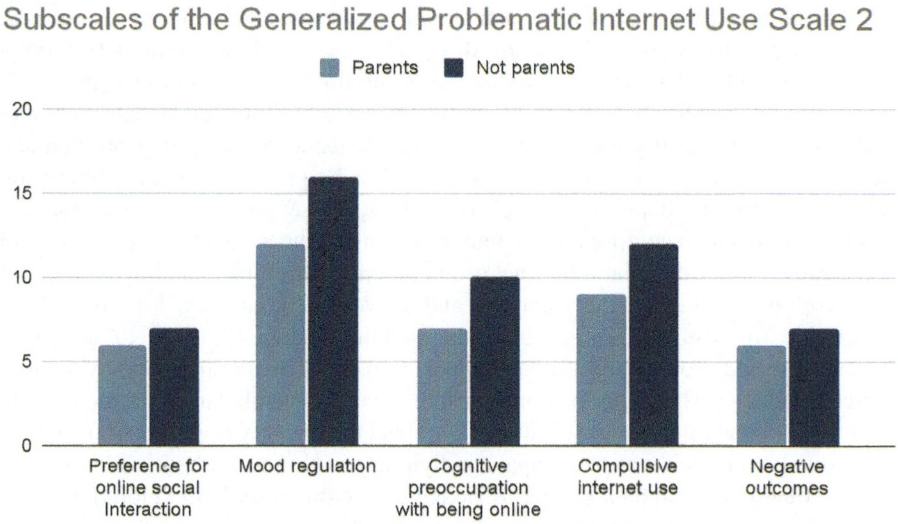

Fig. 17.4 Results of the GPIUS-2 subscales

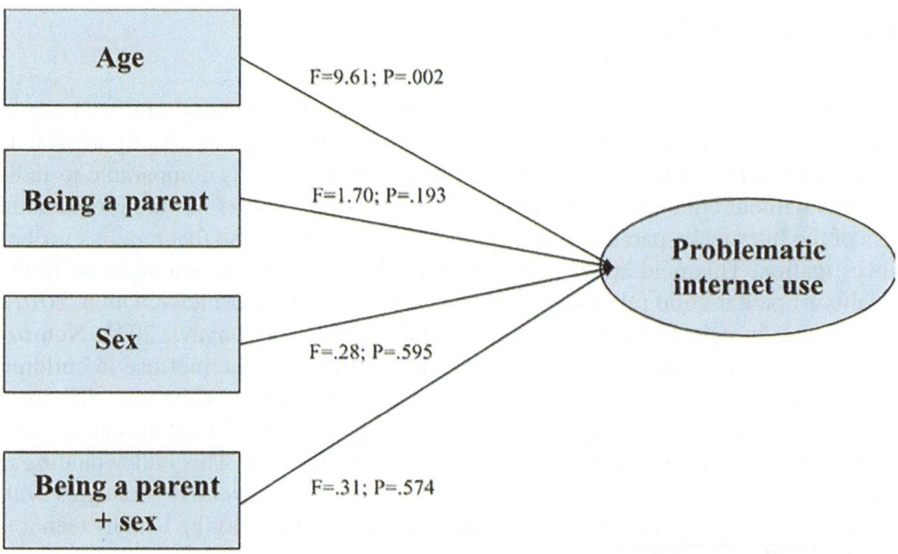

Fig. 17.5 Regression analysis

Based on these findings, several noteworthy considerations emerge. Parenthood encompasses a multitude of changes and responsibilities, and it is understandable that parents encounter challenges in managing their time and reconciling familial demands with Internet usage. The results indicate that Internet usage seems to maintain a consistent pattern after becoming a parent, with variations mainly observed in the type of activities engaged in, such as dating websites and gaming. In essence, there appears to be a shift toward different types of Internet activities post-parenthood, rather than a notable reduction or modification in overall usage.

Should Internet use become problematic, the repercussions can be detrimental to both parents and their children. Previous studies have indicated that problematic Internet use among parents is associated with a heightened risk of problematic Internet use in their offspring (Lam & Wong, 2015; Mun & Lee, 2021). Consequently, it is crucial to gain a comprehensive understanding of the motivations, patterns, and consequences of problematic Internet use in parents. This understanding is essential for developing effective interventions and preventive strategies. Moreover, it is imperative to raise awareness about the potential adverse effects of excessive Internet use and provide appropriate support to parents in adopting healthy technological practices. This support should ensure a harmonious balance between online activities and parental responsibilities. Given that the primary objective of the aforementioned study was not to compare individuals with and without children, it is evident that this is still an area of knowledge that requires further exploration. Such exploration would aim to address intervention and prevention measures effectively.

Final Considerations

Recent research has revealed the numerous impacts of problematic Internet use in adults (Lopes et al., 2022; Pettorrusso et al., 2020; Faghani et al., 2020), as well as indicating that parents have been using smartphones at levels comparable to individuals without children (Almeida et al., forthcoming). Therefore, the problematic use of the Internet by parents has emerged as a research demand that requires further investigation. This field appears to have multiple effects, such as a decrease in the quality of parent-child relationships (Nourozi et al., 2021; Kushlev & Dunn, 2019), an increase in behavioral problems among children (Farajdonyavi, 2022; Nourozi et al., 2021), and a higher risk of developing problematic Internet use in children (Lam & Wong, 2015; Mun & Lee, 2021). Hence, it is crucial for the scientific community to comprehensively explore this issue, aiming to understand the causes, patterns, and consequences of parents' problematic Internet use. This understanding is fundamental for developing effective interventions and preventive strategies with the goal of mitigating the potential negative impacts and promoting healthy technology use in the parental context.

References

Anderson, E. L., Steen, E., & Stavropoulos, V. (2017). Internet use and problematic internet use: A systematic review of longitudinal research trends in adolescence and emergent adulthood. *International Journal of Adolescence and Youth, 22*(4), 430–454). Routledge. https://doi.org/10.1080/02673843.2016.1227716

Andrade, A. L. M., Scatena, A., Bedendo, A., Enumo, S. R. F., Dellazzana-Zanon, L. L., Prebianchi, H. B., de Lara Machado, W., & de Micheli, D. (2020). Findings on the relationship between Internet addiction and psychological symptoms in Brazilian adults. *International Journal of Psychology, 55*(6), 941–950. https://doi.org/10.1002/ijop.12670

Andreassen, C. S., Billieux, J., Griffiths, M. D., Kuss, D. J., Demetrovics, Z., Mazzoni, E., & Pallesen, S. (2016). The relationship between addictive use of social media and video games and symptoms of psychiatric disorders: A large-scale cross-sectional study. *Psychology of Addictive Behaviors, 30*(2), 252–262. https://doi.org/10.1037/adb0000160

Augner, C., Vlasak, T., Aichhorn, W., & Barth, A. (2022). Tackling the 'digital pandemic': The effectiveness of psychological intervention strategies in problematic internet and smartphone use—A meta-analysis. *Australian & New Zealand Journal of Psychiatry, 56*(3), 219–229.

Boer, M., Stevens, G. W. J. M., Finkenauer, C., de Looze, M. E., & van den Eijnden, R. J. J. M. (2021). Social media use intensity, social media use problems, and mental health among adolescents: Investigating directionality and mediating processes. *Computers in Human Behavior, 116*, 106645. https://doi.org/10.1016/j.chb.2020.106645

Cantwell, R. (2021). Mental disorder in pregnancy and the early postpartum. *Anaesthesia, 76*, 76–83.

Caplan, S. E. (2010). Theory and measurement of generalized problematic internet use: A two-step approach. *Computers in Human Behavior, 26*(5), 1089–1097. https://doi.org/10.1016/j.chb.2010.03.012

Casaló, L. V., & Escario, J. J. (2019). Predictors of excessive internet use among adolescents in Spain: The relevance of the relationship between parents and their children. *Computers in Human Behavior, 92*, 344–351. https://doi.org/10.1016/j.chb.2018.11.04

Chee, R. M., Capper, T. S., & Muurlink, O. T. (2023). The impact of social media influencers on pregnancy, birth, and early parenting experiences: A systematic review. *Midwifery, 120*, 103623. https://doi.org/10.1016/j.midw.2023.103623

Chou, W. J., Liu, T. L., Yang, P., Yen, C. F., & Hu, H. F. (2015). Multi-dimensional correlates of internet addiction symptoms in adolescents with attention-deficit/hyperactivity disorder. *Psychiatry Research, 225*(1–2), 122–128. https://doi.org/10.1016/j.psychres.2014.11.003

Davis, R. A. (2001). Cognitive-behavioral model of pathological internet use. *Computers in Human Behavior, 17*(2), 187–195. https://doi.org/10.1016/S0747-5632(00)00041-8

Davis, R. A., Flett, G. L., & Besser, A. (2002). Online Cognition Scale (OCS)[Database record]. APA PsycTests.

Demirtaş, O. O., Alnak, A., & Coşkun, M. (2021). Lifetime depressive and current social anxiety are associated with problematic internet use in adolescents with ADHD: A cross-sectional study. *Child and Adolescent Mental Health, 26*(3), 220–227. https://doi.org/10.1111/camh.12440

Djafarova, E., & Trofimenko, O. (2017). Exploring the relationships between self-presentation and self-esteem of mothers in social media in Russia. *Computers in Human Behavior, 73*, 20–27. https://doi.org/10.1016/j.chb.2017.03.021

Elhai, J. D., Yang, H., & Montag, C. (2021). Fear of missing out (FOMO): Overview, theoretical underpinnings, and literature review on relations with severity of negative affectivity and problematic technology use. *Revista Brasileira de Psiquiatria (Sao Paulo, Brazil: 1999), 43*(2), 203–209. https://doi.org/10.1590/1516-4446-2020-0870

Erickson, N., Julian, M., & Muzik, M. (2019). Perinatal depression, PTSD, and trauma: Impact on mother–infant attachment and interventions to mitigate the transmission of risk. *International Review of Psychiatry, 31*(3), 245–263.

Faghani, N., Akbari, M., Hasani, J., & Marino, C. (2020). An emotional and cognitive model of problematic internet use among college students: The full mediating role of cognitive factors. *Addictive Behaviors, 105*, 106252. https://doi.org/10.1016/j.addbeh.2019.106252

Farajdonyavi, S. (2022). Predicting Children's Behavioral Problems Based on Mothers' Problematic Use Of Virtual Social Networks. *Technology and Scholarship in Education, 1*(2), 27–33.

Gong, Z., Wang, L., & Wang, H. (2021). Perceived stress and internet addiction among Chinese college students: Mediating effect of procrastination and moderating effect of flow. *Frontiers in Psychology, 12*. https://doi.org/10.3389/fpsyg.2021.632461

Gratz, K. L., & Roemer, L. (2004). Multidimensional assessment of emotion regulation and dysregulation: Development, factor structure, and initial validation of the difficulties in emotion regulation scale. *Journal of psychopathology and behavioral assessment, 26*, 41–54.

Griffiths, M. D., & Mamun, M. A. (2020). Internet addiction among young Bangladeshi adults: Critical commentary on Hassan et al. In *Journal of the Egyptian Public Health Association* (Vol. 95, p. 26). Springer Science and Business Media Deutschland GmbH. https://doi.org/10.1186/s42506-020-00054-x

Kushlev, K., & Dunn, E. W. (2019). Smartphones distract parents from cultivating feelings of connection when spending time with their children. *Journal of Social and Personal Relationships, 36*(6), 1619–1639.

Lam, L. T., & Wong, E. M. (2015). Stress moderates the relationship between problematic internet use by parents and problematic internet use by adolescents. *Journal of Adolescent Health, 56*(3), 300–306.

Li, L., Griffiths, M. D., Niu, Z., & Mei, S. (2020). Fear of missing out (FoMO) and gaming disorder among Chinese university students: Impulsivity and game time as mediators. *Issues in Mental Health Nursing, 11*, 1104. https://doi.org/10.1080/01612840.2020.1774018

Liu, Y. L. (2020). Maternal mediation as an act of privacy invasion: The association with internet addiction. *Computers in Human Behavior, 112*, 106474. https://doi.org/10.1016/j.chb.2020.106474

Lopes, L. S., Valentini, J. P., Monteiro, T. H., Costacurta, M. C. F., Soares, L. O. N., Telfar-Barnard, L., & Nunes, P. V. (2022). Problematic social media use and its relationship with depression or anxiety: A systematic review. *Cyberpsychology, Behavior and Social Networking, 25*(11), 691–702. https://doi.org/10.1089/cyber.2021.0300

Lovibond, P. F., & Lovibond, S. H. (1995). The structure of negative emotional states: Comparison of the Depression Anxiety Stress Scales (DASS) with the Beck Depression and Anxiety Inventories. *Behaviour research and therapy, 33*(3), 335–343.

Lukavská, K., Vacek, J., & Gabhelik, R. (2020). The effects of parental control and warmth on problematic internet use in adolescents: A prospective cohort study. In. *Journal of Behavioral Addictions, 9*(3), 664–675). Akademiai Kiado Rt. https://doi.org/10.1556/2006.2020.00068

Lup, K., Trub, L., & Rosenthal, L. (2015). Instagram #Instasad?: Exploring associations among Instagram use, depressive symptoms, negative social comparison, and strangers followed. *Cyberpsychology, Behavior, and Social Networking, 18*(5), 247–252. https://doi.org/10.1089/cyber.2014.0560

Marques, R., Monteiro, F., Canavarro, M. C., & Fonseca, A. (2018). The role of emotion regulation difficulties in the relationship between attachment representations and depressive and anxiety symptoms in the postpartum period. *Journal of Affective Disorders, 238*, 39–46.

Milani, L., Camisasca, E., Ionio, C., Miragoli, S., & Di Blasio, P. (2020). Video games use in childhood and adolescence: Social phobia and differential susceptibility to media effects. *Clinical Child Psychology and Psychiatry, 25*(2), 456–470. https://doi.org/10.1177/1359104519882754

Mun, I. B., & Lee, S. (2021). How does parental smartphone addiction affect adolescent smartphone addiction?: Testing the mediating roles of parental rejection and adolescent depression. *Cyberpsychology, Behavior, and Social Networking, 24*(6), 399–406.

Nakayama, H., Ueno, F., Mihara, S., Kitayuguchi, T., & Higuchi, S. (2020). Relationship between problematic internet use and age at initial weekly internet use. *Journal of Behavioral Addictions, 9*(1), 129–139. https://doi.org/10.1556/2006.2020.00009

Norouzi, Z., Roshan Chesli, R., & Farahani, H. (2021). Predicting the Behavior Problems in Children Aged 3–5 Years According to Mothers' Technoferenc and Problematic Internet use By them. *Rooyesh-e-Ravanshenasi Journal (RRJ), 9*(11), 87–96.

Odaci, H., & Çelik, Ç. B. (2013). Who are problematic internet users? An investigation of the correlations between problematic internet use and shyness, loneliness, narcissism, aggression and self-perception. *Computers in Human Behavior, 29*(6), 2382–2387. https://doi.org/10.1016/j.chb.2013.05.026

Peterka-Bonetta, J., Sindermann, C., Elhai, J. D., & Montag, C. (2019). Personality associations with smartphone and internet use disorder: A comparison study including links to impulsivity and social anxiety. *Frontiers in Public Health, 7*(JUN). https://doi.org/10.3389/fpubh.2019.00127

Pettorruso, M., Valle, S., Cavic, E., Martinotti, G., di Giannantonio, M., & Grant, J. E. (2020). Problematic internet use (PIU), personality profiles and emotion dysregulation in a cohort of young adults: Trajectories from risky behaviors to addiction. *Psychiatry Research, 289*, 113036. https://doi.org/10.1016/j.psychres.2020.113036

Piteo, E. M., & Ward, K. (2020). Review: Social networking sites and associations with depressive and anxiety symptoms in children and adolescents—A systematic review. In *Child and adolescent mental health* (Vol. 25, pp. 201–216). Blackwell Publishing Ltd.. https://doi.org/10.1111/camh.12373

Rocha, N. A. C. F., Dos Santos Silva, F. P., Dos Santos, M. M., & Dusing, S. C. (2020). Impact of mother-infant interaction on development during the first year of life: A systematic review. *Journal of child health care: for professionals working with children in the hospital and community, 24*(3), 365–385. https://doi.org/10.1177/1367493519864742

Rosen, L. D., Lim, A. F., Felt, J., Carrier, L. M., Cheever, N. A., Lara-Ruiz, J. M., Mendoza, J. S., & Rokkum, J. (2014). Media and technology use predicts ill-being among children, preteens and teenagers independent of the negative health impacts of exercise and eating habits. *Computers in Human Behavior, 35*, 364–375. https://doi.org/10.1016/j.chb.2014.01.036

Sakakihara, A., Haga, C., & Osaki, Y. (2019). Association between mothers' problematic internet use and the thinness of their children. *Cyberpsychology, Behavior, and Social Networking, 22*(9), 578–587.

Sánchez-Fernández, M., & Borda-Mas, M. (2022). Problematic smartphone use and specific problematic internet uses among university students and associated predictive factors: A systematic review. *Education and Information Technologies, 28*, 7111. https://doi.org/10.1007/s10639-022-11437-2

Sechi, C., Loi, G., & Cabras, C. (2021). Addictive internet behaviors: The role of trait emotional intelligence, self-esteem, age, and gender. *Scandinavian journal of psychology, 62*(3), 409–417.

Starcevic, V. (2013). Is Internet addiction a useful concept? *Australian and New Zealand Journal of Psychiatry, 47*(1), 16–19. https://doi.org/10.1177/0004867412461693

Tsai, J. K., Lu, W. H., Hsiao, R. C., Hu, H. F., & Yen, C. F. (2020). Relationship between difficulty in emotion regulation and internet addiction in college students: A one-year prospective study. *International Journal of Environmental Research and Public Health, 17*(13), 1–11. https://doi.org/10.3390/ijerph17134766

van Dijk, R., van der Valk, I. E., Vossen, H. G. M., Branje, S., & Deković, M. (2021). Problematic internet use in adolescents from divorced families: The role of family factors and adolescents' self-esteem. *International Journal of Environmental Research and Public Health, 18*(7). https://doi.org/10.3390/ijerph18073385

Wang, Qian, B., Yao, N., Qi, Zhou, X., Liu, J., & Lv, Z. T. (2017). The association between attention deficit/hyperactivity disorder and internet addiction: A systematic review and meta-analysis. *BMC Psychiatry, 17*(1). https://doi.org/10.1186/s12888-017-1408-x

Yen, J. Y., Yeh, Y. C., Wang, P. W., Liu, T. L., Chen, Y. Y., & Ko, C. H. (2018). Emotional regulation in young adults with internet gaming disorder. *International Journal of Environmental Research and Public Health, 15*(1). https://doi.org/10.3390/ijerph15010030

Zhou, R., Fong, P. S. W., & Tan, P. (2014). Internet use and its impact on engagement in leisure activities in China. *PLoS One, 9*(2). https://doi.org/10.1371/journal.pone.0089598

Chapter 18
Educational Intervention on Children's Digital Media Use: Empowering Caregivers, Healthcare Professionals, and Educators

Maíra Lopes Almeida, Gabriela Vescovi, Manoela Yustas Mallmann, Bruna Gabriella Pedrotti, Laura Canani da Rosa, Sofia Sebben, and Giana Bitencourt Frizzo

Introduction

The use of digital media is a recent and common phenomenon in family life. Mobile devices like *tablets* and *smartphones* have become part of the routine, keeping people constantly connected. The American survey Common Sense Media, conducted in 2020, showed that this use tends to vary in the early years of life, so that in the first 2 years, babies use an average of 49 minutes of screens per day, but this time jumps to 2 hours and 30 minutes between 2 and 4 years of the child (Rideout & Robb, 2020). In addition, most parents do not usually report concerns about the amount of screen time, the quality of the content accessed, and the impact of this use on child development. This same survey indicated that 97% of families with children up to 8 years old had at least one cell phone, while the use of *tablets* reached 75% (Rideout & Robb, 2020). Also, children are introduced to technologies at an increasingly early age, with data indicating that 4-month-old babies already make some use of digital media (AAP, 2016; Kabali et al., 2015).

The numbers highlight the frequent use of screens by families, including babies (Brito et al., 2017). However, pediatric societies recommend that children up to 2 years old are not exposed to screens, and, if they do, from 18 months, it is indicated that the use occurs in the presence of a caregiver (AAP, 2016). The guidelines are based mainly on the lack of consensus about the risks and benefits of screens for child development.

M. Lopes Almeida (✉) · G. Vescovi · M. Y. Mallmann · B. G. Pedrotti · L. C. da Rosa
S. Sebben · G. B. Frizzo
Institute of Psychology and the Postgraduate Program in Psychology (PPGPSICO) of Universidade Federal do Rio Grande do Sul, Porto Alegre, Rio Grande do Sul, Brazil
e-mail: mairaalmeida@ufg.br; gabriela-vescovi@saude.rs.gov.br; laura.canani@ufrgs.br; sofia.colognese@ufrgs.br; giana.frizzo@ufrgs.br

G. B. Frizzo (ed.), *Digital Media and Early Child Development*,
https://doi.org/10.1007/978-3-031-69224-6_18

The risks pointed out in the literature relate to impairments in the ability to self-regulate, in the development of language, cognition, and attention (Radesky et al., 2014), as well as behavioral difficulties (McDaniel & Radesky, 2018). Intense media use by children is also associated with obesity, sedentary lifestyle (AAP, 2016; Domingues-Montanari, 2017), and sleep problems (Cheung et al., 2017). The benefits are related to the possibility of bringing distant family members closer through video calls, providing moments of leisure and entertainment to the family, as well as an opportunity for exchanges and learning for the baby, mainly after 2 years and with the assistance of a caregiver to make sense of the content watched (AAP, 2016; Coyner et al., 2017).

It should be noted that habits regarding screen use are already established in early childhood, which highlights the need for prevention and early intervention in order to create healthier routines at this stage of development (McArthur et al., 2020). Internationally, these interventions have become more common (Wu et al., 2016). However, in Brazil, a literature review pointed to a lack of research in the area, so that no intervention was found (Frizzo et al., 2017). In general, studies that describe the step-by-step process of developing an intervention, especially in a systematic way, are rare in the literature. However, they are very important in order to preliminarily assess the feasibility and validity of proceeding, or not, with the main intervention (Durgante & Dell'aglio, 2018). Thus, the previous studies conducted by the research group helped to guide important aspects for the planning of a specific intervention on the use of digital media for the Brazilian context (Frizzo et al., 2017).

With this in mind, the research group initiated, in 2018, a scientific dissemination project. Initially, a video series titled "Babies & Technologies" was produced, available on YouTube. The video series consists of 11 episodes and has interesting results, with positive feedback from the general public. In this context, the development process of the pilot study of the intervention that will be addressed in this article began.

According to the current scenario of digital media use in early childhood, parents, caregivers, health professionals, and educators may question how to use these devices in the best possible way, minimizing risks and maximizing benefits. We start from the principle that educational intervention is an effective means to transmit knowledge about the use of digital media in early childhood, as Pedrotti (2019) puts it.

Therefore, the process of construction and implementation of an educational intervention on the use of digital media by babies will be presented. It is intended to show how the intervention was evaluated based on the knowledge acquired about the theme, as well as the satisfaction with participation. Therefore, the objective of this chapter is to present the educational intervention that we developed on the use of digital media by babies, in addition to describing the criteria we used to evaluate the quality of this intervention, based on the acquisition of knowledge and satisfaction of the participants. In addition, the intervention was first carried out live in person and later transformed into an asynchronous and online mode.

Development of the Intervention

The first step to developing the intervention involved discussions among our team to define and elaborate the intervention. At this planning stage, the research group consisted of five doctoral students, one master's student, and one undergraduate scholarship holder. A doctoral student was responsible for the planning along with an undergraduate in Psychology, a scientific dissemination scholarship holder. According to the main objective, it was expected to carry out an educational intervention with the population in a systematic way, that is, to compile the evidence on the use of digital media by babies into a model of continued learning. Therefore, a lecture format with four meetings was chosen.

After choosing the format, the themes to be worked on were defined. The criterion used was the analysis of the views and engagement of the "Babies & Technologies" series videos on the group's YouTube channel. Thus, four main themes were selected: (1) how to make good use of technologies with the baby; (2) caregiver-child relationship and technologies; (3) the influence of screens on sleep; and (4) the influence of screens on learning.

During this planning stage, some steps prior to execution stood out: the selection of instruments for intervention evaluation and a pre-application of the intervention with a small group (Robson & McCartan, 2016; Runfola et al., 2014). In addition to the theoretical discussions that supported all the elaboration, these stages are crucial for interventions and cannot be neglected, as they guide the understanding of what will be carried out and allow for adaptations before the start (Durgante & Dell'aglio, 2018; Robson & McCartan, 2016).

For the choice of instruments, it was necessary to define which aspects would be relevant to consider that the objectives of the intervention were met. In the discussion for this definition, it was concluded that the aspects to be evaluated related to the knowledge that the individual acquired due to participation in the intervention and satisfaction with the course. Thus, the second step was to conduct a review of the scientific literature on questionnaires that assessed these points.

In the case of the first aspect, no studies were found that had addressed the topic in the same format or with similar topics (Schmidt et al., 2012; Wahi, 2011; Wu et al., 2016). Thus, from a literature review and the knowledge acquired about the theme in the group's previous research, a questionnaire was created to be applied before the start of the lectures and reapplied at the end of the meetings. It is important to note that this questionnaire was constructed based on the scientific literature on the topic, discussed by the postgraduate students in the research group, and reviewed by *experts* who did not participate in the creation of the questionnaire in the initial stage (the coordinating professor and a postdoctoral researcher specialist in the theme).

This instrument titled "*Questionnaire on knowledge about the use of digital media by babies*"[1] is composed of 12 items that contain questions to be answered

[1] The questionnaire is available upon reasonable request from the corresponding author [MLA].

with "yes" or "no." The questions cover topics addressed in the lectures, such as "is babies' exposure to TV associated with problems in sleep quality and routine?", "are there official recommendations from pediatric societies for the use of technologies by babies?", and others. In the end, there was an open question: "Anything else you would like to add?"

Regarding satisfaction with the course, the review pointed to a questionnaire used in continuing education courses with a format similar to the educational intervention. This scale is based on the model of Kirkpatrick and Kirkpatrick (2016), which defines satisfaction as the first of four consecutive stages for the evaluation of continuing education: "reaction," "learning," "behavior," and "results." Satisfaction is synonymous with "reaction" and is an important construct of the learning context, which allows the transfer of skills, knowledge, and competences. In this model, satisfaction is considered as an attitude and is evaluated at three levels: affective, cognitive, and behavioral.

According to this theoretical framework, the questionnaire is titled "*Affective - Behavioral - Cognitive - Satisfaction Questionnaire*," which was developed in English and is composed of 11 items arranged on a 5-point Likert scale (Meng et al., 2018). In the end, the scores are added up, and higher scores indicate greater satisfaction. The scale is divided into three subscales: affective, behavioral, and cognitive. Some examples of the topics addressed in the items are (a) affective (3 items—15), the positive emotional tone during the lectures and the motivation of the speaker; (b) behavioral (2 items), the availability of the material used in the lecture and the preparation of the speaker for the meeting; and (c) cognitive (6 items), whether the knowledge was passed on clearly and whether it is considered that knowledge was acquired. Adequate psychometric properties were presented, such as evidence of face validity; construct validity, which indicated the existence of three factors; and internal consistency of the subscales evaluated by means of Cronbach's alpha, which ranged from 0.60 to 0.83.

Upon identifying that the scale would be useful to collaborate with the intervention, the steps recommended by Borsa et al. (2012) for cross-cultural adaptation of instruments were followed. Initially, contact was made with the authors responsible for the scale (Meng et al., 2018), who authorized the translation, adaptation, and validation of the scale by the research group. After obtaining this authorization, two people responsible for the intervention performed the first translation of the scale, which was evaluated by our team. From this, a synthesis was obtained through consensus, which then underwent a new evaluation. This version was evaluated by the coordinator of the research group, who had not had contact with the original scale and translations until that moment. Once the final version of the instruments was defined, the other fundamental step of planning was carried out: the pre-application of the intervention with a small group to identify possible implementation obstacles.

Dissemination of the Intervention and Pre-application of the Intervention in a Small Group

The group's social networks, the university's, and publication in the local newspaper were the means chosen for the dissemination that took place in September 2019, about a month before the start of the course. Some images were disseminated with the main information about the intervention, such as date, time, location, topics covered, and instructions for registration. In addition, an event was created on Facebook. Immediately, the group noticed the population's interest in the course. Other media, such as news websites and a local newspaper, invited the researchers for reports on the topic, and soon all the spots were filled. In 2 weeks, more than 200 registrations were obtained.

A pilot study, preliminary to the intervention, was developed as a *feasibility test*, with a small group at the public daycare center administered by the university. This event took place 1 month before the start of the intervention and had nine participants, including three caregivers of children who attended the daycare and six teachers. The meeting was designed to briefly cover all four contents. It was also possible to test the interactive digital platform Mentimeter. This platform allows for an interactive presentation between participants and speakers, such as creating a word cloud, surveys, questions and answers, polls, and others. In the end, an open questionnaire was handed out and answered anonymously about what improvements the participants suggested for the meeting and the contents. The responses were all positive, with thanks to the researchers and indicating greater interest in continuing to discuss the subject. Thus, after finalizing the choice, creation, and adaptation of the instruments, course promotion, and pre-application of the intervention, the implementation of the intervention began, which will be detailed below.

Implementation of the Intervention

The intervention was implemented in four weekly meetings, once a month, and in the evening. The meetings were face-to-face, in a university classroom, and averaged 2 hours in duration. A postgraduate student from the research group and an undergraduate student coordinated each meeting.

In this implementation, it is noteworthy that, initially, the main difficulty encountered was the high number of registrants. With the wide dissemination, more than 200 people registered, exceeding the initial planning that expected around 25 people. To solve this problem, emails were sent to those interested in order to confirm participation. As the number of confirmation responses obtained was close to the expected number, the initial planning was maintained in terms of operational issues, such as room and printing of instruments. The meetings followed the following protocol (Table 18.1).

Table 18.1 Description of the educational intervention protocol

Meeting	Objective	Activity	Guidance
First meeting: How to make good use of digital media Estimated time: 40 minutes	Familiarize participants with the theme and offer practical information on how to make good use with children	Part I: Application of instruments Part II: Presentation of recent data on the phenomenon and particularities of the use of digital media in the age group of 0 to 3 years Part III: Positioning of different pediatric societies Part IV: Means suggested by the scientific literature on how to make a healthy use of these media with children were reported	After briefly presenting the introductory part, it is suggested to emphasize the means reported by the scientific literature for healthy use in the family. Online materials can be made available to participants, such as a digital media use plan to be filled out and implemented by family members
Second meeting: Caregivers and digital media relationship Estimated time: 40 minutes	Highlight the importance of the initial caregiver-child bond and the influence that digital media exert in this context	Part I: Theoretical aspects about the importance of initial bonds for healthy child development Part II: Known impacts of the use of digital media on the caregiver-child relationship Part III: Report of the group's research on support network and interventions to reduce screen time	Although the interventions reported in the scientific literature for reducing screen time in young children are international, it is interesting to present some possible and effective practices. A list of suggestions of what was found to be effective can be made available to participants, for example, delivering a list of alternatives for playing with babies
Third meeting: Digital media and the effects on sleep Estimated time: 40 minutes	Inform about the physiological processes of sleep and the damages that digital media have on sleep, both in babies and adults	Part I: The importance of sleep for child development Part II: Impacts of digital media on sleep and possible hypotheses for this impact Part III: Guidelines for parents and health professionals on how to maintain a good sleep routine in the digital context	Some resources were used, such as presenting the circadian cycle in the theoretical part. In addition, sleep hygiene guidelines were provided, equipping them to think about their family's sleep hygiene. For professionals, a script with suggestions of topics for evaluating sleep in children can be provided, such as bedtime routines and daytime activities
Fourth meeting: Digital media and babies' learning Estimated time: 40 minutes	Present the stages of cognitive development, the effects that technology has on babies' cognitive functions, and guide participants to promote healthy cognitive development in children	Part I: What cognitive development is and how learning occurs in early childhood was presented Part II: Effects of digital media on learning Part III: Guidelines on how to promote healthy cognitive development in the current context Part V: Course closure Part IV: Application of instruments	After the theoretical part, some guidelines were provided on how to improve the co-use of digital media with children, for example, how to enhance moments of joint use with the child, encouraging them to ask questions, talking about what they are watching, and others

It is important to note that, at all meetings, selected videos from the web series "Babies & Technologies" were shown, and at the end of each meeting, there was a moment for discussion and clarification of doubts with the help of the digital platform Mentimeter. Also, complementary materials were sent by email, chosen according to the emerging subjects in the discussions and the demands of the participants. For example, a list of alternatives for playing with the children links to videos on the subject and others.

In the implementation of this intervention, it was found difficult to make scientific language more accessible to the population. However, this is a crucial ethical task for researchers in psychology (Cassepp-Borges, 2009). Although the research was known to the speakers, turning this into practical propositions required additional effort. It was noted that the final moment, in which proposals and professional tips were presented, usually attracted much attention, such as what had been done in interventions to reduce screen time in other countries and reported in the scientific literature.

Despite the wide dissemination and more than 200 registrations, another difficulty encountered was the number of participants. This number drastically reduced when confirming by email and even more in face-to-face meetings. A decrease in the frequency of registrants was also observed throughout the lectures. The first meeting had 28 participants, the second and third with 22, and the last with 16. Although the final number is still close to the initially planned number, it is important to consider in future interventions that even greater investment in dissemination is made, besides tracking participants' reasons for dropping out.

Even with these challenges, a great interest of the participants in the theme was observed. During the meetings, the reports of numerous situations experienced in professional and family daily life that ratified the scientific evidence presented by the speakers were common. When mentioning their own experiences, it was possible to notice an existing demand to know alternatives that can contribute to a healthier use of screens with babies. As the speakers presented some possibilities, the participants thought together and formulated other solutions to the issues that were being discussed, positively complexifying the strategies and reflections on the subject. In addition, they always requested that extra materials be sent to help them in the endeavor to reduce or make better use of these technologies.

In general, the participants were health or education professionals and caregivers of a child. This confluence of professional and personal roles meant that the intervention was not only a transfer of theoretical-practical knowledge, but also reflective. At various times, reflections on the use of digital media by themselves or their family were reported, especially in meetings that emphasized the importance of the adult's mode of use for the child's use. In this way, it is understood that the intervention fulfilled more than the function of transmitting knowledge, providing a space for considerations about the roles that digital media can play for the adult, children, and their families.

Evidence of the Intervention

For the evaluation of the intervention, the following instruments were considered: *Questionnaire on knowledge about the use of digital media by babies* and *Affective-Cognitive-Behavioral Satisfaction Questionnaire*. At the first meeting, before the start of the lectures, the Knowledge Questionnaire was handed out for participants to fill out. Then, each participant was assigned a code, and a questionnaire was for later comparison. At the last lecture, the instrument was reapplied along with the Satisfaction Questionnaire. The data were then tabulated, typed, and analyzed using the statistical program *Statistical Package for the Social Sciences* (SPSS) version 24.

The sample consisted of 16 participants who filled out all the questionnaires, with 14 identifying as women and 2 as men. Most were health professionals ($n = 6$) or education ($n = 5$), followed by education students ($n = 2$), mothers ($n = 2$), and a health student. The intervention started with 28 participants and ended with 16, recording a loss of 43%. A meta-analysis indicated that intervention studies on digital media use do not refer to the participant loss rate (Friedrich et al., 2014). However, the number found in this study is in accordance with other intervention studies that obtained rates that varied between 0% and 78.2% (Van der Mispel et al., 2017).

Initially, the instruments were evaluated quantitatively, and then the questions answered by the participants were included in the Knowledge Questionnaire. A descriptive statistical analysis of the two questionnaires was carried out. The analysis of the instruments also aimed to evaluate whether there was a statistically significant difference in the scores of the *Knowledge Questionnaire* after participation in the educational intervention. Due to the non-normal distribution of the data, the Wilcoxon test for paired samples was applied with the aim of evaluating the difference in the instrument's scores at the two moments pre-intervention and post-intervention. The Mann-Whitney test was also used to check if there were differences in the participants' satisfaction level regarding the number of lectures attended (presence at the four meetings or less).

The descriptive statistical analysis showed that the average obtained in the *Affective-Cognitive-Behavioral Satisfaction Questionnaire* in relation to the intervention was 52.6 (SD = 2.50) out of a total of 55 points. This value is considered high (Meng et al., 2018), indicating a good level of participant satisfaction with the course. Regarding the subscales, it was noted that the behavioral dimension had the highest satisfactory level ($M = 9.5$; SD = 0.89) out of a total of 10 points, followed by the cognitive dimension ($M = 29.30$; SD = 1.35) out of a total of 30 points and affective ($M = 8.87$; SD = 0.95) out of a total of 15 points. In the Mann-Whitney test, no statistically significant differences were found in the level of satisfaction with regard to the number of lectures attended ($U = 44, 00$; $p = 0.150$). Other educational interventions with a number of meetings close to four also recorded similar results regarding satisfaction (Silva et al., 2018; Torquato et al., 2019).

Regarding the knowledge acquired, a statistically significant difference was found in the scores of the *Knowledge Questionnaire* applied before and after

Table 18.2 Comparison between knowledge about the use of digital media in early childhood for participants of the face-to-face course (negative ranks, *mean* = 3.00; positive ranks, *mean* = 6.30)

Variable	Intervention	Mean	Standard deviation	Median	*p* value
Knowledge about digital media in early childhood (face-to-face course)	Pre	9.06	1.56	9.5	0.007
	Post	10.5	0.81	10	

participation in the educational intervention with a high effect size ($r = -0.67$). This data reveals that the intervention is promising and is encouraging, as previous studies have shown that the educational intervention model is effective not only for transmitting knowledge but also for reducing excessive screen use by teenagers and for increasing physical activities in childhood, indirectly reducing screen time (Gholamian et al., 2019; Harrison et al., 2006), as can be seen in Table 18.2.

In addition, a qualitative stage was considered in which participants were asked in writing if they would like to add anything. At this stage, the responses indicated that the participants considered the experience positive. The results even showed a request for the continuation of the meetings in the following year. Some reports evidenced this positive evaluation, for example: "*I will take everything I learned; the course changed my view on the use of screens*" *(P14)* and "*I would like future lectures on the subject*" (P9).

Thus, the analysis of the data indicates that the educational intervention on the use of digital media in early childhood achieved the initial objectives of transmitting theoretical-practical knowledge while constituting a satisfactory experience for the participants. Notably, the use of digital media by babies, as a recent and growing phenomenon, makes these interventions increasingly necessary.

Connected and Online Babies: A Response to the COVID-19 Pandemic

From March 2020, face-to-face activities were suspended at the university due to the outbreak of the COVID-19 pandemic. As a result, plans to hold new in-person editions of the intervention were suspended. With all activities happening remotely, it was decided in a meeting by the team to adapt the educational intervention to an online format. It was hoped to offer scientific information to families and professionals at a time when the use of digital media was skyrocketing (Nyström et al., 2020; Sá et al., 2021).

The online course was developed by the same team that conducted the in-person intervention, plus two postgraduate students in psychology. The contents were fully adapted to the online format. A postgraduate student and a scientific initiation scholarship holder were responsible for assisting their colleagues in the construction of the online course, from how to present the information clearly and dynamically to

Table 18.3 Comparison between knowledge about use of digital media in early childhood for participants of the online course

Variable	Intervention	Mean	Standard deviation	Median	*p* value
Knowledge about digital media in early childhood (online course)	Pre	13.2	1.22	13.0	<0.001
	Post	14.1	1.24	14.0	

reviewing the developed content. After a new literature review, updates on the topic were included, including important information related to the context of the pandemic.

The course was divided into modules: an initial module, with an introduction to the content; six modules divided on the following themes: "The use of digital media during the COVID-19 pandemic"; "The baby's relationship with its caregivers and digital media"; "Digital media, sleep, and vision"; "Digital media and feeding"; "Digital media and learning" and "How to make good use of digital media"; and a final module to conclude the course. In addition to the online format, other modifications were made since the initial intervention. The online course was made entirely self-applicable, asynchronous, and with various materials, such as texts, booklets, interactive images, animated videos, and recorded video lessons. The participants' doubts were answered in a forum open to participants weekly. The workload was also increased, being 20 hours/lesson, along with the availability of several supplementary materials.

Subsequently, the course was advertised on the research group's social networks and the researchers' personal profiles. More than 200 people signed up for the course, offered free of charge by the university. In total, 176 people answered the *Questionnaire on knowledge about the use of digital media by babies* that allowed access to the course content. Of these, 94 people answered the same questionnaire at the course's end, signaling the content's completion. For the online version, the adapted questionnaire came to have 17 questions (including 3 questions about feeding and 2 about the COVID-19 pandemic), each worth one point. The data from the 94 participants were analyzed in the same way as reported for the in-person course. The results are in Table 18.3.

It is possible to note that there was a significant difference in the participants' knowledge before and after the course, with the effect size being considered high ($r = -0.64$). We conclude that the online version of the course was also very promising, as it expanded access compared to the in-person intervention, generating similar results in terms of knowledge acquisition by the participants.

Final Considerations

In the present study, it was possible to analyze the process of construction and implementation of the pilot study of an educational intervention on the use of digital media by babies (in both in-person and online versions), as well as the evaluation of the knowledge acquired on the topic and the participant's satisfaction with the intervention, in a systematic way. The positive evaluation of the participants about the intervention stands out, with high satisfaction rates, as well as good results regarding its effectiveness in the acquisition of knowledge by the participants.

This experience allowed us to identify relevant information to be considered when developing educational interventions on the use of digital media by babies, in addition to adapting to Brazilian Portuguese a satisfaction scale that proved suitable for evaluating the intervention. Although the intervention was developed and carried out in a Brazilian context, it is plausible to think that it could also be applied to other contexts. Both the difficulties encountered and the potentialities identified in this study can elucidate necessary improvements for greater reach and better adherence of participants. However, this study innovatively contributed by elucidating the creation, evaluation, and dissemination of an intervention not presented in Brazil until then. In conclusion, it proved feasible and promising in its objectives and results, and it is hoped that it can contribute to advancing this theme.

Acknowledgments The original version of this chapter was written in Portuguese and translated into English with the help of artificial intelligence. A subsequent human revision was done primarily in terms of content.

Part of this work is published in the format of an article in the journal Revista da SPAGESP, with reference Almeida, M. L., Rosa, L. C., Vescovi, G., Pedrotti, B. G., Mallmann, M. Y., & Frizzo, G. B. (2022). Educational intervention on the use of media in early childhood. *Revista da SPAGESP, 23*(1), 103–116, and authorized the partial reproduction of the content for this chapter.

References

American Academy of Pediatrics, Council on Communications and Media. (2016). Media and young minds. *Pediatrics, 138*(5), 1–8. https://doi.org/10.1542/peds.2016-2591

Borsa, J. C., Damásio, B. F., & Bandeira, D. R. (2012). Adaptação e validação de instrumentos psicológicos entre culturas: Algumas considerações. *Paidéia (Ribeirão Preto), 22*(53), 423–432. https://doi.org/10.1590/S0103-863X2012000300014

Brito, R., Franscisco, R., Dias, P., & Chaudron, S. (2017). Family dynamics in digital homes: The role played by parental mediation in young children's digital practices around 14 European countries. *Contemporary Family Therapy, 39*, 271–280. https://doi.org/10.1007/s10591-017-9431-0

Cassepp-Borges, V. (2009). Devolução de dados por correio eletrônico: Uma alternativa para pesquisas quantitativas. *Avaliação Psicológica, 8*(1), 149–152. Recuperado de http://pepsic.bvsalud.org/scielo.php?script=sci_abstract&pid=S1677-04712009000100015&lng=pt&nrm=iso&tlng=pt

Cheung, C. H. M., Bedford, R., Saez de Urabain, I. R., Karmiloff-Smith, A., & Smith, T. J. (2017). Daily touchscreen use in infants and toddlers is associated with reduced sleep and delayed sleep onset. *Scientific Reports, 7*(46104), 1–7. https://doi.org/10.1038/srep46104

Coyner, S. M., Radesky, J., Collier, K. M., Gentile, D. A., Linder, J. R., Nathanson, A. I., Rasmussen, E. E., Reich, S. M., & Rogers, J. (2017). Parenting and digital media. *Pediatrics, 140*(2), 112–116. https://doi.org/10.1542/peds.2016-1758N

Domingues-Montanari, S. (2017). Clinical and psychological effects of excessive screen time on children. *Journal of Paediatrics and Child Health, 53*, 333–338. https://doi.org/10.1111/jpc.13462

Durgante, H., & Dell'Aglio, D. D. (2018). Critérios metodológicos para a avaliação de programas de intervenção em psicologia. *Avaliação Psicológica, 17*(1), 155–162. https://doi.org/10.15689/ap.2017.1701.15.13986

Friedrich, R. R., Polet, J. P., Schuch, I., & Wagner, M. B. (2014). Effect of intervention programs in schools to reduce screen time: A meta-analysis. *Jornal de Pediatria, 90*(3), 232–241. https://doi.org/10.1016/j.jped.2014.01.003

Frizzo, G., Bandeira, D., Lewandowski, D., Azevedo, E. C., Mendonça Filho, E., Mallmann, M., … Silva, M. (2017). Infants, families, and the use of technologies: A multi-method study for child development. Unpublished Research Project.

Gholamian, B., Shahnazi, H., & Hassanzadeh, A. (2019). The effect of educational intervention based on BASNEF model for reducing internet addiction among female students: A quasi-experimental study. *Italian Journal of Pediatrics, 45*(1), 164. https://doi.org/10.1186/s13052-019-0761-4

Harrison, M., Burns, C. F., McGuinness, M., Heslin, J., & Murphy, N. M. (2006). Influence of a health education intervention on physical activity and screen time in primary school children: 'Switch Off–Get Active'. *Journal of Science and Medicine in Sport, 9*(5), 388–394. https://doi.org/10.1016/j.jsams.2006.06.012

Kabali, H. K., Irigoyen, M. M., Nunez-Davis, R., Budacki, J. G., Mohanty, S. H., Leister, K. P., & Bonner, R. L. (2015). Exposure and use of mobile media devices by young children. *Pediatrics, 136*(6), 1044–1050. https://doi.org/10.1542/peds.2015-2151

Kirkpatrick, J. D., & Kirkpatrick, W. (2016). *Four levels of training evaluation* (3rd ed.). ATD Press.

McArthur, B. A., Browne, D., Tough, S., & Madigan, S. (2020). Trajectories of screen use during early childhood: Predictors and associated behavior and learning outcomes. *Computers in Human Behavior, 113*, 106501. https://doi.org/10.1016/j.chb.2020.106501

McDaniel, B. T., & Radesky, J. S. (2018). Technoference: Parent distraction with technology and associations with child behavior problems. *Child Development, 89*(1), 100–109. https://doi.org/10.1111/cdev.12822

Meng, M., Peter, D., Mattner, F., Igel, C., & Kugler, C. (2018). Development and psychometric pilot-testing of a questionnaire for the evaluation of satisfaction with continuing education in infection control nurses. *Nurse Education in Practice, 31*, 77–82. https://doi.org/10.1016/j.nepr.2018.05.003

Nyström, C. D., Alexandrou, C., Henström, M., Nilsson, E., Okely, A. D., Wehbe El Masri, S., & Löf, M. (2020). International study of movement behaviors in the early years (SUNRISE): Results from SUNRISE Sweden's pilot and COVID-19 study. *International Journal of Environmental Research and Public Health, 17*(22), 8491. https://doi.org/10.3390/ijerph17228491

Pedrotti, B. G. (2019). Como prescindir das novas tecnologias no cuidado e na interação com os bebês? [How to do without new technologies in the care and interaction with babies?] (Dissertação de Mestrado [Master's thesis], Universidade Federal do Rio Grande do Sul). Universidade Federal do Rio Grande do Sul, Porto Alegre. Recuperado de https://www.lume.ufrgs.br/handle/10183/202058.

Radesky, J. S., Silverstein, M., Zuckerman, B., & Christakis, D. A. (2014). Infant self-regulation and early childhood media exposure. *Pediatrics, 133*(5), 1172–1178. https://doi.org/10.1542/peds.2013-2367

Rideout, V., & Robb, M. B. (2020). *The common sense census: Media use by kids age zero to eight, 2020*. Common Sense Media. Disponível em: https://www.commonsensemedia.org/sites/default/files/research/report/2020_zero_to_eight_census_final_web.pdf

Robson, C., & McCartan, K. (2016). *Real world research: A resource for users of social research methods in applied settings* (4th ed.). Wiley.

Runfola, C. D., Zucker, N. L., Holle, A. V., Mazzeo, S., Hodges, E. A., Perrin, E. M., et al. (2014). NURTURE: Development and pilot testing of a novel parenting intervention for mothers with histories of an eating disorder: Nurture pilot testing. *International Journal of Eating Disorders, 47*(1), 1–12. https://doi.org/10.1002/eat.22178

Sá, C. S. C., Pombo, A., Luz, C., Rodrigues, L. P., & Cordovil, R. (2021). COVID-19 social isolation in Brazil: Effects on the physical activity routine of families with children. *Revista Paulista de Pediatria, 39*, e2020159. https://doi.org/10.1590/1984-0462/2021/39/2020159

Schmidt, M. E., Haines, J., O'Brien, A., McDonald, J., Price, S., Sherry, B., & Taveras, E. M. (2012). Systematic review of effective strategies for reducing screen time among young children. *Obesity, 20*(7), 1338–1354. https://doi.org/10.1038/oby.2011.348

Silva, F. B., Gondim, E. C., Henrique, N. C. P., Fonseca, L. M. M., & de Mello, D. F. (2018). Intervenção educativa com mães jovens: Aquisição de saberes sobre cuidados da criança. *Acta Paulista de Enfermagem, 31*(1), 32–38. https://doi.org/10.1590/1982-0194201800006

Torquato, I. M. B., Collet, N., Forte, F. D. S., França, J. R. F. D. S., Silva, M. D. F. D. O. C., & Reichert, A. P. D. S. (2019). Effectiveness of an intervention with mothers to stimulate children under two years. *Revista Latino-Americana de Enfermagem, 27*, e3216. https://doi.org/10.1590/1518-8345.3176.3216

Van der Mispel, C., Poppe, L., Crombez, G., Verloigne, M., & De Bourdeaudhuij, I. (2017). A self-regulation-based eHealth intervention to promote a healthy lifestyle: Investigating user and website characteristics related to attrition. *Journal of Medical Internet Research, 19*(7), e241. https://doi.org/10.2196/jmir.7277

Wahi, G. (2011). Effectiveness of interventions aimed at reducing screen time in children: A systematic review and meta-analysis of randomized controlled trials. *Archives of Pediatrics & Adolescent Medicine, 165*(11), 979. https://doi.org/10.1001/archpediatrics.2011.122

Wu, L., Sun, S., He, Y., & Jiang, B. (2016). The effect of interventions targeting screen time reduction: A systematic review and meta-analysis. *Medicine, 95*(27), e4029. https://doi.org/10.1097/MD.0000000000004029

Chapter 19
Supporting Parents and Caregivers: Guidelines and Interventions on Screen Exposure in the Early Years

Débora Becker and Tagma Marina Schneider Donelli

Introduction

Over the last decade, mobile connectivity has increased around the world. By the end of 2022, more than 5.4 billion people had used a mobile service, primarily smartphones, with mobile Internet access (GSMA, 2023). Along with the expansion of mobile technology, screen time is also increasing worldwide. Problematic use of screens is a reality among adult and child populations once children are exposed to different screens by adults, mainly during their first 6 months (Becker & Donelli, 2024; Kabali et al., 2015; Kiliç et al., 2019), suffering all the effects of early screen exposure.

Screen time is defined as the amount of time someone spends per day watching screens, such as smartphones, computers, television, and other electronic devices. The literature points out that screen time or screen usage generates interaction disruptions, interfering negatively with social relationships and physical and mental health. In the domain of parenting, interruptions caused by parental usage of digital media during interactions with family members are called *technoference* (McDaniel & Coyne, 2016), a recent phenomenon that may negatively impact the quality of interpersonal relationships, including parent-infant interactions (Becker, 2020; Wolfers et al., 2020). The dyadic interaction can hardly be affected once parents use technology during caregiving (Becker, 2020; McDaniel, 2019; Wolfers et al., 2020).

Screens, in general, impact children's development in different domains, such as emotional, cognitive, physical, and social domains. Concerning language development, children may face difficulties with language acquisition, presenting delays in those skills. Visual problems were also reported because of excessive screen

D. Becker (✉) · T. M. Schneider Donelli
Psychology Graduate Program—Universidade do Vale do Rio dos Sinos—UNISINOS University, São Leopoldo, RS, Brazil
e-mail: debbecker@edu.unisinos.br; tagmad@unisinos.br

G. B. Frizzo (ed.), *Digital Media and Early Child Development*,
https://doi.org/10.1007/978-3-031-69224-6_19

exposure. Screens may also affect children's circadian rhythm, impacting sleep quality and emotion regulation. Moreover, screen time is related to hyperactivity, sedentary behaviors, and obesity (Coyne et al., 2017; Kozeis, 2009; Stiglic & Viner, 2019). So, with a growing number of children under the age of 3 being exposed to screens worldwide in the last decade, concerns about child development have become more imminent, being intensively discussed in academic and clinical fields.

Families nowadays are suffering the side effects of excessive screen exposure. Over the past few years, children have been exposed to screens more than ever, which was enhanced during the last years due to the COVID-19 pandemic (Bergmann et al., 2022; Bergonsi et al., 2022; Portinho et al., 2023). However, individuals' average screen time is unlikely to drop to pre-pandemic levels. So, how can we establish guidance and support for families, especially those with small children, from now on? How can we make guidelines that are effective and accessible? How can interventions strengthen parent-infant bonds and reduce screen time in families?

To address these challenges, policymakers are updating relevant policies to address current needs. Similarly, considering the role of early interventions in the quality of dyadic interactions and the presence of digital media in family surroundings, interventions focused on parental skills can be strategic prevention tools targeting screen usage in families. Screen usage among adults and children is a public health issue and demands attention. Therefore, this chapter will present guidelines released in several countries and discuss the need for parental interventions as a complementary strategy to target the audience.

Guidelines on Screen Time Across the Globe

Nowadays, children under 3 are often seen being entertained with screens in playgrounds and restaurants worldwide. Some parents use their phones and televisions as digital pacifiers to entertain children and face stress and lack of a social support network (Becker & Donelli, 2024; Radesky et al., 2016). Facing this reality and considering what research is highlighting as an alert for child development in different countries, parenting guidelines, which oriented parents regarding child development, have been updated to encompass screen exposure. The studies that explored screen time during childhood have focused more on sedentary behavior, which is responsible for the increase in obesity among children and adolescents (Vasques et al., 2012). Most guidelines are based on these studies, focusing on the importance of physical activity and screen time reduction during childhood and adolescence. Therefore, in 2019, the World Health Organization (WHO) released guidelines on physical activity, sedentary behavior, and sleep for children under 5 (WHO, 2019).

Guidelines are essential strategies to disseminate evidence-based information, as many parents and caregivers are not well-informed about the health-related effects of screen exposure in a child's development, especially during early years, and misinformation may lead to increased screen availability to children. With the exemption of video calls, children should not be exposed to screens before the age of 2

(WHO, 2019). However, the literature shows that children are exposed very early, stressing parental misinformation and low access to the current guidelines (Becker, 2020; McArthur et al., 2022).

In the United States of America, the American Academy of Pediatrics (AAP, 2016) released a guide to oriented parents through screen time. The AAP guidelines are recognized worldwide and used as an example in different countries. The AAP does not recommend screen exposure under 18 months and highlights the importance of parental mediation when screens are involved. In the United Kingdom, the guidelines of the Royal College of Paediatrics and Child Health (RCPCH, 2019) go in the opposite direction of the guidelines from the AAP and WHO and recommend family control of a child's screen time, considering the needs of each child, which sounds more easily implemented for some families. However, flexible recommendations demand parental psychoeducation about potential screen exposure adverse effects on a child's development.

In some countries, the world's first 24-hour movement guidelines are being followed. It consists of a guide to parents and caregivers with a picture of a 24-hour day period for a child. It was released in 2016 by Canada (Tremblay et al., 2016), followed by Australia and South Africa (Draper et al., 2020; Tooth et al., 2019) and other countries around the globe. It includes information about playing, sitting, and lying down time, sleep routine, and screen time. These guidelines do not recommend sedentary screen engagement for children under 2, matching the WHO (2019) recommendations.

In India, which is one of the most populous countries with high levels of media consumption (Joseph et al., 2022), the guidelines were released by the Indian Academy of Pediatrics (IAP, 2021) and focus on potential risks of screen exposure in physical, mental, social, and scholastic domains. As stated by the IAP, children should not get screen exposure under 2 years of age once there is a higher risk of exposure to violent and sexual content, such as inadequate advertisements, and an increase in sleep disorders. The Indian guidelines also include a topic about adult digital hygiene and the role model parents play to their children, which seems an important aspect to be explored in this parental supportive material (IAP, 2021; Gupta et al., 2022). In Japan, the recommendations followed a different path once the Japanese guideline suggested limiting screen exposure to 2 hours per day for children of age 2 (Arai et al., 2023).

In Spain, the Spanish Pediatric Association (AEP, 2023) developed a Family Digital Plan (Plan Digital Familiar), which families can customize. There is a version for pediatricians that oriented professionals to offer family support favoring families' digital health habits and children's and caregiver's mental health. The Spanish guide acts as supportive material for families with children, highlighting no screen time during the first 2 years of life, no screens during mealtimes and before bedtime, and the importance of parental presence during interactions with screens, who must set limits and supervise the children. Moreover, the Spanish guide includes scientific explanations about early screen exposure, answering questions such as the following: According to science, why should we not expose a baby to a screen? What kind of activities should we avoid? The guide also includes a blank space for parents to use to report the recommendations they consider relevant and are not contemplated in the manual. Germany recommends that parents refrain from exposing children under 3 to screens and children from 3 to 6 may only be exposed to screens for up to 30 min per day (Hebestreit & Sina, 2024), which is aligned with research findings about the side effects of early exposure. Italy, like most countries in Europe, follows AAP and WHO recommendations (Bozzola et al., 2018).

Latin American countries like Argentina, Brazil, and Chile also follow an approach aligned with the AAP guidelines and WHO recommendations. The Argentinian Society of Pediatrics (SAP, 2020) recommends not exposing children under 2 to screens, except for video calls. The Argentinian guideline highlights that when needed, adults should consider the type of content and prioritize educative and interactive content when the adult is present to supervise the child. In 2020, the SAP introduced guidelines for the recreational use of screens, considering the needs of families during the COVID-19 pandemic. The Brazilian Society of Pediatrics (SBP) recommends avoiding passive screen exposure for children under 2 years old, especially during mealtime and before bedtime (SBP, 2019). On the other hand, Chile released an activity guide with a list of activities that can replace screens and promote child entertainment (CCC, 2018). The Chilean manual also includes reflective questions for children and specific questions targeting parents and caregivers, such as: "How many hours do we spend viewing television at home?"

The guidelines this chapter reviewed generally caution screen time for children and adolescents, except for Chilean, Indian, and Spanish guides, which emphasized the salient role of caregivers and screen exposure in the early years. It is essential to consider that parents and caregivers are also connected in family and scholarly surroundings. The introduction of the topic of adult screen usage during caregiving and the impacts of screens on the parent-child relationship should be considered in the developing recommendations, pointing out the negative repercussions of adult screen usage on the dyadic interactions, as highlighted by different authors (Becker, 2020; Becker & Donelli, 2024; McDaniel, 2019; Wolfers et al., 2020). Moreover, it is essential to stress the possible repercussions of early exposure in a child's development, especially concerning their socio-emotional development.

Despite the efforts of pediatric societies around the world and the WHO, the studies pointed out that most parents do not adhere to screen use recommendations and are misinformed about the side effects of screen exposure (Becker & Donelli, 2024; Durham et al., 2021; Lammers et al., 2022; McArthur et al., 2022; Roman-Vinas et al., 2016). According to Lammers et al.'s (2022) study exploring parental awareness and adherence to the AAP recommendations, mothers who did not adhere to the recommendations presented more infant screen time per day in comparison with mothers who adhere to the recommendations. Compared to unaware mothers, mothers who are aware of the AAP recommendations were more likely to limit screen time for their children. Muppalla et al.'s (2023) review on effects of screen time on child development underscored the essential role parents play in managing screen time in childhood. Bozzola et al. (2018) stressed the repercussions of early digital media exposure in different domains of child development and the pediatricians' role in advising families with young children regarding this. However, as highlighted by Becker and Donelli (2024) and Lammers et al. (2022), some parents believe that early screen exposure may be crucial for child's development, ignoring the recommendations of no screen time at an early age. All these aspects reinforce the necessity to provide parents and caregivers with evidence-based information about the side effects of screen exposure in child development and during interactions, encouraging parents to stimulate children with activities that do not encompass screens.

Based on recent research findings, the recommendation of no screen time for infants should be included in all guidelines. However, the guidelines should encompass, in an accessible language, information about how to use screens healthily when needed since the recommendation to avoid screens does not seem plausible for most parents, especially those families who do not have a support network. Using evocative vocabulary and images can be helpful in clarifying the topics of interest. The guidelines should include topics such as calming the child down without screens and a list of playtime activities that may replace technology with the child, as highlighted in the Chilean activity manual (CCC, 2018) since parents expected some oriented guidance to calm down the child and entertain, which are the most common reasons for parents offer devices to infants as suggested in some studies (Becker & Donelli, 2024; Radesky et al., 2016). The topic of "technoference" should also be part of the manuals to inform parents about technology's repercussions on personal relationships and to educate parents to use screens with awareness since adults' usage of screens can influence children's screen usage (Coyne et al., 2017).

Furthermore, as stated in the Indian guidelines (IAP, 2021), new guides can explore adult digital hygiene. More than this, national campaigns in the media and in primary healthcare should be run, encompassing the reality of families, the cultural aspects, the patterns of screen usage, and other singularities that vary around the globe. Moreover, to make orientations more effective and to increase parental adherence to the guidelines, interventions focusing on caregivers' skills may be a feasible strategy to improve the quality of early relationships as soon as educating parents and caregivers to deal with screens nowadays.

Why Focus on Caregiver Skills Through Interventions?

A child is not alone in the world. When a child is born, they are in contact with another human being who will provide the biological and emotional support necessary to survive outside the woman's body. The child needs a human's constant presence during their early years and to be seen by this figure to feel protected and ready to explore the world. When we consider protecting a child, we must also consider protecting their caregivers.

- Who takes care of the child's caregivers?
- How can unhealthy caregivers provide good care?

It is stressed that during the early years, the child's caregiver plays a vital role in developing the child's independence and emotional bonds. Caregivers are expected to provide love, awareness, emotional availability, responsiveness, sensitivity, and other abilities or characteristics that may nurture the foundation of early relationships, performing a crucial role in a child's sense of security (Biringen & Easterbrooks, 2012; Donelli et al., 2020). Parental sensitivity, for example, plays a fundamental role in a child's emotion regulation, especially stress regulation. Moreover, sensitive parenting may decrease the risk of psychopathologies during childhood (Cooke et al., 2022). Sensitive caregivers may also present a good mentalization ability, which consists of understanding oneself and others regarding underlying mental states, such as feelings and desires (Fonagy & Allison, 2012). Parents with a satisfactory mentalization ability may facilitate a child's socioemotional development, emotional self-regulation, and the development of a secure attachment (Slade, 2005).

In the domain of mentalization, parental reflective functioning is considered a critical human capacity that enables social relationships. Once the ability to recognize emotions in others is an essential step in social interactions, as stated by Mayes and Cohen (2002), parental reflective functioning capacity is essential to maintaining infant-caregiver healthy relationships, being considered a more significant predictor of infant attachment (Barlow et al., 2020). However, when parents are under stress and immersed in screens, those skills may be impaired, negatively affecting the child's socioemotional development, including the development of the child's reflective functioning ability.

Connecting adults may present decreased sensitivity and responsiveness levels, such as increased hostility, observed during parent-infant interactions (Becker, 2020). Moreover, as already mentioned before, studies have shown the negative impacts of excessive or inappropriate screen exposure on a child's social, emotional, cognitive, and motor skills acquisition (Coyne et al., 2017; Muppalla et al., 2023), pointing out the need of intervening at an early stage. Therefore, adults need to be educated to use screens in a good and safe way, keeping in mind protecting a child's timing since many parents seem not to realize that early screen exposure may impact a child's interactions with peers, caregivers, and the environment where they are exploring the world by creating connections with the real life (Becker & Donelli, 2024). Furthermore, many adults do not know that screen usage may affect family routines and social interactions, including their interactions with their children. By targeting parents' and caregivers' behaviors through interventions, we are favoring caregiver-child bonds and reverberating positively on the child's socioemotional development and healthier screen usage habits in the future.

Early Intervention Programs

When discussing early intervention programs, we consider providing adequate early support to children and their families, focusing on health prevention and promotion strategies. Interventions targeting families aim to prevent adverse outcomes and promote positive outcomes in a family context (Donelli et al., 2020; Zeanah & Zeanah, 2019). Intervention programs focusing on the early years and parenting are effective, as highlighted in different studies (Byrne et al., 2018; Donelli et al., 2020; Rutherford & Mayes, 2019; Slade et al., 2020; Taubner et al., 2013). Most of the programs reported in the literature were run in Europe and North America. They were built from a mentalization approach, focusing on improving parental skills, including parental reflective functioning. Furthermore, early intervention programs based on mentalization are seen as practical strategies to offer the best beginning of life possible to children to decrease infant's disorganized attachment and improve parental reflective functioning (Barlow et al., 2020; Donelli et al., 2020). Moreover, these interventions can reduce levels of parental stress and decrease the levels of parental substance use (Rutherford & Mayes, 2019), reinforcing the importance of these programs when screen time is in focus since screen usage, when problematic, may present similar patterns with substance use.

In a general overview, there is an incipience of studies focusing on interventions targeting early screen usage in family and scholarly surroundings, despite a higher incidence of screen usage in these environments and by this audience (Boonmun et al., 2023; Jones et al., 2021). Most of the programs target adolescents and older children's screen time and focus on behavior-change techniques to regulate screen time, as highlighted by Jones et al. (2021) in a review, stressing the scarcity of interventions focusing on young children and their parents and caregivers.

In Australia, the intervention Family@play, delivered to parents of 2–3-year-old infants (Hinkley et al., 2015), was accessed and showed promising results. It consists of an intervention based on social cognitive and family systems theory to reduce a child's screen time. The intervention comprises six sessions, encompassing themes such as media recommendations, managing high-risk situations, and strategies to reduce screen time. Similarly, an intervention focusing on parents and infant kindergarten caregivers was proposed and accessed in southern Brazil (Becker & Donelli, 2023). The intervention used conversation groups and psychoeducation activities. The intervention was built on a mentalization approach, focusing on parental skills, such as parental reflective functioning and sensitivity. The intervention encompassed three sessions (three sessions with the parents and three sessions with the kindergarten caregivers), with 60 min for each session. The following themes were approached during the sessions: (a) Technology in a familiar context/a school context, encompassing questions such as the following: How does technology pervade the family surroundings? How and how early is the infant introduced in the digital world? What are the most common reasons for handling screens for an infant? What are the most common reasons adults stay connected when interacting with their children? (b) Child as a digital native, focusing on challenges of educating children nowadays, how the interactions are happening in an environment with screens, establishing limits, seeking information, and replacing screens with other activities. An overview of research on the topic conducted in recent years was presented during the encounters. Videos of adults and children engaging with screens (available on the Internet) were accessed to generate discussions about screens. As highlighted by the authors (Becker & Donelli, 2023), parents and caregivers reported that the intervention was an important strategy to change some behaviors and attitudes toward screen usage at home and school. The participants evaluated the intervention as a tool to reflect on the interaction with the child and to access evidence-based information, such as the current guidelines and the side effects of technology. The participants also pointed out the possibility of seeing the child more clearly as a subject with different needs as necessary to change some screen usage patterns.

In early interventions, home visiting programs are recognized as effective for family well-being and improving health outcomes, especially for at-risk populations. These interventions may be a strategy to be used with existing guidelines since they promote guidance and education to families, especially those living in a vulnerable context. Avellar and Supplee (2013) highlighted that those programs may positively resonate with family functioning and positive outcomes in child development when targeting early years. An example is the Minding the Baby (MTB) program, which was developed to support high-risk new mothers and their babies. The MTB is a longitudinal intervention based on attachment theory and consists of weekly home visits carried out by an interdisciplinary team (Slade et al., 2020). Mothers are encouraged to be aware of their child's physical and mental states to help them respond appropriately to their child's needs. According to Sadler et al. (2013), the MTB program positively impacts children's attachment development and parenting since the program has shown an increase in secure attachment rates and a decrease in disorganized attachment rates. Moreover, mothers presented higher sensitivity and availability to the child, positively impacting the family organization.

Another mentalization-based program recognized for its effectiveness is the Lighthouse Parenting Program (LPP). The LPP consists of a mentalization-based intervention aiming to prevent child maltreatment. The program was developed in the UK and promotes sensitive parenting by strengthening reflective functioning in parents (Byrne et al., 2018). The original program used psychoeducational activities and has been applied in Western countries. In Brazil, the LPP-adapted version of the Brazilian cultural context included screen usage topics in some sessions. A pilot study pointed out improvements in parental self-efficacy and reflective functioning, such as decreased parental anxiety, stress, and problematic smartphone usage (Becker et al., in prep). A randomized controlled trial is being planned to evaluate the effectiveness of the Brazilian version.

Conclusions

Regarding infants, the guidelines, in general, highlight the amount of time infants should be exposed to screens as soon as they stress the need to consider the content of the videos and the parental mediation during the exposure. However, most parents need information beyond time limits and expect to receive more concrete tips about how to proceed with early screen exposure. It is essential to consider that each country has different needs and realities when planning policy. For example, families with a lower parental educational level may need help accessing this content and following the recommendations, highlighting the importance of individual guidance by pediatricians and primary healthcare services. The language used in the guidelines and interventions must be meaningful and understandable for the target audience, contemplating the cultural aspects of each country or region. Therefore, cultural adaptation of guidelines, such as AAP and WHO recommendations, is required. Moreover, the communication must be effective, highlighting the need for reliable channels to spread the content. Accessible channels, such as mass media, local radio, local and national news media, websites, and social media, can reach different populations.

At this time, most interventions focusing on screen time were developed targeting older children and adolescents, stressing a need for interventions to educate and support parents of young children dealing with the technological world. More than this, since an infant's mental health is critically influenced by the quality of care offered by children's caregivers during early years, interventions with the potential to explore parental skills seem to be an essential tool to improve caregiver-child emotional bond and reduce screen time among adults and children. Psychoeducational strategies should be considered to improve parental adherence to the guidelines, and to target this aim, interventions appear as complementary and reachable strategies, especially those based on the mentalization approach, which focuses on early relationships and presents favorable outcomes.

Additional research about early screen exposure and digital media usage during caregiving is needed to provide more evidence to support the policy. More studies exploring the parental view about the phenomena are also required, especially since the beginning of the COVID-19 pandemic, which incorporated more technology into the family context and changed human relationships. By listening to parents, we can gain an overview of families' realities and better understand what they are seeking and which kind of information will be helpful for them. Based on parental reports, the guidelines and interventions can be structured to align with parental demands, respecting their reality and encompassing culture, beliefs, and values.

References

American Academy of Pediatrics [AAP] Council on Communications and Media. (2016). Media and young minds. *Pediatrics, 138*(5).

Arai, Y., et al. (2023). Association between children's difficulties, parent-child sleep, parental control, and children's screen time: A cross-sectional study in Japan. *Pediatric Reports, 15*(4), 668–678. https://doi.org/10.3390/pediatric15040060

Asociación Española de Pediatria [AEP]. (2023). *Plan digital familiar*. https://plandigitalfamiliar.aeped.es/plandigitalfamiliar.php

Avellar, S., & Supplee, L. (2013). Effectiveness of home visiting in improving child health and reducing child maltreatment. *Pediatrics, 132*(2), S90–S99. https://doi.org/10.1542/peds.2013-1021G

Barlow, J., Sleed, M., & Midgley, N. (2020). Enhancing parental reflective functioning through early dyadic interventions: A systematic review and meta-analysis. *Infant Mental Health Journal, 42*(1), 21–34. https://doi.org/10.1002/imhj.21896

Becker, D. (2020). *Digital technologies in the context of mother-baby and father-baby interactions: An exploratory approach*. Master's dissertation. Universidade do Vale do Rio dos Sinos, UNISINOS.

Becker, D., & Donelli, T. M. S. (2023). Impressões de pais e educadores sobre a exposição do bebê as telas? Um relato de experiência. *Revista SPAGESP, 23*, 128–142.

Becker, D., & Donelli, T. M. S. (2024). "It doesn't always work, but it helps": Parental perceptions of infants' screen exposure. *Psicologia em Estudo, 29(1). https://doi.org/10.4025/psicolestud.v29i1.54957*

Becker, D., Donelli, T.M.S., Byrne, G., Rutherford, H., & Taubner, S. (in prep). *Cultural adaptation of the lighthouse parenting program in Brazil: Targeting mothers with strong social vulnerability*.

Bergmann, C., Dimitrova, N., Alaslani, K., et al. (2022). Young children's screen time during the first COVID-19 lockdown in 12 countries. *Scientific Reports, 12*, 2015. https://doi.org/10.1038/s41598-022-05840-5

Bergonsi, F.; Becker, D.; Paiani, R.L. & Donelli, T.M.S. (2022) *O bebê em isolamento social e à exposição às mídias digitais: um estudo exploratório*. 29. Mostra de iniciação científica e tecnológica UNISINOS. http://www.guaritadigital.com.br/casaleiria/unisinos/eventos/mostra2022/234/index.html

Biringen, Z., & Easterbrooks, M. A. (2012). Emotional availability: Concept, research, and window on developmental psychopathology. *Development and Psychopathology, 24*(1), 1–8.

Boonmun, W., et al. (2023). A program for parents' screen time reduction for preschool children: A quasi-experimental study. *PRIJNR, 27*(2), 368–380. https://he02.tci-thaijo.org/index.php/PRIJNR/article/view/260440

Bozzola, E., Spina, G., Ruggiero, M., Memo, L., Agostiniani, R., Bozzola, M., Corsello, G., & Villani, A. (2018). Media devices in pre-school children: The recommendations of the Italian pediatric society. *Italian Journal of Pediatrics, 44*(1), 69. https://doi.org/10.1186/s13052-018-0508-7

Byrne, G., Sleed, M., Migley, N., Fearon, P., Mein, C., Bateman, A., & Fonagy, P. (2018). Lighthouse parenting Programme: Description and pilot evaluation of mentalization-based treatment to address child maltreatment. *Clinical Child Psychology and Psychiatry*, 1–14.

Chile Crece Contigo [CCC]. (2018). *Niños y Niñas frente a las pantallas*. http://www.bibliotecaminsal.cl/wp/wp-content/uploads/2018/01/070.CNTV_guia-ninos_ninas-frente-a-las-pantallas-REF.pdf

Cooke, J. E., Deneault, A. A., Devereux, C., Eirich, R., Fearon, R. M. P., & Madigan, S. (2022). Parental sensitivity and child behavioral problems: A meta-analytic review. *Child Development, 93*(5), 1231–1248. https://doi.org/10.1111/cdev.13764

Coyne, S. M., Radesky, J., Collier, K. M., Gentile, D. A., Linder, J. R., Nathanson, A. I., Rasmussen, E. E., Reich, S. M., & Rogers, J. (2017). Parenting and digital media. *Pediatrics, 140*, s112–s116.

Donelli, T. M. S., Schaefer, M. P., Mortari, E. M., Trage, F., Becker, D., Kunzler, M., Alves, A. A., & Bittencourt, A. C. O. (2020). Interventions for promoting parental reflective functioning. In S. M. F. Enumo, T. L. Dias, & F. P. Ramos, (org.) (Eds.), *Intervenções psicológicas para promoção de desenvolvimento e saúde na infância e adolescência. 1ed* (Vol. 1, pp. 15–357). Appris.

Draper, C. E., et al. (2020). The South African 24-hour movement guidelines for birth to 5 years: An integration of physical activity, sitting behavior, screen time, and sleep. *Journal of Physical Activity and Health, 17*(1), 109–119. https://doi.org/10.1123/jpah.2019-0187. Erratum; PMID: 31877557.

Durham, K., et al. (2021). Digital media exposure and predictors for screen time in 12-month-old children: A cross-sectional analysis of data from a German birth cohort. *Frontiers in Psychiatry, 12*. https://doi.org/10.3389/fpsyt.2021.737178

Fonagy, P., & Allison, E. (2012). In N. Midgley & I. Vrouva (Eds.), *What is mentalization? The concept and its foundations in developmental research* (pp. 11–34). Minding the child: Mentalization-based interventions with children, young people and their families.

GSMA Intelligence [GSMA]. (2023). *The mobile economy 2023*. https://data.gsmaintelligence.com/research/research/research-2023/the-mobile-economy-2023

Gupta, P., et al. (2022). IAP guideline committee on digital wellness and screen time in infants, children and adolescents. Indian academy of pediatrics guidelines on screen time and digital wellness in infants, children and adolescents. *Indian Pediatrics, 59*(3), 235–244.

Hebestreit, A., & Sina, E. (2024). Wirkungen digitaler Medien auf die Gesundheit von Kindern und Jugendlichen mit Schwerpunkt auf dem Verzehr ungesunder Lebensmittel. *Bundesgesundheitsbl, 67*, 292–299. https://doi.org/10.1007/s00103-024-03834-4

Hinkley, T., Cliff, D. P., & Okely, A. D. (2015). Reducing electronic media use in 2–3 year-old children: Feasibility and efficacy of the family@play pilot randomised controlled trial. *BMC Public Health, 15*, 779. https://doi.org/10.1186/s12889-015-2126-2

Indian Academy of Pediatrics [IAP]. (2021). *Screen time guidelines for parents*. Available from: https://iapindia.org/pdf/Screentime-Guidelines-for-Parents-Ch-005.pdf

Jones, A., Armstrong, B., Weaver, R. G., Parker, H., von Klinggraeff, L., & Beets, M. W. (2021). Identifying effective intervention strategies to reduce children's screen time: A systematic review and meta-analysis. *International Journal of Behavioral Nutrition and Physical Activity, 16*(18), 1–126. https://doi.org/10.1186/s12966-021-01189-6. PMID: 34530867; PMCID: PMC8447784.

Joseph, H. B., Sandhiya, K., & Shetty, A. P. (2022). Touch screen device usage and its effect on sleep among young children: Do parents delude younger generation deliberately? Time to ruminate and impede this technological harm. *Indian Journal of Community Medicine, 47*, 360–363.

Kabali, H. K., Irigoyen, M. M., Nunez-Davis, R., Budacki, J. G., Mohanty, S. H., Leister, K. P., & Bonner, R. L. (2015). Exposure and use of mobile media devices by young children. *Pediatrics, 136*(6), 1044–1050.

Kılıç, A. O., et al. (2019). Exposure to and use of mobile devices in children aged 1-60 months. *European Journal of Pediatrics, 178*(2), 221–227.

Kozeis, N. (2009). Impact of computer use on children's vision. *Hippokratia, 13*(4), 230–231.

Lammers, S. M., Woods, R. J., Brotherson, S. E., Deal, J. E., & Platt, C. A. (2022). Explaining adherence to American Academy of Pediatrics screen time recommendations with caregiver awareness and parental motivation factors: Mixed methods study. *JMIR Pediatrics and Parenting, 5*(2), e29102. https://doi.org/10.2196/29102

Mayes, L., & Cohen, D. (2002). The Yale Child Study Center guide to understanding your child. In *Healthy development from birth to adolescence*. Little Brown.

McArthur, B. A., Volkova, V., Tomopoulos, S., & Madigan, S. (2022). Global prevalence of meeting screen time guidelines among children 5 years and younger: A systematic review and meta-analysis. *JAMA Pediatrics, 176*(4), 373–383. https://doi.org/10.1001/jamapediatrics.2021.6386

McDaniel, B. T. (2019). *Parent distraction with phones, reasons for use, and impacts on parenting and child outcomes: A review of the emerging research*. Human Behavior and Emerging Technologies.

McDaniel, B. T., & Coyne, S. M. (2016). "Technoference": The interference of technology in couple relationships and implications for women's personal and relational well-being. *Psychology of Popular Media Culture, 5*(1), 85–98.

Muppalla, S. K., Vuppalapati, S., Reddy Pulliahgaru, A., & Sreenivasulu, H. (2023). Effects of excessive screen time on child development: An updated review and strategies for management. *Cureus, 15*(6), e40608. https://doi.org/10.7759/cureus.40608

Portinho, D. F., Becker, D., Schaefer, M. P., Paiani, R., & Donelli, T. M. S. (2023). *A pandemia de COVID-19 e suas repercussões na rotina de famílias com bebês: uso de telas e saúde mental*. Congresso SOCERGS.

Radesky, J. S., et al. (2016). Parent perspectives on their mobile technology use: The excitement and exhaustion of parenting while connected. *Journal of Developmental &Behavioral Pediatrics, 37*(9), 694–701.

Roman-Vinas, B., Chaput, J.-P., Katzmarzyk, P., Fogelholm, M., Lambert, E., Maher, C., & Tremblay, M. (2016). Proportion of children meeting recommendations for 24-hour movement guidelines and associations with adiposity in a 12-country study. *International Journal of Behavioral Nutrition and Physical Activity*. https://doi.org/10.1186/s12966-016-0449-8

Royal College of Paediatrics and Child Health [RCPCH]. (2019). *The health impacts of screen time: a guide for clinicians and parents*. https://www.rcpch.ac.uk/sites/default/files/2018-12/rcpch_screen_time_guide_-_final.pdf

Rutherford, H. J. V., & Mayes, L. C. (2019). Parenting stress: A novel mechanism of addiction vulnerability. *Neurobiology of Stress, 10*, 100172. https://doi.org/10.1016/j.ynstr.2019.100172

Sadler, L. S., Slade, A., Close, N., Webb, D. L., Simpson, T., Fennie, K., & Mayes, L. C. (2013). Minding the Baby: Enhancing reflectiveness to improve early health and relationship outcomes in an interdisciplinary home visiting program. *Infant Mental Health Journal, 34*(5), 391–405. https://doi.org/10.1002/imhj.21406

Slade, A. (2005). Parental reflective functioning: An introduction. *Attachment & Human Development, 7*(3), 269–281. https://doi.org/10.1080/14616730500245906

Slade, A., Holland, M. L., Ordway, M. R., Carlson, E. A., Jeon, S., Close, N., Mayes, L. C., & Sadler, L. S. (2020). *Minding the Baby®*: Enhancing parental reflective functioning and infant attachment in an attachment-based, interdisciplinary home visiting program. *Development and Psychopathology, 32*(1), 123–137.

Sociedad Argentina de Pediatria [SAP]. (2020). Uso de pantallas en tiempos del Coronavirus. Recomendaciones elaboradas por el Comité Nacional de Crecimiento y Desarrollo y la Subcomisión de Tecnologías de Información y Comunicación. https://www.sap.org.ar/uploads/archivos/general/files_uso-pantallas-epocacovid_1589324474.pdf

Sociedade Brasileira de Pediatria [SBP]. (2019). In: http://www.sbp.com.br

Stiglic, N., & Viner, R. M. (2019). Effects of screentime on the health and well-being of children and adolescents: A systematic review of reviews. *BMJ Open, 9*, e23191.

Taubner, S., Munder, T., Unger, A., & Wolter, S. (2013). Zur Wirksamkeit präventiver Früher Hilfen in Deutschland–ein systematisches Review und eine Metaanalyse [Effectiveness of early prevention programs in Germany: a systematic review and a meta-analysis]. *Praxis der Kinderpsychologie und Kinderpsychiatrie, 62*(8), 598–619.

Tooth, L., Moss, K., Hockey, R., & Mishra, G. D. (2019). Adherence to screen time recommendations for Australian children aged 0–12 years. *Medical Journal of Australia, 211*(4), 181–182.

Tremblay, M. S., Carson, V., Chaput, J.-P., et al. (2016). Canadian 24-hour movement guidelines for children and youth: An integration of physical activity, sedentary behaviour, and sleep. *Applied Physiology, Nutrition, and Metabolism, 41*, S311–S327.

Vasques, C., Mota, M., Correia, T., & Lopes, V. (2012). Prevalence of overweight/obesity and its association with sedentary behavior in children. *Revista Portuguesa de Cardiologia, 31*(12), 783–788. https://doi.org/10.1016/j.repce.2012.11.009

Wolfers, L. N., Kitzmann, S., Sauer, S., & Sommer, N. (2020). *Phone use while parenting: An observational study to assess the association of maternal sensitivity and smartphone use in a playground setting*. Computers in Human Behavior. Advance Online Publication. https://doi.org/10.1016/j.chb.2019.08.013

World Health Organization (WHO). (2019). Retrieved from: https://www.who.int/news-room/detail/24-04-2019-to-grow-up-healthy-children-need-to-sit-less-and-play-more

Zeanah, C., & Zeanah, P. (2019). *Infant mental health: The science of early experience*. Guilford Press.

Index

G. B. Frizzo (ed.), *Digital Media and Early Child Development*, https://doi.org/10.1007/978-3-031-69224-6

The manufacturer's authorised representative in the EU is Springer Nature Customer Service Centre GmbH, Europaplatz 3, 69115 Heidelberg, Germany. If you have any concerns regarding our products, please contact ProductSafety@springernature.com

Printed and bound by CPI Group (UK) Ltd, Croydon, CR0 4YY
28/09/2026
02224081-0013